Endurance Sports Nutrition

THIRD EDITION

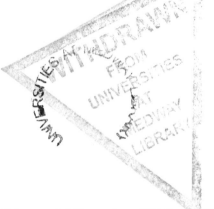

Suzanne Girard Eberle, MS, RDN, CSSD

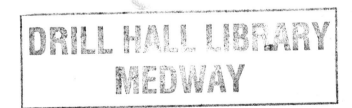

Human Kinetics

Library of Congress Cataloging-in-Publication Data

Eberle, Suzanne Girard, 1962- author.
  Endurance sports nutrition / Suzanne Girard Eberle, MS, RDN, CSSD. -- Third edition.
    pages cm
  Includes bibliographical references and index.
  1. Athletes--Nutrition. I. Title.
  TX361.A8E39 2014
  613.7--dc23

                              2013019506

ISBN-10: 1-4504-3215-8 (print)
ISBN-13: 978-1-4504-3215-3 (print)

This publication is written and published to provide accurate and authoritative information relevant to the subject matter presented. It is published and sold with the understanding that the author and publisher are not engaged in rendering legal, medical, or other professional services by reason of their authorship or publication of this work. If medical or other expert assistance is required, the services of a competent professional person should be sought.

The web addresses cited in this text were current as of June 2013, unless otherwise noted.

Acquisitions Editor: Justin Klug; **Developmental Editor:** Carla Zych; **Assistant Editors:** Rachel Fowler and Elizabeth Evans; **Copyeditor:** Joy Wotherspoon; **Indexer:** Nan Badgett; **Permissions Manager:** Martha Gullo; **Graphic Designer:** Nancy Rasmus; **Graphic Artist:** Tara Welsch; **Cover Designer:** Keith Blomberg; **Photograph (cover):** Peter Blakeman/Action Plus/Icon SMI; **Photographs (interior):** © Human Kinetics, unless otherwise noted; **Photo Asset Manager:** Laura Fitch; **Visual Production Assistant:** Joyce Brumfield; **Photo Production Manager:** Jason Allen; **Art Manager:** Kelly Hendren; **Associate Art Manager:** Alan L. Wilborn; **Illustrations:** © Human Kinetics, unless otherwise noted; **Printer:** Sheridan Books

Printed in the United States of America   10 9 8 7 6 5 4 3 2 1

The paper in this book is certified under a sustainable forestry program.

Human Kinetics
Website: www.HumanKinetics.com

United States: Human Kinetics
P.O. Box 5076
Champaign, IL 61825-5076
800-747-4457
e-mail: humank@hkusa.com

Canada: Human Kinetics
475 Devonshire Road Unit 100
Windsor, ON N8Y 2L5
800-465-7301 (in Canada only)
e-mail: info@hkcanada.com

Europe: Human Kinetics
107 Bradford Road
Stanningley
Leeds LS28 6AT, United Kingdom
+44 (0) 113 255 5665
e-mail: hk@hkeurope.com

Australia: Human Kinetics
57A Price Avenue
Lower Mitcham, South Australia 5062
08 8372 0999
e-mail: info@hkaustralia.com

New Zealand: Human Kinetics
P.O. Box 80
Torrens Park, South Australia 5062
0800 222 062
e-mail: info@hknewzealand.com

E5780

To the trees and the clouds: Thank you for the shade.

CONTENTS

PART II Nutrition Plans for Specific Events and Conditions

PREFACE

We ask a lot of our bodies. This is especially true of endurance athletes (people who live by the mantra "no guts, no story"), who often find it challenging to do things in moderation. And if you're like most of the athletes I work with, you probably expect your body to simply show up and do whatever it is you want it to. In reality, however, our body gets the final say. Our ability to go long, whether we run, cycle, swim, hike, ski, or row, is a gift. None of us is entitled to do these activities, even if we're really good at them. The key is to work with your body by giving it what it needs, so you are able to consistently perform to your best. In other words, when it comes to your body, you need to feed it, rest it, and take care of it.

My first career or day job was as an elite professional runner. After running competitively in high school and college, I was good enough to keep pursuing this path. I ran around the world, including representing the United States three times on national teams. Currently, I'm a board certified sports dietitian and nutrition coach. I counsel teen and adult athletes of all shapes, sizes, and athletic abilities on mastering high-performance eating habits. It's simple—if you're relying on your body to perform, you're an athlete! It doesn't matter if you're a shoo-in to make the podium or if you simply want to survive and cross the finish line—you're an athlete.

The first task, and it's often the hardest, is simply making it to the starting line. By eating smart, you will have greater energy to train, suffer fewer injuries, get sick less often, and recover more quickly. You'll also enjoy a saner relationship with food and have an easier time reaching and maintaining an appropriate, healthy weight. Eating smart, after all, is not about eating right, being perfect, or becoming a gourmet chef. It's about making daily food choices and establishing regular eating habits that are based on balancing nutrition with convenience and pleasure. Putting the science (yes, nutrition is a science) into practice during your chosen endeavor sets you up to perform better and to enjoy the adventure or race more. (Or at least as much as possible.)

This sports nutrition book is unique in two aspects. First, it's not just another general sports nutrition book. It's geared specifically to the endurance athlete. If you train for and participate or compete in endurance-based events or would like to do so in the future—whether you run a 10K, finish an Ironman, cycle across your state, or race against others across the entire country—you have nutrition needs that differ from those of athletes in power, stop-and-go, and team sports. Because most active people don't have the time or the scientific background to keep up with the ever-evolving field of sports nutrition, I've done it for you. Part I of this book offers eight chapters that deliver practical endurance-specific nutrition information that you can apply the next time you open the refrigerator door, hear about a new supplement, worry about your weight, or wonder, now that you've signed up, how you're ever going to go that far or last that long. Even if friends and family, a coach, or your teammates consider you nutritionally challenged, you will be ready to pursue smarter eating habits after reading these chapters.

Second, I've drawn on my background as both a sports dietitian and a successful endurance athlete to sort through what sports science professionals recommend versus what works in real life. Armed with my professional expertise and personal experiences, I've partnered with some of the best endurance athletes in the country so that as you read, you are learning from the best.

Some themes ring loud and clear to the top-notch runners, cyclists, triathletes, adventure racers, rowers, open water swimmers, mountaineers, and winter athletes involved in Nordic and backcountry skiing that I counsel. They know their bodies extremely well. They always go into an endurance event or race with a well-thought-out nutrition game plan. Most important, they are always thinking about their food, fluid, and electrolyte needs while on the move.

In part II (chapters 9 through 16), I coach you through the unique nutrition challenges endurance athletes face in shorter-range, long-distance, ultra, and multiday events and races in order to go longer as well as faster. Included are strategies for dealing with challenging conditions such as altitude and extreme heat or cold. Regardless of your sport or activity—running, cycling, mountain biking, triathlon, adventure racing, hiking, mountaineering, Nordic skiing, open water swimming, or rowing—your job is to go into the endeavor with a well-conceived nutrition game plan. Regardless of your goal—hoping just to finish or going farther and faster than ever before—your job is to monitor your food, fluid, and electrolyte needs while on the move. What bright athlete wouldn't want to have an endurance-minded nutrition coach by his or her side?

This book is offered to you, the endurance athlete, as food for thought. Dig in!

ACKNOWLEDGMENTS

Many, many thanks to acquisitions editor Justin Klug and to developmental editor Carla Zych for their expert guidance and extraordinary patience.

I continue to be grateful to the gifted athletes who again shared their time and wisdom for this edition as well as all those who continue to seek my advice. Special thanks to Michael for answering all queries regarding anything to do with cycling, to Gil, my personal soccer coach, for providing hours of instruction and entertainment, and lastly, to John, my husband and best friend, for reading every word.

PART I

Nutrition Strategies for Endurance Athletes

1

Eating Smart, Training Smart, Racing Smart

Many athletes put a lot of emphasis on the pre-event meal, believing it is the key element to performance. It is important to remember that food eaten throughout the training week and food and fluid consumed during the event is just as important.

Source: Australian Institute of Sport, 2009, Eating before exercise. [Online]. Available: www.ausport. gov.au/ais/nutrition/factsheets/competition_and_training/eating_before_exercise [April 12, 2013].

Eating for endurance sports is an art and a science. The everyday fluid and fuel needs of an endurance athlete can vary tremendously, especially when compared to athletes involved in power and team sports. As an endurance athlete, you put yourself at a real disadvantage if you think that you can eat like your buddies who play a pickup game a few days a week or if you wait until race day to focus on the nutrition piece of the performance equation. Furthermore, if you believe that only elite-level runners, cyclists, open water swimmers, rowers, triathletes, adventure racers, hikers, mountaineers, and backcountry and Nordic skiers benefit from paying attention to what they eat, think again. Regardless of your age or athletic ability, three factors figure prominently in your success: genetics, training, and nutrition. You can't do anything about your genes, so to improve, you must concentrate on the other two (along with getting adequate rest and recovery and having strong mental skills, too, of course).

Indeed, what and how you eat, from one day to the next, and your ability to train are inextricably linked. The people who are most successful at completing endurance endeavors, such as running a marathon or tackling a half Ironman, are those who consistently train smart. And training smart hinges on eating smart, day in and day out. Whether you want to place or just want to finish, you must establish high-performance eating habits that support what you're personally trying to accomplish each day, en route to your long-term goal. How else do you think that you can tackle an early morning swim workout, work a full day, and then put in a quality bike ride or run in the evening? And then get up the next day and do it again? Just as important, how can you feel strong and confident and enjoy every passing mile (or at least most of them) while you're doing it?

Eating a well-balanced diet doesn't guarantee success. Poor eating habits, however, will literally stop you in your tracks, or at least slow you down. Our daily food choices fuel our training sessions, provide critical nutrients required for muscle repair and recovery, and either support or stress our immune and endocrine (hormonal) systems. Frequent poor training days, recurrent colds, and lingering overuse injuries signal that your nutrition program is out of sync with your training program. If you're a competitive athlete, you obviously must think about what to eat and drink on race day. But what about your food choices on all the other days? Even if you race every weekend—52 times a year—that leaves 313 other days that dramatically influence your ability to be successful!

Besides being good for you, the foods that you choose to eat from day to day must also be tasty and satisfying; otherwise, you won't eat them. The key is to master an eating style that fulfills both these needs—high-performance foods that supply key nutrients and fuel your body (foods that you need) and foods that feed your mind (foods that you want). In addition, unless you like to spend time in the kitchen or can afford to hire a personal chef, you probably want to figure out how to eat smart without wasting valuable time or energy.

Evaluating Your Typical Food Choices

You may already know something about what constitutes a healthy training or day-to-day diet for an endurance athlete. Maybe you know a lot. Regardless, looking at what you're actually eating is always a worthy endeavor. Knowledge about a topic doesn't automatically translate into practice. Being aware of and owning your current eating habits will help you answer for yourself the plea I most often hear from athletes: "Just tell me what to eat!"

Keep It Simple

First, familiarize yourself with My Plate (see figure 1.1), a visual reminder of a healthy diet based on a familiar image—a place setting for a meal. Use My Plate as a template for building a smart, well-balanced sports diet. It organizes foods by the nutrients that they contain into five food groups: fruits, vegetables, grains (complex carbohydrates), dairy, protein foods, and a separate category for the modest amount of healthy fat (oils) that we need daily. My Plate also reminds us of the role of what I refer to as fun foods. These are foods such as chips, alcohol, and candy that should be enjoyed in moderation because they supply solid fats and added sugars (SoFAS), and thus calories, but few or no nutrients. The message is simple. Fill your plate, at mealtimes and snacks, with high-performance (nutrient-dense) food-group foods. Include fun foods and extras, as warranted, to help meet daily energy (caloric) needs and to ensure that eating is a pleasurable experience. How much you need to eat is particular to you, and heavily depends on how much you move. This is good news for endurance athletes: Those who move more get to eat more!

As you take a closer look at My Plate, you may wonder where some foods fit.

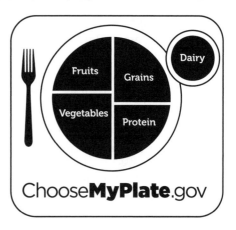

FIGURE 1.1 High-performance eating habits require you to balance eating foods you want with the foods you need. Use My Plate to guide your daily choices.

U.S. Department of Agriculture

Fruits: all fresh, frozen, canned, and dried fruits as well as 100 percent fruit juices.

Vegetables: all fresh, frozen, canned, and dried vegetables as well as vegetable juices.

Grains: all foods made from wheat, rice, oats, cornmeal, barley, or another cereal grain, such as bread, pasta, oatmeal, breakfast cereals, tortillas, and grits. Grain group foods are divided into two subgroups, whole grains and refined grains. Whole grains, such as whole wheat flour, bulgur, oatmeal, whole cornmeal, and brown rice, contain the entire grain kernel—the bran, germ, and endosperm—and are nutritionally superior.

Protein foods group: meat, poultry, fish and seafood, eggs, peanut butter, tofu and other processed soy products (tempeh, veggie burgers, and TVP); also, a quarter-cup of cooked dry beans or peas is considered a 1-ounce (30 g) equivalent.

Dairy group: all fluid milk products and foods made from milk that retain their calcium content, such as yogurt, cheese, and cottage cheese. Foods made from milk that have little to no calcium, such as cream cheese, cream, and butter, are not included. Fortified soy milk (soy beverage) is included here because it provides a nutrition profile that is similar to cow's milk, particularly in its calcium, vitamin D, vitamin A, potassium, and protein content. (Calcium-fortified rice and almond milks are included, too; however, keep in mind that these varieties supply far less protein than a cup of cow's milk.)

Oils (not a food group, but oils provide essential nutrients): fats from many different plants that are liquid at room temperature, such as canola, corn, olive, soybean, and sunflower oil. Other foods naturally high in oils also fit best here, including nuts, seeds, and nut butters; flaxseed, olives, and avocados; fattier fish and foods that are mainly oil, such as mayonnaise, certain salad dressings, and soft margarines.

Fun foods and extras (enjoy as long as food group recommendations are met and overall calorie needs are not exceeded): coffee and tea, soda, fruit-flavored drinks, alcohol, cream cheese, butter and stick margarine, jam and jelly, nondairy creamer, condiments, sour cream, sugar, honey, maple syrup, pickles, sauces, gravy, bacon, fatty deli meats, hot dogs, sausage, French fries, onion rings, chips or crisps and other snack foods, oil-popped popcorn, candy, chocolate, sherbet, gelatin desserts, high-fat ice cream and frozen yogurt, cookies, doughnuts, muffins, pastries, cakes, and pies.

Rate Your Own Plate

Before you read any further, take 10 minutes and look at what a typical eating day means for you. First, recall what you had to eat (and drink) yesterday, from the time you arose until you went to bed, so that you can evaluate your choices and see how they compare to the My Plate guidelines. If yesterday was unusual—if, for example, you were ill or traveling—choose another, more typical day. Refer to figure 1.2, and use my favorite personal recording format to track the foods and beverages that you consumed in that 24-hour period. First, record the approximate time at which you ate or drank something. Next, write down the item in the second column, followed by the amount or portion you ate (using household measurements, such as cups or ounces), and in the last column, list the appropriate food group(s) or category this food or beverage belongs to as well as the number of My Plate servings it represents. For example, if you stopped on the way to work for a bagel with cream cheese and a container of orange juice, your food record would look like the example in figure 1.2.

FIGURE 1.2   Sample Food Journal Entry

Date: _____ Day of the week: _____

Time	Food/Beverage	Portion	Food Group(s) & Number of Servings
7:30 am	Bagel	1 large (4 oz)	Grains 4
	Orange juice	Medium (12 oz)	Fruit 1.5
	Cream cheese	Large smear	Extras

Don't forget to include snacks, beverages, and foods that you ate on the move, such as the energy bar that you downed in the car on the way home or the cheese and crackers that you grabbed while passing through the kitchen. Be sure to separately record condiments or major additions to foods, such as the Parmesan cheese (dairy) that you covered your plate of spaghetti with or the olive oil (oils) in which you soaked your bread. Obviously, we most often eat mixed foods, such as pizza, beef stew, chili, and Chinese food. Mixed foods represent more than one food group or category. When keeping food records, you need focus only on the major ingredients. A bean and cheese burrito, for example, would count in the grains group (tortilla, rice), dairy group (cheese), and protein foods group (beans).

To calculate the number of food group servings you consumed, compare the amount that you ate (portion size) with standard My Plate serving sizes (see table 1.1). For example, a large bagel counts as four grains, since the average bakery or grocery-store bagel weighs 4 ounces (112 g) (1 oz, or 28 g, of bread is equal to one serving). For a mixed food (a small burrito, for example), a good estimate would be two and one-half grains (small 6 in.,

TABLE 1.1 What Counts as a Serving?

Grains group	What counts as an ounce?
Bread	1 regular slice, 1 small slice French
Tortilla	1 small (6 in., or 15 cm, diameter) flour or corn, 1/4 large (12 in., or 30 cm, diameter)
Roll, biscuit	1 small (2 in., or 5 cm, diameter)
Bagel	1 mini (2.5 in., or 6.5 cm, diameter), 1/4 large
Hamburger bun, English muffin	1/2 bun or muffin
Ready-to-eat cereal	~1 cup flakes or rounds
Pasta, rice	1/2 cup, cooked (1 oz or 30 g)
Bulgur, millet, buckwheat, and other whole grains	1/2 cup, cooked
Oatmeal	1/2 cup, cooked, 1 packet instant, 1 oz (1/3 cup) dry–regular or quick
Small crackers	5 whole wheat, 2 rye crispbreads, 7 round or square
Pancake	1 pancake (4.5 in., or 11.5 cm, diameter)
Muffins	1 small (2.5 in., or 6.5 cm, diameter), 1/3 large (3.5 in., or 9 cm, diameter)
Popcorn	3 cups, popped, 1/2 mini microwave bag or 100-calorie bag, popped

> continued

< continued, **Table 1.1**

Vegetable group	What counts as a cup?
Raw, leafy greens (lettuce, spinach, and so on)	In general, 2 cups raw
Greens (collard, turnip, kale)	1 cup cooked
Spaghetti sauce	1 cup
Raw or cooked vegetable	In general, 1 cup
Tomato or vegetable juice	1 cup (240 ml)
Carrots	2 medium
Baked or boiled potato	1 medium (2.5–3 in., or 6.5–8 cm, diameter)
Winter squash (acorn, butternut, Hubbard)	1 cup cubed, cooked
Mashed potatoes	1 cup
Sweet potato	1 large baked (at least 2.25 in., or 6 cm, diameter), 1 cup sliced or mashed, cooked
Corn	1 cup or 1 large ear (8–9 in., or 20–23 cm)
Fruit group	**What counts as a cup?**
Commonly eaten fruit	1 small apple, 1 large orange or peach, 2 large plums, 12 strawberries, 32 seedless grapes
Banana	1 large (8 in., or 20 cm)
Applesauce	2 (4 oz, or 112 g) snack containers
Sliced or chopped, raw or cooked, canned fruit	1 cup
Cantaloupe (rock melon)	1 large wedge (1/4 of medium melon)
Grapefruit	1 medium
100% fruit juice	1 cup
Dried fruit	1/2 cup
Dairy group	**What counts as a cup?**
Milk	1 cup (250 ml), 1/2 cup evaporated milk
Yogurt	1 cup, 1 regular container
Hard cheese (cheddar, mozzarella, Swiss, Parmesan)	1.5 oz (42 g)
Shredded cheese	1/3 cup
Ricotta cheese	1/2 cup
Processed cheese (e.g., American)	2 oz (56 g)
Cottage cheese	2 cups
Fat-free or low-fat frozen yogurt or ice cream	1 cup frozen yogurt, 1 1/2 cups ice cream
Pudding made with milk	1 cup
Calcium-fortified soy milk	1 cup

Protein foods group	What counts as an ounce equivalent?
Meats: cooked lean beef, pork, or ham	1 oz, 1/3 to 1/2 small lean hamburger
Poultry: cooked chicken or turkey (without skin)	1 oz, 1/3 chicken breast
Seafood: cooked fish or shellfish	1 oz, 1/4 of 1 can of tuna, drained 1/4 to 1/6 salmon steak
Cooked beans (e.g., kidney, black) and cooked peas (e.g., chickpeas, lentils)	1/4 cup, 1/2 cup lentil or bean soup
Baked or refried beans	1/4 cup
Hummus	2 tbsp
Tofu	1/4 cup (~2 oz, or 56 g)
Tempeh	1 oz, cooked
Soybeans	1/4 cup roasted, 1/2 soy or bean burger patty, 1 falafel patty
Egg	1, 1.5 egg whites
Peanut butter or almond butter	1 tbsp
Oils	**What counts as a teaspoon?**
Soft margarine (trans-fat free)	Count 1 tbsp as 2+ tsp
Mayonnaise	Count 1 tbsp as 2+ tsp
Vegetable oils	Count 1 tbsp as 3 tsp
Salad dressing	Count 1 tbsp as 2+ tsp
Olives	Count 8 large as 1 tsp
Avocado	Count 1/2 medium as 3 tsp
Mixed nuts, peanuts, cashews, almonds	Count 1 oz as 3 tsp
Sunflower seeds	Count 1 oz as 3 tsp
Peanut butter	Count 2 tbsp as 4 tsp
Extras and fun foods	
Regular soft drink	12 oz (350 ml) can = +135 cal
Wine	1 glass or 5 oz (150 ml) = +120 cal
Beer, regular	1 12 oz (350 ml) can = +155 cal
Butter or stick margarine	1 tbsp = +100 cal
Cream cheese	1 tbsp = +40 cal
Cheese sauce	1/4 cup = +75 cal
Croissant	1 medium (2 oz) = +230 cal
French fries (chips)	1 medium order = +430 cal
Fruit-flavored drink	1 cup = +130 cal

or 15 cm, tortilla; 3/4 cup of rice), one dairy (1 oz, or 28 g, of cheese), and two protein foods (1/4 cup of cooked dried beans is one serving; 1/2 cup would be two). Tally up the number of servings that you ate in each food group or category and put a circle around the number. Be sure to monitor the extras that provide relatively few, if any, nutrients and often are sources of solid fats and added sugars.

Keeping the particular needs of endurance athletes in mind, I've modified the My Plate system slightly. Because of their similar nutrition profiles, I place starchy vegetables (like potatoes, sweet potatoes, winter squash, and corn) in the grains group, and I put nuts and seeds in the oils category, rather than thinking about them as a lean-protein source. (One ounce, or 28 grams, of nuts provides 14 to 18 grams of fat and only 4 to 6 grams of protein.) Beans and peas (such as kidney, black, and garbanzo beans; black-eyed and split peas; and lentils) are unique foods. They are excellent sources of plant protein, fiber, folate, and potassium, along with some iron and zinc, and credible nutrition experts, myself included, highly recommend that everyone eat them frequently. If you regularly eat meat, poultry, and fish, or if your plate includes an adequate serving of another protein-rich food, I would count beans and peas in the grains group. Vegetarians, vegans, and other people who seldom eat meat, poultry, or fish would count them in the protein foods group.

Granted, one day of tracking what you eat doesn't give you a complete picture of your eating habits. You may be pleasantly reassured, however, at how well you're meeting your nutrition needs. You may also be prompted to rethink some of your current choices. Because both male and female endurance athletes come in all sizes and shapes, and because we participate in events ranging from running a 10K to cycling across the country, our fuel (caloric) needs vary widely.

Using the Choose My Plate System

Further assessment of your 24-hour food intake requires that you now estimate your individual calorie needs and determine the corresponding number of servings from each food group or category that you personally require. While doing this based on just one day's intake is certainly beneficial, you'll learn much more by keeping a food journal.

Nutrition-wise, what's most important is the big picture—not any single food, meal, or day. To get a better handle on your typical eating habits, keep a written record of what you eat for at least three consecutive days (two weekdays and one weekend day) or, if you're really committed, for a full week. Record your choices (items and portion sizes) daily and calculate the corresponding number of food group or category servings. (Your recording system can be as simple or sophisticated as you like; refer back to figure 1.2.) Keeping a food journal helps you identify true habits and patterns. For example, perhaps you undereat during the day and then backload calories in at night, or you diet during the week, only to splurge on weekends. Additionally, a food journal can help you see that you miss out on key nutrients if you routinely skimp on or eliminate entire food groups.

One of my clients, a health-conscious 22-year-old runner, came for a nutrition checkup before heading back to college. A vegetarian, she was worried that she wasn't getting enough protein to perform at her best and help her team return to the national championships. Keeping a food journal for just three days enabled her to assess for herself that her protein intake was too low. She responded by deciding to consume an ample lunchtime serving of a protein-rich food, such as hard-boiled eggs, lentil soup, or tofu. She was also shocked to see that over three days she had actually consumed very few vegetables!

The value of using the Choose My Plate system to guide your daily food choices is that you don't need to worry about individual nutrients. Who has time to track the 40-plus nutrients that our bodies need daily? Remember, each food group (and the oils) contains foods that are high or rich in a unique package of nutrients. Just by eating balanced meals and snacks (made from a variety of foods from all five food groups and a modest amount of healthy fat) most of the time, you will very likely get the nutrients that you need. Learning to achieve and maintain a balance between eating high-performance foods that you need and the extras that you want has other rewards too. You'll feel satisfied and will have plenty of energy to do what you want to do, and you won't waste precious time and mental energy being preoccupied or obsessed with food. Last but not least, you won't need to worry about throwing your system off balance by taking supplements that can contain too much of certain nutrients and not enough of others.

A quick nutrition checkup can be, at times, particularly useful. You'll want to adjust your daily diet, for example, whenever you step up your training. Just like keeping a daily training log, a food journal can help you (or a sports dietitian) assess what is working and what isn't. Additionally, anytime your training is going poorly, be sure to evaluate both your diet and your training log. Poor food choices, such as failing to eat enough carbohydrate-rich foods to fully replete your glycogen stores or consuming too few calories because you want to drop a few pounds, can leave you feeling unusually fatigued and stale in a matter of days. On the other hand, consuming an iron-poor diet may not slow you down for a few weeks to a few months, however, you will feel the negative effects of depleted iron reserves eventually. A constant battle with one injury after another may also be linked with poor eating habits. Athletes who routinely exercise with low muscle glycogen stores incur more injuries. Finally, if you're trimming calories to lose weight, make sure that you don't trim vital nutrients by eliminating entire food groups. Keeping a food journal will, at the very least, help you become more aware of what you're eating, and it's been repeatedly shown to help those trying to lose weight.

Estimate Your Daily Calorie Needs

Determining the amount of energy, or calories, your body requires on a daily basis is as much art as it is science. Obsessively counting calories isn't necessary, and it frequently does more harm than good. Simply estimating your daily calorie needs, however, can quickly help you better understand your fuel needs as an endurance athlete. Use the following simple method to estimate the range of calories that you need daily. (A more sophisticated method designed for endurance athletes is presented in chapter 2. For individualized information, consult with a sports dietitian or visit www. choosemyplate.gov.)

Less active: little or no purposeful exercise, such as when you're taking a break from training or recuperating from an injury or illness

Body weight in pounds × 13.5 to 15 calories per pound (body mass in kilograms × 29 to 33 calories per kilogram) = _____ calories

Light to moderately active: approximately 45 to 60 minutes a day of purposeful exercise (moderate intensity), most days of the week

Body weight in pounds × 16 to 20 calories per pound (body mass in kilograms × 36 to 44 calories per kilogram) = _____ calories

Very active: approximately 60 to 120 minutes a day of purposeful exercise (moderate intensity), most days of the week

Body weight in pounds × 21 to 25 calories per pound (body mass in kilograms × 46 to 55 calories per kilogram) = _____ calories

Extremely active: training for an ultraendurance event, such as an Ironman triathlon or 100-mile (160 km) ultra run

Body weight in pounds × 25 to 30 calories or more per pound (body mass in kilograms × 55 to 66 calories or more per kilogram) = _____ calories

Note that fitness enthusiasts and athletes commonly overestimate their physical activity level. Don't select a category based solely on the hardest day of your week. The high ends of the calorie ranges equate to consistently training or working out at moderate intensity or higher five to six days per week. Additionally, the mid to higher ends of the ranges apply to male athletes and the lower to mid ranges to active female athletes.

Translate Calories Into Daily Food Amounts

Once you've estimated the amount of calories you require to meet your nutrient needs, maintain your current weight, and adequately fuel your workouts, turn your attention to table 1.2. Use it as a guide to translate calories into food amounts so that you know how much you actually need to eat. Compare the circled values on your one-day or 24-hour food record with the recommended food group targets in table 1.2. (Note: Some endurance athletes may require more than 3,200 calories daily while racing or during periods of high-volume training.)

TABLE 1.2 Translating Calories Into Daily Food Amounts

Total calories needed*	Fruits (cups)	Vegetables (cups)	Grains	Protein foods	Dairy (cups)**	Oils (tsp)	Daily calories from extras and fun foods***
1,600 (6,690 kJ)	1.5	2	5 oz-eq	5 oz-eq	3	5	132 (540 kJ)
1,800 (7,525 kJ)	1.5	2.5	6 oz-eq	5 oz-eq	3	5	195 (815 kJ)
2,000 (8,360 kJ)	2	2.5	6 oz-eq	5.5 oz-eq	3	6	267 (1,115 kJ)
2,200 (9,200 kJ)	2	3	7 oz-eq	6 oz-eq	3	6	290 (1,210 kJ)
2,400 (10,030 kJ)	2	3	8 oz-eq	6.5 oz-eq	3	7	362 (1,515 kJ)
2,600 (10870 kJ)	2	3.5	9 oz-eq	6.5 oz-eq	3	8	410 (1,715 kJ)
2,800 (11,700 kJ)	2.5	3.5	10 oz-eq	7 oz-eq	3	8	426 (1,780 kJ)
3,000 (12540 kJ)	2.5	4	10 oz-eq	7 oz-eq	3	10	512 (2,140 kJ)
3,200 (13,375 kJ)	2.5	4	10 oz-eq	7 oz-eq	3	11	648 (2,710 kJ)

*1 calorie = 4.18 kJ

**Teens, young athletes up to age 24, and women who are pregnant or breastfeeding need 3 or more servings daily (300 mg of calcium per serving) from the dairy group.

***Consume enough total calories to maintain a healthy weight by choosing more energy-dense (higher-calorie) items from the five food groups, eating more servings from the five food groups, consuming more healthy oils, and enjoying more extras and fun foods. Athletes who eat a balanced diet and still have trouble meeting their daily energy needs can obtain additional calories from high-carb drinks, meal replacement beverages, and energy bars.

Adapted from the U.S. Department of Agriculture Center for Nutrition Policy and Promotion, 2012, USDA food patterns. [Online]. Available: www.cnpp.usda.gov/Publications/USDAFoodPatterns/USDAFoodPatternsSummaryTable.pdf [April 12, 2013].

Assessing Your Current Eating Habits

Consider the following points as you assess not only your one-day food record, but also what is most important to you nutrition-wise—the big picture. Remember, the effectiveness of your eating style doesn't hinge on any one food, meal, or even day of eating; rather, it's determined by your usual or typical food choices over the course of several days.

Balance

First, a smart sports diet is well balanced. Does your plate typically hold wholesome, carbohydrate-rich foods, such as brown rice, whole grains, whole wheat pasta, and whole-grain breads and cereals (as well as potatoes, sweet potatoes, and corn)? These foods provide complex carbohydrate, B vitamins, fiber, and numerous other nutrients, while contributing little or no fat.

Carbohydrate provides the most readily available form of energy our bodies need to fuel endurance sports and activities. Glycogen (carbohydrate stored in the liver and muscles), for example, is the primary fuel that our muscles rely on whenever we exercise more intensely. These same glycogen reserves also help decide the length of time we can exercise continuously. Accomplished endurance athletes have learned (often the hard way) to consume enough carbohydrate daily to adequately replace the muscle glycogen that is used up during workouts. Otherwise, they begin to feel sluggish or unmotivated, and they are slower to recover and vulnerable to more injuries. Maintaining a normal training pace (or even getting out the door) on subsequent days also feels harder. A regular eating schedule, based on meals and snacks built on whole grains, bread, cereal, rice, and pasta, as well as an ample amount of carbohydrate-rich fruits, vegetables, beans or peas, and low-fat milk and yogurt, is the key to ensuring that approximately 60 percent of your total daily calories come from carbohydrate—the foundation of any serious endurance athlete's diet. Eating a higher-carbohydrate diet daily, as compared to stuffing pasta down the night before a race, is also a far better strategy if your goal is to train consistently day after day.

As important as it is, endurance athletes cannot live on carbohydrate alone. In fact, many endurance athletes suffer from carbohydrate overload. Their diets are out of balance: too much carbohydrate and too little protein. As endurance athletes, our bodies require quality protein from the foods that we eat for numerous reasons: to build, maintain, and repair muscle fibers damaged during daily exercise; to help injuries heal promptly; to make hemoglobin, which carries oxygen to exercising muscles; to form antibodies to fight off colds, infections, and other more serious diseases; to produce enzymes and hormones that help regulate critical energy processes in the body; and to help meet energy (caloric) needs in the latter stages of ultraendurance events. Up to 20 percent of your total daily calories should come from protein.

Lean meats, chicken, fish, eggs, beans and peas (black, kidney, pinto, and so on), peanut butter, and soy foods such as tofu, tempeh, and edamame supply protein as well as varying amounts of two other key nutrients—iron and zinc. Low-fat dairy foods supply high-quality protein as well as significant doses of calcium, a nutrient needed for healthy nerves, muscles, and bones. How well are you doing at meeting your protein needs by eating lean protein–rich foods daily? Five to 7 ounces of meat (140–200 g), or the equivalent, and 3 cups (750 ml) of milk a day, or the equivalent, cover the minimum needs of most endurance athletes. Athletes often go to one extreme or another when it comes to these two groups—protein foods and dairy foods. Some have little trouble exceeding their requirements, thanks to supersized burgers and pints of ice cream. Others, concerned about eating a meat-free diet or reducing their fat intake, skimp on or eliminate animal products with little regard for finding alternatives. In either case, the athlete is no longer eating a smart, well-balanced sports diet.

Do you routinely fill one-half of your plate with colorful fruits and vegetables? Nonfat and chock-full of vitamins A and C, fiber, and a host of other health-promoting phytochemicals, fruits and vegetables are truly nature's vitamin pills. Nutrition researchers and health professionals don't always come to the same conclusion on what we should eat for optimal health; however, one guideline exists that they do agree on: Eat more fruits and vegetables. That's because the scientific evidence is clear and overwhelming. Filling up on fruits and vegetables can help you maintain a healthy weight and reduce your risk of diet-related chronic diseases, such as diabetes, heart disease, stroke, and some cancers. Besides, consuming 6 to 9 cups of fruits and vegetables daily is far tastier and much more effective (not to mention more enjoyable) than hoping you've guessed right about which supplements to take.

Fat, by the way, is an appropriate and necessary part of a healthy sports diet. Besides providing a concentrated dose of energy or calories, the fat supplied by the foods we eat has other important roles. Consuming fat enables your body to absorb and transport fat-soluble vitamins (A, D, E, and K) and ensures that you get an adequate amount of linoleic acid, an essential fatty acid (the body cannot make it) needed for growth and healthy skin and hair. Including enough fat also helps us feel satisfied, so that we're not preoccupied with thoughts about food. A smart, well-balanced sports diet obtains at least 20 percent of its total calories from fat. If you're an elite swimmer, distance runner, triathlete, or cyclist who requires in excess of 4,000 calories a day, you may need to consume a greater percentage of your calories as fat in order to meet your high energy needs. How well are you doing at including enough healthy fat daily as vegetable oil, salad dressing, fattier fish, trans-fat-free margarine, avocados, olives, and nuts (5 to 11 teaspoons, or 25 to 55 milliliters, a day covers most endurance athletes)?

Extras are foods that offer little in the way of nutrition, such as coffee and soda, as well as fun foods that supply more calories, unhealthy solid fats, or added sugars than they do nutrients. These foods round out an overall healthy diet and can help endurance athletes meet their high energy requirements. Go ahead and enjoy the taste, pleasure, and psychological boost that these foods provide. Problems arise when extras and fun foods routinely take over the plate and squeeze out healthier food group options, or when distorted fears about these foods lead to or further unhealthy eating behaviors such as restrictive eating followed by bingeing.

Variety

A healthy sports diet is full of variety. No single food, or food group for that matter, can supply the 40 or more nutrients that we need (see appendix B for vitamins and minerals needed for optimal health and performance). Each food group contains foods that are particularly rich in a unique package of nutrients. Fruits and vegetables, for example, serve up mainly vitamins A, C, and fiber, whereas dairy foods supply protein, calcium, vitamin D (milk and yogurt), and riboflavin. You can get your calories from anywhere. Not so for nutrients. Eliminating entire groups of food puts you at risk for being low in certain essential nutrients needed for good health and optimal athletic performance. Check your plate—do all five food groups appear daily?

Additionally, eating a varied diet also refers to including as many different foods as possible from each of the five food groups. For example, if you always have apple juice for breakfast and snack on a banana, you've missed opportunities to boost your vitamin C intake, as well as experiment with other great-tasting foods rich in vitamin C, such as cantaloupe (rock melon) and tangerine juice. (Apple juice provides no vitamin C unless it's been fortified, and bananas, although rich in potassium, carbohydrate, and fiber, provide minimal amounts of vitamin C.)

Keep in mind that some foods are nutritional powerhouses compared with others. Although you can certainly meet your carbohydrate needs by eating bagels, plates of spaghetti, and an energy bar or two, your health and performance (never mind your taste buds) would undoubtedly benefit from including more whole grains, such as oatmeal for breakfast, brown rice or couscous for dinner, and whole wheat fig bars as a snack.

Taking a multivitamin can help ensure that you get an adequate intake of most nutrients, but it's no guarantee that the nutrients will be as well absorbed as those from food are. And vitamin supplements don't supply all the health benefits, such as fiber, phytochemicals, and other yet undiscovered nutritional boosters, contained in food. How much effort do you typically make daily to eat a variety of foods from *within* each of the five food groups?

Moderation

Moderation is the final piece of a healthy sports diet. Good at doing things in extreme, endurance athletes often struggle with eating in moderation. Many shun nutrient-rich foods because such foods also contain fat, or they continually rely on sugar and caffeine for a pickup instead of obtaining the energy that they need from real foods. No foods are good or bad for you; your overall diet is what counts. Eating a single food, a specific type of energy bar, for example, won't save an otherwise poor diet. At the same time, eating a bowl of premium high-fat ice cream or a fast-food meal won't erase all your healthier choices.

Think about your personal day-to-day eating habits. Do you simply avoid many foods or even eliminate entire food groups? Or do you substitute healthier versions (less fat and sodium, fewer calories, and so on) or work at incorporating appropriate alternatives? If you choose not to eat dairy foods, for example, do you replace milk and yogurt with fortified soy or rice versions, as well as eat plenty of dark green leafy vegetables to boost your calcium intake? If you frequently struggle to maintain a healthy weight or are simply trying to eat more healthfully, do you work at including more fiber-rich fruits, vegetables, and whole grains daily? Or do you simply try to stay away from foods high in unhealthy fats and added sugar, like chips, muffins, and chocolate? Keep in mind when assessing your fat intake that you need to consider any significant amounts in other food group choices (for example, oatmeal versus a croissant? Grilled chicken breast or fried chicken?), as well as the amount that extras and fun foods contribute.

For many athletes, performing a diet makeover or losing weight without skimping on good nutrition hinges on cutting out excess fat. A gram of fat supplies 9 calories (37 kilojoules) compared with the 4 calories (17 and 16 kilojoules) contained in a gram of protein or carbohydrate. (A gram of alcohol supplies 7 calories, or 29 kilojoules.) But this doesn't mean you should bypass a sandwich and a glass of low-fat milk to eat an entire box of fat-free cookies! A healthy sports diet includes moderation, and that means having a positive relationship with food and striving to fit in all foods.

Getting the Most Out of Food Nutrition Labels

Being able to decipher food nutrition labels is the next best thing to having a personal sports dietitian accompany you to the grocery store. Read on for some tips on how to make food labels work for you (see figure 1.3).

1. First, always check the listed serving size. Compare it to the amount that you actually consume. Adjust the rest of the listed nutrition information accordingly. For example, if you eat twice as much as the listed serving size, double the values given. Use labels to compare similar food products because they generally have the same listed serving size.

Serving Size: Always check the serving size first. All the nutritional info that follows relates to this standard amount. If you eat more or less than the serving size listed, adjust the numbers accordingly.

Calories: The total number of calories (from fat, carbohydrate, and protein) provided by one serving.

Total Fat: Listed in grams for one serving. Includes mono- and polyunsaturated fat, saturated fat, and trans fat. (5 grams = 1 tsp.)

Saturated Fat: Eating too much of this unhealthy fat can raise blood cholesterol levels.
Trans Fat: Has been determined to be as heart unhealthy as saturated fat, or more so; recommended daily limit is less than 1% of total calories.

Cholesterol: Cholesterol in foods you eat can raise your blood cholesterol level. For healthy adults, ≤ 300 mg per day is recommended. For adults with high blood cholesterol, ≤ 200 mg per day is recommended.

Sodium: Can exacerbate high blood pressure in susceptible individuals. For healthy adults, < 2,300 mg per day is recommended. Endurance athletes may need more at times.

Total Carbohydrate: Listed in grams. Includes all carbohydrate sources: complex carbohydrates (in grains, beans, etc.), sugars, and dietary fiber.

Calories from Fat: A quick comparison with "Calories" tells you how fatty the food is. The closer the two numbers, the higher the fat content.

% Daily Value: An easy way to see how a food fits into your overall diet. (Labels use a 2,000-calorie diet as a standard.)

Dietary Fiber: 5 g or more per serving = high fiber. 2.5 g to 4.9 g per serving = good source of fiber.

Sugars: Includes naturally occurring sugars found in milk and fruit, so limit only sugars from empty calorie foods such as soda or candy and foods with excessive amounts of added sugar, such as high-fructose corn syrup. (4 grams = 1 tsp.)

Beneficial Nutrients: Obtaining 100% of each daily usually requires eating a combination of healthy foods. Don't expect one food to do it all!

Reference Values: Based on 2,000-calorie and 2,500-calorie diets. This information remains the same on every label, so you don't need to read it every time.

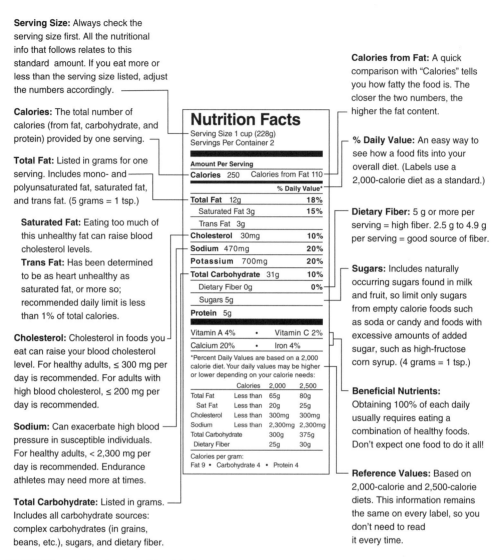

FIGURE 1.3 Use food nutrition labels to select high-performance foods that provide power nutrients and to determine which foods to limit or consume in moderation.

2. Don't confuse *calories from fat* with *total fat* or percent of calories from fat. *Calories from fat* tells you the calories that come from fat and, when compared to *calories*, how fatty a food is (in figure 1.3, a 1-cup serving provides 110 calories from fat, which is almost 50 percent of the 250 calories a serving provides). *Total fat* gives you the grams of fat in a serving (in this example, 1 cup provides 12 grams). To determine the percentage of calories from fat, divide *calories from fat* by *calories* and multiply by 100 (in this example, 110 / 250 × 100 = 44 percent of calories from fat).

3. Use *percent daily value* (% DV) to quickly assess whether a serving is high or low in nutrients. A low percent daily value (5 percent or less) means that the food provides a small amount or is a poor source of a nutrient, whereas a higher percent daily value means that it contributes a large amount (based on a 2,000-calorie diet). Check if the food is a good source (at least 10 percent) or an excellent source (20 percent or more) of key nutrients that most endurance athletes need more of—fiber, vitamins A and C, calcium, and iron. Aim to select foods that together provide 100 percent or more of these nutrients (or average close to 100 percent over a few days). For nutrients to eat in moderation, such as fat, saturated fat, trans fat, cholesterol, and sodium, choose foods that together provide 100 percent or less of the daily value.

4. Scan the ingredients list (required on most packaged foods) for information on ingredients that you may be trying to eat more of (whole wheat, for instance) and others that you want to avoid or limit for health, religious, or other reasons. Labels list ingredients by weight from most to least, and must now clearly indicate whether the food contains any of eight major allergens: milk, eggs, fish, shellfish, tree nuts, peanuts, wheat, or soybeans.

Building the Best Training Diet: Simple Solutions for Busy Endurance Athletes

You're not alone if your plate doesn't always measure up to the standard. Athletes of all abilities, from beginners to world class, routinely shortchange their health and performance by not paying enough attention to their daily food choices (what to eat) and their typical eating patterns (how to eat). This section focuses on what foods to eat (see chapter 8 for advice on how to eat) and provides quick solutions for even the busiest or most nutritionally challenged endurance athlete. The bottom line—don't count calories. Instead, make your calories count! (See appendix B for a quick review of the functions, required amounts, and best food sources of key vitamins and minerals.)

Make at Least Half Your Grains Whole

Very few athletes struggle to rack up enough grain servings. We like bread, cereal, rice, and pasta, and those foods tend to be affordable, easy to prepare, and readily available. In addition, modest serving sizes add up quickly. Consuming at least half as whole grains, however, is often another matter. Grains group foods (as well as starchy vegetables, dried beans and peas, and low-fat milk and yogurt) supply complex carbohydrates that feed the brain and replenish the glycogen used by working muscles and are superior to the carbohydrate provided by processed foods, such as candy bars, snack items, desserts, and soft drinks. It's wise to be discerning about the type and amount of carbohydrate that you eat (because all carbohydrates are not created equal); however, you don't need to fear or avoid carbohydrate-rich foods altogether. Whole grains supply more fiber, vitamin E, vitamin B_6, zinc, copper, manganese, and potassium than do refined grains. In addition, whole grains help fill you up, without filling you out.

The following are simple solutions for making at least half your grains whole.

- Choose whole wheat bread more often than you do white, wheat, multigrain, rye, or pumpernickel. Look for whole wheat (the key word is *whole*) as the first ingredient listed, or at least listed before any other flour. Try whole wheat tortillas, bagels, pitas, and waffles too.

- Experiment with whole wheat pasta and other whole grains, such as couscous, bulgur, kasha, quinoa, and brown rice. Buy prepackaged, quick-cooking (15 minutes or less) whole-grain mixes or premade salads featuring whole grains.

- Eat a whole-grain breakfast cereal (hot or cold) like oatmeal, Wheatena, Ralston, Roman Meal, Shredded Wheat, Grape Nuts, Cheerios, Wheaties, or Total. Bran cereals like Raisin Bran, All-Bran, or 100% Bran count, too.

- Eat more whole-grain crackers and whole-grain crispbreads.

- Choose brown rice over white rice as often as you can.

- When baking at home, substitute whole wheat flour for half (or more) of white flour in recipes.

Focus on Fruits and Vary Your Vegetables

Shortchanging yourself by barely squeezing in the recommended amounts every now and then means you're missing out on essential nutrients, like naturally occurring antioxidants, vitamins A and C. Besides, if you aren't eating these wholesome, fiber-rich foods, what are you filling up on? The trick—think color! Eat a rainbow every day: red, orange, deep yellow, dark green, blue, and purple.

Power Foods: Fruits and Vegetables

High in vitamin A: apricots, cantaloupe, carrots, kale, collards, romaine lettuce, spinach, sweet potatoes, winter squash

High in vitamin C: broccoli, cabbage, bell peppers, cantaloupe, grapefruit, kiwi, mangoes, oranges, spinach, strawberries, tomatoes

High in fiber: apples, bananas, berries, carrots, cherries, dates, figs, pears, spinach, sweet potatoes

---

Here are simple solutions for varying your veggies:

- Drink tomato or 100 percent vegetable juice. Keep individual-sized servings on hand.

- Include a cup (250 ml) of vegetable soup with lunch.

- Instead of another pale green, nutrition-poor dinner salad, order or serve vegetable-based soup.

- Buy fresh, ready-to-eat varieties, such as prepackaged baby carrots and sugar snap peas and prewashed salad, in a bag, or pick up precut favorites from the salad bar. Keep a favorite low-fat dressing on hand for dipping and dressing salads.

- Stock up on frozen or canned vegetables. Toss them into whatever else you're making or heating up during the last few minutes—spaghetti sauce, soup, stew, casseroles, or mashed potatoes.

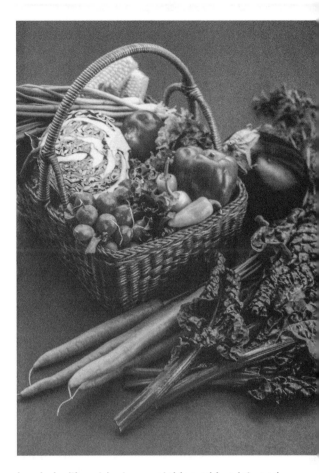

Loaded with nutrients, vegetables add variety and flavor to meals and snacks.
© PhotoDisc

- Prepare vegetables in a few minutes or less using the microwave or a vegetable steamer with an automatic timer. Super-short cooking times mean that fewer nutrients are lost.

- Bake a potato or sweet potato in the microwave. Add your favorite low-fat topping.

- Eat more of the ones that you like, especially if you eat vegetables at only one meal.

- Choose fast food with veggies—vegetarian pizza, Chinese stir-fry, vegetable curries, and so on.

- Always serve (or order) two vegetables at dinner.

- Learn to like vegetables that you hated as a kid. When you find yourself smiling and having a good time during a meal, take one bite (no more) of a veggie that you dislike. Do this at least a half dozen times, a few days to a week or more apart. After not experiencing misery or adverse reactions (like being sent to your room) several times, your brain may decide that this food isn't so bad after all.

The following tips will help you put a smart focus on fruit. Keep in mind that studies repeatedly show we're more likely to eat fruit if we don't have to prepare it first.

- Start early. Drink 8 ounces (240 ml) of 100 percent fruit juice or add fruit (fresh, frozen, or canned) to your morning meal. Try a banana, peach, or berries on cereal, pancakes, or waffles, or stir extra fruit into yogurt.
- Keep dried fruit, such as raisins, dates, dried apples, cherries, and apricots, stashed in your desk drawer, car, and sports bag.
- Keep bananas in the refrigerator (only the skins turn black) so that they ripen more slowly.
- Stock up weekly with ready-to-eat fresh fruit, prepackaged or from the salad bar.
- Make or choose desserts that emphasize the fruit, such as fruit parfaits, tarts, or crustless pies.
- Buy frozen berries and use them as a topping for ice cream, frozen yogurt, or plain cakes, or to make fruit parfaits.

Go Lean With Protein

Making sure day-to-day protein choices are lean and of high quality is another area where both endurance athletes and active women can short-change themselves. Athletes need ample amounts of protein, iron, and zinc to consistently train and perform at a high level. Iron is needed for forming hemoglobin and myoglobin, the oxygen-carrying compounds in blood and muscles. Iron-deficiency anemia results when iron levels are too low to produce healthy red blood cells, leading to fatigue and subpar performances. Zinc is required for fighting off infections and helping wounds and injuries heal properly, including the cellular microdamage caused by logging an ambitious number of daily training miles.

Animal foods, such as red meat, dark poultry, and seafood, provide the most readily absorbable form of iron (heme

---

Power Nutrient: Iron

Animal sources

Beef, pork, lamb, liver, and other organ meats

Poultry (especially dark meat)

Fish and shellfish

Plant sources

Dark leafy greens: spinach, beet, collard, and turnip greens; Swiss chard

Tomato and prune juice

Dried fruit: apricots, raisins

Legumes: chickpeas; black, kidney, lima, navy, and pinto beans

Lentils

Soy foods: tofu, tempeh, textured vegetable protein, soy milk

Whole-grain and enriched breads and cereals (including hot cereals, such as oatmeal and Cream of Wheat)

Wheat germ

iron) and zinc. Boost your absorption of nonheme iron from plant foods by eating a food rich in vitamin C at the same time. Have a glass of orange juice, for example, with your morning bowl of oatmeal. If you're eating enough protein, you are most likely getting enough zinc. Coffee and the tannins in tea (regular and decaffeinated) block the absorption of iron and zinc from foods, so drink these beverages between meals, not with them.

Incorporate these simple strategies to ensure you go lean with protein:

> ### Power Nutrient: Zinc
>
> **Animal sources**
>
> Shellfish: oysters, crab, shrimp, clams
>
> Red meat: beef, pork, lamb, liver, and other organ meats
>
> Poultry
>
> Fish
>
> Dairy foods: milk, yogurt, cheese
>
> **Plant sources**
>
> Legumes: chickpeas; kidney, lima, navy, and pinto beans; split peas
>
> Lentils
>
> Spinach
>
> Soy foods: tofu, tempeh, textured vegetable protein
>
> Peanut butter
>
> Peanuts, cashews, Brazil nuts
>
> Sunflower seeds
>
> Whole-grain and enriched breakfast cereals, including oatmeal
>
> Wheat germ

- Choose lean cuts of meat (rounds and loins, such as tenderloin, sirloin, and round steak) and trim all visible fat. Choose the leanest ground beef that you can afford or substitute ground turkey breast instead. Buy boneless, skinless poultry or remove the skin.

- Use low-fat cooking methods, such as baking, broiling, and grilling. A 3-ounce (85 g) serving of meat is only the size of a deck of cards.

- Eat more fish. Preparing fish takes only minutes. Or buy ready-to-eat shellfish, such as precooked shrimp. Don't like fish? Order it when you dine away from home, from someone who is an expert at preparing it.

- Eat more beans. Keep several canned varieties on hand, buy beans from a salad bar to add to salads, or serve as a side dish instead of potatoes or rice. Choose soups made from beans or peas (minestrone, split pea, black bean, or lentil) and try at least one meatless meal a week, such as tacos or burritos stuffed with beans, vegetarian chili, or black beans with rice.

- Don't shy away from eggs. Inexpensive and easy to prepare, eggs provide the highest quality protein. At 213 milligrams of dietary cholesterol per egg, most endurance athletes can afford to follow the American Heart Association guidelines and include eggs (daily recommended cholesterol limit is less than 300 milligrams of cholesterol for people with normal levels of bad LDL cholesterol) as part of an overall heart healthy diet. Choose egg whites or egg substitutes (such as Egg Beaters) to get protein without the fat and cholesterol.

- Toss tofu (rich in high-quality protein and a good source of iron, magnesium, and zinc) into soups, stews, and lasagna, mash it with cottage cheese and seasonings to make a sandwich spread or dip, or blend it with lemon juice and salt for a baked-potato topping.

- Other time-savers include canned tuna (packed in water) or chicken, precubed meat for kebabs and stir-fries, precooked rotisserie chickens, frozen veggie burgers or garden burgers, and edamame (preboiled soybeans).

- Include a source of lean, quality protein at each meal. Don't eat your grains plain. Smear your bagel with peanut butter, toss baked beans over noodles, and add precooked seafood to your favorite sauce and pour it over pasta, rice, or couscous.

Get Your Calcium-Rich Foods

If the foods you eat don't supply the calcium your body needs, it steals from the only source it has—your bones! To reduce your risk of osteoporosis later in life, optimize your bone mass when you can, which is up to about age 25; after that, the goal becomes holding on to what you have. Because many endurance athletes hit their stride later in life, every day counts in consuming enough calcium.

If you choose not to drink milk or consume dairy foods, you need to incorporate other calcium-rich foods into your daily diet. Aim for at least 1,000 milligrams of calcium daily (1,300 milligrams for younger athletes age 9 to 18 and 1,200 milligrams for adults over age 50). It's easy to determine how much calcium a serving of a particular food provides. Check the food's nutrition label and add a zero to the listed percent daily value for calcium. For example, a food supplying 25 percent of the daily value provides 250 milligrams of calcium.

Follow these simple strategies to boost your calcium intake from low-fat, calcium-rich foods:

- Drink milk whenever you can—any variety will do, but choose low-fat milk as often as you can. Drink low-fat milk shakes, fruit smoothies, lattes, and flavored milks (check the dairy case for chocolate and other varieties or stir in flavored syrups). Enjoy pudding or custard for dessert.

- Prepare foods such as hot chocolate, oatmeal, or tomato soup with low-fat milk rather than water.

- Snack on yogurt or use it to make a salad dressing or vegetable dip.

- Add a slice or two of low-fat cheese to a sandwich or burger, snack on low-fat string cheese or a slice of cheese pizza, and sprinkle low-fat Parmesan or mozzarella cheese on foods.

- Don't let less nutritious beverages, such as soda (diet and regular), coffee, tea, iced tea, lemonade, and fruit drinks squeeze milk out of your diet.

- If you suffer from lactose intolerance, try drinking or eating a limited amount (one-half cup) of milk or ice cream at a time. Have it with a meal, not on an empty stomach. Experiment with lactose-reduced and lactose-free milk and milk products or take lactase tablets before you consume dairy foods. You can also substitute soy, rice, or almond milk (choose a brand fortified with calcium and vitamin D) for regular milk. Yogurt and natural-aged hard cheeses, such as cheddar and Swiss, tend to produce fewer symptoms.

- To boost your calcium intake beyond that supplied by dairy foods, verify that your tofu is prepared with calcium sulfate (check the label) and add or substitute other calcium-fortified foods, such as breakfast cereals, orange juice, and soy, rice, or almond milk. Eat plenty of dark green leafy vegetables, such as kale, collard, and turnip greens; bok choy; and broccoli. (Don't count on the calcium in spinach because the body absorbs it poorly.)

> **Power Nutrient: Calcium***
>
> 1 cup (250 ml) of milk (nonfat, low fat, or whole)
>
> 1 cup of yogurt
>
> 1.5 oz (42 g) of cheese
>
> 2 cups of cottage cheese
>
> 1 1/2 cups of ice cream or frozen yogurt
>
> 1 cup of fortified soy, rice, or almond milk
>
> 1 cup of fortified orange juice
>
> 1 1/2 cups of cooked collards, turnip greens, or kale
>
> 3 cups of cooked broccoli
>
> 1 1/2 cups of baked beans
>
> 5 oz (140 g) of firm tofu (prepared with calcium sulfate)
>
> 1/2 cup of soy nuts
>
> 4 oz (112 g) of canned salmon with bones
>
> 1 3.75 oz can (105 g) of sardines with bones
>
> *Note:* Contains at least 300 mg per serving.

Choose Healthy Fats (Oils) Over Unhealthy Fats

As previously discussed, a smart sports diet contains an adequate amount of fat. And just as not all carbohydrates are created equal, nor are fats. The goal is to include enough of the healthier fats and limit the unhealthy offenders—the saturated fats and trans fats. High-fat foods that are liquid (or soft) at room temperature, like vegetable oils and soft-spread margarine, are favored because they contain more heart-healthy monounsaturated fat and little or no saturated or trans fat. The same is true for the fat in nuts, seeds, avocados, olives, and fattier fish. Saturated and trans fat are the bad guys that tend to clog arteries, raise cholesterol levels, and lower the body's level of HDL, or good, cholesterol. The American Heart Association recommends a daily trans-fat limit of 1 percent of total calories, or 2 grams for those eating 2,000 calories a day. (Be aware of your portion sizes on anything labeled "0 Trans Fats!" Foods are allowed to have as much as a half gram of trans fat per single serving and still carry this label.)

All fats are energy dense. At 9 calories per gram (when looking at food labels, think of 5 grams of fat as being equal to a teaspoon), only the most physically ambitious endurance athletes can get away with eating all the fat that they want. Severely restricting or trying to avoid eating fat altogether, though, can lead to serious problems. For most athletes, however, attempting to eat a diet too low in fat simply backfires. They eventually feel deprived and unsatisfied, and compensate by overeating, either bingeing on high-fat foods or just eating too much in general.

Rely on these simple solutions for incorporating healthier fats (in modest amounts) over unhealthy fats into your diet:

- Top salads with low-fat salad dressings and use low-fat dressings as a dip for vegetables.
- Switch to a liquid or soft-spread (tub) margarine.
- Experiment and find a low-fat cheese and ice cream that you like.
- Read the food nutrition label on items traditionally high in trans fats—cookies, crackers, cakes, muffins, preprepared cake mixes, pancake mixes, donuts, hard taco shells, packaged or microwave popcorn, and frozen dinners—and choose brands that don't use trans fats and are low in saturated fat. For baked goods without food labels, scan the ingredients list and choose varieties those that don't contain the words "partially hydrogenated."
- Eat fattier fish (rich in heart-healthy omega-3 fatty acids), like salmon, herring, sardines, striped bass, trout, halibut, or albacore tuna, at least twice a week.
- Limit saturated fat (which tends to be solid at room temperature) by doing the following consistently: Trim visible fat on meats, remove the skin from chicken and turkey, select the leanest ground beef that you can afford, swap ground turkey breast for other ground meats, and eat smaller portions of major offenders—bacon, sausage, hot dogs, fatty deli meats, and ribs—and eat them less frequently.
- Eat fried food, especially fried fast food (including French fries, fried-fish sandwiches, and chicken nuggets), as infrequently as possible—save those foods for special occasions.
- Substitute a small handful of nuts (1 ounce, or 30 grams) for foods higher in unhealthy fats, like chips or crisps, candy bars, crackers, and many types of energy bars.

Taste and Savor Extras and Fun Foods

Who better to enjoy sweets, treats, and some extra fat and sugar than endurance athletes putting in the miles? Occasional, even daily, indulgences can support both your body and your spirit. After all, being a smart eater involves choosing foods that not just meet your daily nutrition or physical needs, but also leave you feeling satisfied. In other words, food is not the enemy. Eating is supposed to be a pleasant and enjoyable experience. Despite poplar opinion, eating foods high in fat or sugar and otherwise low in nutrients does not cause people to automatically or instantly gain weight. Routinely eating calories from any food when you're no longer physically hungry (when your body no longer needs food) causes weight gain. Extras and fun foods become a problem only when those foods consistently squeeze out healthier options or when they contribute to excess calories being consumed.

On the other hand, just because you work out doesn't mean that you can simply tune out and pay little to no attention to what you eat. It's unlikely you'll be able to eat whatever food you want in whatever amount you want (or are served, if you often dine away from home) all the time. Consuming too much fat or too much of the wrong kind of fat (saturated and trans fats), going overboard on cholesterol and sodium, or just eating more calories than you require to keep your weight in a healthy range increases your risk for heart disease, diabetes, and some cancers. That sort of diet is also unlikely to do much for your performance. So, budget your calories and decide what luxuries you can afford to include: more food from any food group; soft drinks, wine, beer, candy, desserts, and modest amounts of solid fats like butter and cream cheese; or high-calorie versions of foods, such as fried chicken, cheese sauce, and bacon.

The following are simple solutions to finding a balance when it comes to the extras and fun foods in your diet:

- Snack on real food from the five food groups. Aim to put together snacks that include at least one food group (two is even better). Instead of plowing through a box of cookies, for example, enjoy a reasonable amount with a glass of milk. Better yet, on some occasions, pour a bowl of your favorite whole-grain cereal and add milk.

- Savor your favorites. Slow down and figure out what it is that you really crave or desire. Sit down, serve it on a plate, and consciously enjoy every bite. Rushing can leave you feeling unsatisfied and can cause you to eat more than you really need, as can restricting or depriving yourself for as long as possible.

- Cut down on soft drinks and other caffeinated beverages. Drinking too much coffee, tea, and soft drinks fills you up and may temporarily perk you up, but that's it. Ask yourself whether what you really need is something to eat. Sustainable energy comes from the calories provided by foods and nutritious beverages. On top of that, you can only consume so much fluid, and water, low-fat milk, 100 percent fruit or vegetable juice, herbal tea, and sports drinks (when appropriate) make far healthier choices.

- Make your own healthy soda by mixing 100 percent fruit juice and seltzer, half and half.

- Answer a chocolate craving before it gets out of control—chocolate syrup drizzled on fruit, flavored hot chocolate made with low-fat milk, a couple of small chocolates, or a small piece of the real thing.

- On occasions when fun foods abound, such as buffets, parties, and holiday celebrations, choose one or two items that you really want, enjoy them, and move on. Spend your time and emotions connecting with people instead of worrying or feeling guilty about food.

Fill Up on Smart Fluids

Water is the ultimate nutrient, especially for athletes. Our muscles are 70 to 75 percent water, and it serves as the medium in which the body conducts almost all its activities.

Water performs numerous functions:

- It helps digest food through saliva and stomach secretions.
- Water helps lubricate joints and cushion organs.
- It transports nutrients, hormones, and oxygen through the blood (of which water is the main ingredient) to working muscles, and removes waste products such as carbon dioxide and lactic acid.
- In urine, water carries waste products out of the body.
- In sweat, it helps regulate body temperature, especially during exercise, by absorbing the heat generated by muscles and transporting it to the skin where it can evaporate.

Classic early signs of being underhydrated (even when you're not exercising) include light-headedness or dizziness, headaches, loss of appetite, dark-colored urine, lack of energy, and fatigue. Throughout the day, don't wait until your tongue sticks to the roof of your mouth to think about your fluid needs. Waiting until you're outright thirsty means that you've waited too long. Stay on top of your fluid needs by drinking a minimum of 8 cups (2 L) of fluid a day. Emphasize healthy beverages such as water, 100 percent fruit or vegetable juice, low-fat milk, herbal tea, and, when appropriate (such as before, during, and immediately after exercise), sports drinks. To prevent kidney stones and reduce your risk of colon and bladder cancer, aim to drink at least 4 cups, or half of your daily intake, as water. Alcohol, soda, and other highly caffeinated energy drinks aren't the best hydrating choices. Besides being nutrition zeros, alcohol and large doses of caffeine act as diuretics (they cause you to urinate), and the carbonation in fizzy beverages may cause you to drink less.

Here are simple solutions for increasing your daily fluid intake.

- Begin the day conscious of the need to stay hydrated. Drink an 8-ounce (240 ml) glass of water when you get up in the morning.
- If you take vitamins or other supplements, take them with a full glass of water, not just a few sips.
- Drink at least a cup of water or another healthy beverage with all your meals and snacks.
- For easy access, keep a jug of water on your desk or carry a water bottle with you when traveling or running errands.
- Hydrate before you head out to exercise by drinking water or a sports drink—aim for 2 cups during the 2 hours before exercise.
- Have a large glass of water along with your beer, wine, or other alcoholic drink. An added bonus is that you'll handle the alcohol better.
- Make your own healthy soda by mixing fruit juice and seltzer, half and half.

2

Meeting Energy Demands

Exercise represents one of the highest levels of extreme stresses to which the body can be exposed. For example, in a person who has an extremely high fever approaching the level of lethality, the body metabolism increases to approximately 100 percent above normal; by comparison, the metabolism of the body during a marathon race increases to 2,000 percent above normal.

Source: A. Suleman, K. Riaz, and K.D. Heffner, 2011, Exercise physiology. [Online]. Available: http://emedicine.medscape.com/article/88484-overview [April 12, 2013].

Consuming adequate calories, or fuel, daily sets you up to train successfully—a necessity for those who compete. It's also a must, however, if you just want to feel good while working out. The longer or more strenuous the activity, the more important it is to consume the optimal mix of energy-supplying nutrients—carbohydrate, fat, and protein. As you read in chapter 1, consistently eating well-balanced meals and snacks (in the recommended amounts for you) that contain a variety of foods will most likely supply you with adequate calories, as well as the nutrients required for fueling your typical day-to-day activities. This chapter provides detailed information about obtaining the optimal mix of fuel based on your training and competitive needs as an endurance athlete, which vary significantly from the needs of athletes involved in power or team sports.

This chapter is for athletes who want to delve deeper and understand the underlying physiology of how to best ready their bodies for future endurance endeavors. How you fuel your body directly affects your workouts during the week and your weekend races and endurance adventures (as well as your day-to-day overall health). The type of exercise that you undertake also influences the fuel that your body uses. All of us have heard conflicting advice about eating for endurance activities. What you'll come to understand as the formula for athletic success is this: Carbohydrate makes up the backbone of a smart sports diet; however, protein and fat play crucial roles, too.

The Body's Fuel Sources

Our ability to run, bicycle, ski, swim, and row hinges on the capacity of the body to extract energy from ingested food. As potential fuel sources, the carbohydrate, fat, and protein in the foods that you eat follow different metabolic paths in the body, but they all ultimately yield water, carbon dioxide, and a chemical energy called adenosine triphosphate (ATP). Think of ATP molecules as high-energy compounds or batteries that store energy. Anytime you need energy—to breathe, to tie your shoes, or to cycle 100 miles (160 km)—your body uses ATP molecules. ATP, in fact, is the only molecule able to provide energy to muscle fibers to power muscle contractions. Creatine phosphate (CP), like ATP, is also stored in small amounts within cells. It's another high-energy compound that can be rapidly mobilized to help fuel short, explosive efforts. To sustain physical activity, however, cells must constantly replenish both CP and ATP.

Our daily food choices resupply the potential energy, or fuel, that the body requires to continue to function normally. This energy takes three forms: carbohydrate, fat, and protein. (See table 2.1, Estimated Energy Stores in Humans.) The body can store some of these fuels in a form that offers muscles an immediate source of energy. Carbohydrates, such as sugar and starch, for example, are readily broken down into glucose, the body's principal energy source. Glucose can be used immediately as fuel, or can be sent to the liver and muscles and stored as glycogen. During exercise, muscle glycogen is converted back into glucose, which only the muscle fibers can use as fuel. The liver converts its glycogen back into glucose, too; however, it's released directly into the bloodstream to maintain your blood sugar (blood glucose) level. During exercise, your muscles pick up some of this glucose and use it

TABLE 2.1   Estimated Energy Stores in Humans

Energy source	Storage site	Approximate energy (kcal)
ATP/CP*	Various tissues	5
Carbohydrate	Blood glucose	80
	Liver glycogen	400
	Muscle glycogen	1,500
Fat	Serum free fatty acids	7
	Serum triglycerides	75
	Muscle triglycerides	2,500
	Adipose tissue	80,000+
Protein	Muscle protein	30,000

*ATP/CP = adenosine triphosphate/creatine phosphate

in addition to their own private glycogen stores. Blood glucose also serves as the most significant source of energy for the brain, both at rest and during exercise. The body constantly uses and replenishes its glycogen stores. The carbohydrate content of your diet and the type and amount of training that you undertake influence the size of your glycogen stores.

The capacity of your body to store muscle and liver glycogen, however, is limited to approximately 1,800 to 2,000 calories worth of energy, or enough fuel for 90 to 120 minutes of continuous, vigorous activity. If you've ever hit the wall while exercising, you know what muscle glycogen depletion feels like. As we exercise, our muscle glycogen reserves continually decease, and blood glucose plays an increasingly greater role in meeting the body's energy demands. To keep up with this greatly elevated demand for glucose, liver glycogen stores become rapidly depleted. When the liver is out of glycogen, you'll "bonk" as your blood glucose level dips too low, and the resulting hypoglycemia (low blood sugar) will further slow you down. Foods that you eat or drink during exercise that supply carbohydrate can help delay the depletion of muscle glycogen and prevent hypoglycemia.

Fat is the body's most concentrated source of energy, providing more than twice as much potential energy as carbohydrate or protein (9 calories per gram versus 4 calories each per gram). During exercise, stored fat in the body (in the form of triglycerides in adipose or fat tissue) is broken down into fatty acids. These fatty acids are transported through the blood to muscles for fuel. This process occurs relatively slowly as compared with the mobilization of carbohydrate for fuel. Fat is also stored within muscle fibers, where it can be more easily accessed during exercise. Unlike your glycogen stores, which are limited, body fat is a virtually unlimited source of energy for athletes. Even those who are lean and mean have enough fat stored in muscle fibers and fat cells to supply up to 100,000 calories—enough for over 100 hours of marathon running!

Fat is a more efficient fuel per unit of weight than carbohydrate. Carbohydrate must be stored along with water. Our weight would double if we stored the same amount of energy as glycogen (plus the water that glycogen holds) that we store as body fat. Most of us have sufficient energy stores of fat (adipose tissue or body fat), plus the body readily converts and stores excess calories from any source (fat, carbohydrate, or protein) as body fat. In order for fat to fuel exercise, however, sufficient oxygen must be simultaneously consumed. The second part of this chapter briefly explains how pace or intensity, as well as the length of time that you exercise, affects the body's ability to use fat as fuel.

As for protein, our bodies don't maintain official reserves for use as fuel. Rather, protein is used to build, maintain, and repair body tissues, as well as to synthesize important enzymes and hormones. Under ordinary circumstances, protein meets only 5 percent of the body's energy needs. In some situations, however, such as when we eat too few calories daily or not enough

Fuel Metabolism and Endurance Exercise

Carbohydrate, protein, and fat each play distinct roles in fueling exercise.

Carbohydrate

- Provides a highly efficient source of fuel—Because the body requires less oxygen to burn carbohydrate as compared to protein or fat, carbohydrate is considered the body's most efficient fuel source. Carbohydrate is increasingly vital during high-intensity exercise when the body cannot process enough oxygen to meet its needs.

- Keeps the brain and nervous system functioning—When blood glucose runs low, you become irritable, disoriented, and lethargic, and you may be incapable of concentrating or performing even simple tasks.

- Aids the metabolism of fat—To burn fat effectively, your body must break down a certain amount of carbohydrate. Because carbohydrate stores are limited compared to the body's fat reserves, consuming a diet inadequate in carbohydrate essentially limits fat metabolism.

- Preserves lean protein (muscle) mass—Consuming adequate carbohydrate spares the body from using protein (from muscles, internal organs, or one's diet) as an energy source. Dietary protein is much better utilized to build, maintain, and repair body tissues, as well as to synthesize hormones, enzymes, and neurotransmitters.

Fat

- Provides a concentrated source of energy—Fat provides more than twice the potential energy that protein and carbohydrate do (9 calories per gram of fat versus 4 calories per gram of carbohydrate or protein).

- Helps fuel low- to moderate-intensity activity—At rest and during exercise performed at or below 65 percent of aerobic capacity, fat contributes 50 percent or more of the fuel that muscles need.

- Aids endurance by sparing glycogen reserves—Generally, as the duration or time spent exercising increases, intensity decreases (and more oxygen is available to cells), and fat is the more important fuel source. Stored carbohydrate (muscle and liver glycogen) are subsequently used at a slower rate, thereby delaying the onset of fatigue and prolonging the activity.

Protein

- Provides energy in late stages of prolonged exercise—When muscle glycogen stores fall, as commonly occurs in the latter stages of endurance activities, the body breaks down amino acids found in skeletal muscle protein into glucose to supply up to 15 percent of the energy needed.

- Provides energy when daily diet is inadequate in total calories or carbohydrate—In this situation, the body is forced to rely on protein to meet its energy needs, leading to the breakdown of lean muscle mass.

carbohydrate, as well as during latter stages of endurance exercise, when glycogen reserves are depleted, skeletal muscle is broken down and used as fuel. This sacrifice is necessary to access certain amino acids (the building blocks of protein) that can be converted into glucose. Remember, your brain also needs a constant, steady supply of glucose to function optimally.

The Body's Energy Systems

The first energy system the body relies on is the phosphagen system. A small reserve of ATP and another high-energy compound called creatine phosphate (CP; also called phosphocreatine) is stored within muscles to power activity instantly. This reserve is sufficient to fuel several seconds of short, high-power, all-out efforts, such as when you lift weights or serve a tennis ball. When you perform exercise lasting beyond 10 seconds, however, your body requires an additional energy source for the continual resynthesis of ATP. Fat and glycogen, therefore, represent the major energy sources that the body routinely relies on.

The second energy system that the body relies on is anaerobic glycolysis, a series of biochemical reactions that don't require oxygen to convert the glycogen stored in muscles into useable energy. Carbohydrate is the only nutrient whose stored energy can be used to generate ATP anaerobically (without adequate oxygen). This factor becomes increasingly important during high-intensity exercise of short duration. The anaerobic breakdown of muscle glycogen generates ATP (as well as lactic acid) rapidly for a short amount of time, and it serves as the primary fuel for all-out exercise lasting 1 to 2 minutes, such as running an 800-meter race. During anaerobic metabolism, every molecule of glucose burned yields 2 molecules of ATP.

As an endurance athlete interested in completing longer bouts of exercise, you rely predominantly on a third system known as aerobic metabolism (involves a series of oxygen-requiring reactions) to generate a constant supply of ATP. Endurance and ultraendurance activities require the body to take in more oxygen (hence, your relatively slower pace) so that carbohydrate and fat will be oxidized more completely, yielding a more substantial amount of ATP. During aerobic metabolism, every molecule of glucose oxidized yields 36 ATP (as compared with only 2 ATP when broken down anaerobically). For example, during the first 20 minutes of moderately paced, less-than-all-out exercise, liver and muscle glycogen are broken down to glucose, and the ATP generated supplies about half the energy that the body requires. The breakdown of fat stores supplies the remainder of energy at this time.

Thank goodness for our body's ability to store fat. The complete oxidation of a triglyceride molecule yields 460 ATP! During light to moderate exercise, fat supplies about 50 percent of the energy required. The oxidation of fat gradually increases as moderately paced exercise continues past an hour or two and muscle glycogen stores become more and more depleted. During prolonged exercise, the oxidation of fatty acid molecules can provide nearly 80 percent of the energy that the body needs. The complete breakdown of fatty acids, however, depends in part on the breakdown of carbohydrate. When carbohydrate levels (that is, glycogen and blood glucose) in the body fall, the ability of the body to break down fat for fuel also falls. So, as an endurance athlete, keep the science in mind and remember that fat burns in a carbohydrate flame.

If not enough carbohydrate and fat are present to meet energy needs, the body must turn to using protein for energy. Protein must first be converted into a form that can enter various metabolic pathways to produce ATP aerobically. In some cases, amino acids can be broken down directly in muscles, and the by-products can be converted into glucose and used for energy. In other cases, amino acids are converted into intermediate products in the liver and then broken down through the same pathways as glucose to yield energy.

Energy Demands for Intensity and Duration

Don't fall into the trap of believing that you burn either solely carbohydrate or solely fat when you exercise. In reality, our bodies rely on a mixture of fuels during every activity that we do, from resting on the couch to sprinting toward the finish line. How hard you work (the intensity) and how long you go (the duration) ultimately determine what proportion of fuels is used. At rest, for example, more fat than carbohydrate (blood glucose) is burned to meet energy needs. During low-intensity exercise (about 25 percent of maximal oxygen uptake, or 25 percent of $\dot{V}O_2$max; for more on this topic, see What Is $\dot{V}O_2$max?) such as walking, fat continues to supply more than half of the required energy. At these times, the body favors burning fat as fuel because enough oxygen is available to break it down. Lastly, as long as you consume enough calories and carbohydrate from day to day, your body won't have to resort to using protein to fuel everyday activities or exercise.

If the intensity of the exercise that you perform remains low to moderate (up to 65 percent of maximal oxygen uptake, or $\dot{V}O_2$max), your body relies on a mixture of fat and carbohydrate (glycogen and blood glucose) as fuel. As you pick up the pace (increase the intensity above 70 percent of $\dot{V}O_2$max), you have trouble consuming enough oxygen to meet your needs. Your body responds by relying less on fat for energy, shifting instead to burning more glycogen. First, fat cannot be mobilized (broken down into free fatty acids and brought to the muscle from adipose tissue) or burned quickly enough to meet the energy demands of intense muscle contractions. Second, the burning, or oxidation, of carbohydrate for energy requires less oxygen than does the oxidation of fat, so carbohydrate becomes the preferred fuel whenever oxygen is a limiting factor. On top of that, as lactic acid accumulates (as a by-product of the breakdown of glycogen when enough oxygen isn't

What Is $\dot{V}O_2$max?

$\dot{V}O_2$max is a measurement of aerobic capacity—the ability of the body to take in, transport, and use oxygen. As you exercise more intensely, the rate at which you consume oxygen increases. At some point, however, your body reaches a limit on the amount of oxygen that it can consume, even if the intensity of the exercise continues to increase. This point is known as your maximal oxygen uptake, or $\dot{V}O_2$max. As an indicator of aerobic fitness, $\dot{V}O_2$max can help predict which athletes will perform well in endurance activities. It can't, however, determine who will win.

Two other major factors influence your performance in endurance activities: your ability to perform at a high percentage of your $\dot{V}O_2$max for a prolonged period of time (referred to as your lactate threshold) and your skill or efficiency at performing the exercise. Your lactate threshold is the exercise pace above which lactic acid begins to accumulate significantly in your bloodstream. This occurs when glycogen and glucose are broken down rapidly because sufficient oxygen isn't available (as occurs during anaerobic metabolism). By training smartly, you can push your lactate threshold higher. That means you will be able to perform more intensely before accumulating lactate—a distinct competitive advantage because the buildup of lactate contributes to fatigue. Second, the more skilled or proficient you are at performing a type of exercise, the more economical you are. That is, you require less oxygen to perform the same rate of work (you work at a lower percentage of your maximal $\dot{V}O_2$max), which is another distinct advantage because it helps you conserve energy over the long run.

available), it further hinders the ability of muscles to burn fat. At times of high-intensity, all-out exercise (90 to 95 percent of aerobic capacity), your body relies exclusively on glucose.

You've probably figured out by now that how long you go (duration) is inversely related to how fast you go (intensity). For example, no matter how talented you may be, your average speed in a marathon won't be as fast as it is during a 10K race. Fat becomes more important as a fuel source as the intensity of exercise decreases, which occurs as the distance or time that you exercise increases. The oxidation of fat, for example, contributes up to 70 percent of the energy needed during moderate-intensity exercise lasting 4 to 6 hours. As exercise continues and glycogen stores run low, the breakdown of fat supplies most of the energy needed (see figure 2.1). Because the burning or oxidation of fat supplies ATP at a significantly slower rate, however, you cannot maintain the same intensity or pace. Intensity becomes limited to approximately 60 percent or less of aerobic capacity and only if some carbohydrate is still available.

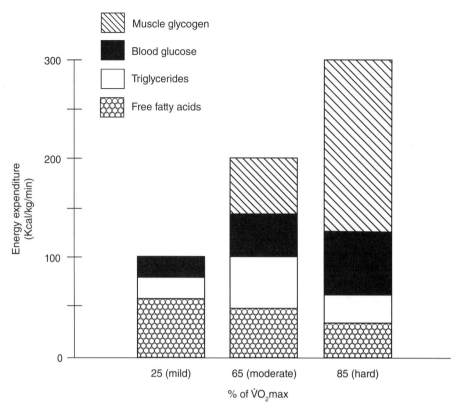

FIGURE 2.1 As exercise intensity increases (your pace quickens or you work harder), the body's dependence on carbohydrate (glycogen and blood glucose) as fuel increases.

Adapted, by permission, from J.A. Romijn, E.F. Coyle, L.S. Sidossis, et al., 1993, "Regulation of endogenous fat and carbohydrate metabolism in relation to exercise intensity and duration," *American Journal of Physiology - Endocrinology and Metabolism* 265(3): E380-E391.

The limiting factor on performance, therefore, even during moderate-intensity exercise, remains the body's limited carbohydrate stores. No matter how ample your fat stores, after you deplete your muscle glycogen stores, you will experience fatigue to some degree and will be unable to sustain your current pace. On top of that, your brain needs a constant supply of glucose. As previously mentioned, if you exhaust your liver glycogen stores and thus cannot maintain an adequate blood sugar level, your body simply shuts down. Remember, too, that a certain amount of carbohydrate breakdown is required for the complete burning of fat as fuel. The longer that you exercise (continuously) past an hour, the more important an outside source of glucose (for example, sports drinks, energy gels, or other carbohydrate-rich foods) becomes to compensate for your dwindling glycogen reserves.

Endurance events, such as marathons and short-course triathlons, and ultraendurance events, such as the Race Across America, a 3,000-mile (4,800 km) coast-to-coast cycling event, and 50- and 100-mile (80 km and 160 km) foot races, provide particularly challenging situations. Elite marathoners typically race at paces equivalent to 86 percent of $\dot{V}O_2$max. Marathoners who finish with times over 3 hours run at 65 percent of $\dot{V}O_2$max—exercise intense enough to require a substantial amount of glycogen for fuel. Glycogen depletion can also be a concern in ultraendurance cycling, such as the Race Across America and multistage events like the Tour de France, because these athletes generally cycle at an intensity greater than 70 percent of $\dot{V}O_2$max. Riders must constantly ingest carbohydrate-rich foods and beverages (before, during, and after their rides) to replenish their glycogen stores.

On the other hand, at the exercise intensities of most ultraendurance running events (less than 60 percent of $\dot{V}O_2$max), such as 50- and 100-mile running races, hypoglycemia, or bonking, is more likely to occur than is glycogen depletion. Well-prepared ultraendurance runners may be very efficient at burning fat as fuel, but their brains still need a constant supply of carbohydrate to function well. As a protective mechanism when muscle and liver glycogen levels run low, the brain shuts down the body until another source of carbohydrate comes along. (See chapter 4 for more on how to avoid hitting the wall and bonking.)

Fulfilling the Demands Efficiently

Endurance athletes vary tremendously in their daily energy needs depending on their size and gender, training program, and their chosen sport. Some athletes may, at times, need as many as 10,000 calories a day! Endurance athletes, in particular, often struggle to consume enough calories to balance the energy demands of day-to-day life and a rigorous training schedule. No magical formulas or foods exist; nevertheless, all athletes can benefit from taking a closer look at the quantity and mix of carbohydrate, fat, and protein in their daily diet.

Carbohydrate Intake

An adequate, continuous supply of carbohydrate is critical for an endurance athlete. You can tap into the power of carbohydrate in four main ways:

- by eating a carbohydrate-rich training diet,
- by taking advantage of the carbohydrate window immediately following exercise,
- by loading up on carbohydrate-rich foods for 3 days before long events and races, and
- by consuming carbohydrate (sports drinks, energy gels, and if appropriate, carbohydrate-rich foods) during exercise.

Athletes who consistently eat a carbohydrate-rich diet have greater muscle glycogen stores to draw on during training and racing efforts. Remember, adequate muscle glycogen stores help delay the onset of fatigue as you pick up the pace or exercise more intensely (as in a 10K running race or a sprint triathlon) or when you exercise longer than 120 minutes (as in a marathon or an Olympic or Ironman distance triathlon). Another bonus is that workouts (and races) will seem easier to complete when you have enough glycogen on board to fuel the entire session.

For fitness enthusiasts who work out consistently for an hour or more daily and athletes who are training purposefully, eating a daily training diet approaching 3 to 4 grams of carbohydrate per pound of body weight (6 to 8 grams per kilogram) speeds up recovery from training bouts, making it easier to get out the door the next day. This also reduces the risk of being sidelined, because athletes who exercise with low muscle glycogen stores tend to incur more injuries. As discussed in chapter 1, breads, cereals, pasta, rice and other grains, fruits and vegetables, cooked beans and lentils, and milk and yogurt are the best options for meeting daily carbohydrate needs. Also useful are sports drinks and energy gels and bars, when used appropriately. Foods that contain a great deal of added sugar, such as cookies and other desserts, ice cream, frozen yogurt, candy, and soft drinks, supply carbohydrate but few nutrients. Eat these foods in moderate amounts to round out or to help fulfill your overall carbohydrate need.

Poor training days or unusual feelings of sluggishness or nonrecovery are often caused by poor eating habits. Why? The effects of glycogen depletion are cumulative. Many devoted exercisers and athletes start out the week strong, only to feel as if they are running on fumes by Thursday. When you don't replenish your glycogen stores on a daily basis, you increase the risk of digging yourself into a hole. Once there, you're forced either to back off or to take time off completely in order to recover. By the way, planned rest days are a good idea. Rest enables your body to catch up and fully replenish its glycogen stores, which takes about 20 hours.

Immediately refueling after intense or prolonged physical efforts is the last step to getting the most benefit out of your training. The first hour following exercise, a period known as the carbohydrate window, is when muscles are most receptive to replacing glycogen. Unfortunately, rather than eating, athletes often spend this window of opportunity showering and racing back to their workplace, socializing, running errands, or commuting. Furthermore, because exercise elevates body temperature, which in turn depresses appetite, you can't rely on feeling hungry to prompt proper refueling.

Within the first 30 minutes following a hard or long workout, get in the habit of immediately consuming a recovery drink that supplies both fluid and carbohydrate, such as a sports drink, fruit juice, or a meal-replacement beverage (even a soft drink will do in a pinch). Aim to consume at least half a gram of carbohydrate per pound (1 to 1.2 grams per kilogram) of body weight within the first 30-minute window, which equates to 50 to 100 grams for most athletes. Ease in carbohydrate-rich foods as soon as you can tolerate them. Popular choices include yogurt, fruit, a low-fat milk shake or smoothie, cereal, bagels, baked potatoes, and energy bars. Be sure that you're putting in carbohydrate, not fat. To determine the carbohydrate content of sports drinks and foods, check food nutrition labels.

In addition, studies repeatedly show that carbohydrate loading, or topping off glycogen stores, prior to continuous exercise lasting 2 hours or longer, significantly enhances performance. This is accomplished by boosting carbohydrate intake to 4 to 5 grams per pound of body weight (8 to 10 grams per kilogram) for at least 3 full days prior to an endurance event or race. Athletes who have trouble eating enough carbohydrate can supplement their food intake with high-carbohydrate or meal-replacement beverages.

Last but not least, sports scientists have firmly established the benefits of consuming a carbohydrate-containing beverage (such as sports drinks) during prolonged exercise (2 hours or more). The ingested carbohydrate (40 to 75 grams per hour) nearly always delays fatigue and boosts performance by maintaining or raising blood glucose levels and by sustaining a high rate of carbohydrate oxidation by muscle. In other words, carbohydrate consumed at this time is an invaluable source of immediate energy that further spares the body's limited glycogen stores. Ingesting carbohydrate may also be beneficial during exercise of shorter duration and greater intensity (e.g., continuous efforts lasting about 1 hour) as well as during intermittent high-intensity efforts (e.g., hill repeats or interval sessions) when the body burns glycogen at a rapid rate. Furthermore, recent research suggests that the ingestion of carbohydrates that use different transporters during exercise may increase total carbohydrate absorption from the intestine. Carbohydrate from a single source, such as glucose or maltodextrins, can only be oxidized at rates of approximately 60 grams per hour. Ingesting a combination of carbohydrates (for example, glucose and fructose), however, allows oxidation rates of 100-plus grams of carbohydrate per hour to be achieved, a significant finding for endurance and ultraendurance athletes. (For more on the role of ingesting multiple carbohydrate sources during exercise, see chapter 4.)

Besides improving performance, consuming carbohydrate during prolonged exercise appears to boost your immune system by preventing precipitous dips in blood sugar. A too-low blood sugar level signals the body to release large quantities of stress hormones, particularly cortisol. Typically elevated after prolonged exercise, cortisol profoundly suppresses immune function. Studies show that taking in plenty of carbohydrate and keeping a steady blood sugar level during exercise also helps to keep the body's cortisol level significantly lower, which may provide just the edge that you need to keep a cold, sore throat, or the flu at bay.

The optimal concentration of carbohydrate-containing drinks intended for use during exercise appears to be 6 to 8 percent, the amount found in most commercially available sports drinks, such as Gatorade and Powerade. (To determine the carbohydrate concentration of your favorite sports drink, divide the number of grams of carbohydrate in an 8-ounce, or 240-millilter, serving by 240 and multiply by 100.) Fruit juice and soft drinks fall outside the established guidelines because they are more concentrated in carbohydrate (as well as low in sodium), which can delay their absorption from the stomach. With a carbohydrate concentration greater than 10 percent, water may actually be drawn into your gastrointestinal tract to dilute the excess carbohydrate, thereby robbing the blood and muscles of valuable water and causing an upset stomach (or something worse). Drinking carbonated drinks during exercise may also upset your stomach. People respond in different ways to carbohydrate-based drinks and foods, however, so some athletes can consume juice and soda with no ill effects.

You may have noticed that sports drinks contain sodium and that some brands taste salty if you drink them when you're not exercising. Sports drinks include sodium for many reasons. Sodium helps speed the rate at which fluid and carbohydrate are emptied from the stomach and absorbed out of the intestinal tract—good news for working muscles and your brain, which need a steady supply of glucose to keep functioning. The presence of sodium also makes you feel thirsty (stimulating you to drink), replaces some sodium lost in sweat, and helps you retain or hold on to the fluids that you ingest.

Fat Intake

Because endurance athletes rely increasingly on fat as an energy source during prolonged bouts of exercise, you may be tempted to eat a high-fat diet to improve your performance. Before you begin fat loading (well-designed studies have participants obtain at least 60 percent of energy or total calories from fat), look at the research. To date, studies reveal that endurance performance (also referred to as time to exhaustion) doesn't seem to be affected in any consistent manner after subjects followed a high-fat diet during an adaptation period lasting from 2 to 7 weeks. Time to exhaustion in laboratory trials has been shown to increase (in one study), remain unchanged, or decrease when subjects were on a prolonged high-fat diet as compared with a carbohydrate-rich diet. Consuming a high-fat diet beyond 4 weeks has been shown definitively to have a detrimental effect on endurance.

For example, in one study, trained cyclists improved their ability to adapt to and use fat as a fuel during exercise (increased fat oxidation) and were able to cycle longer. Their improved performance, however, was not statistically significant. In this case, after 4 weeks on a diet that obtained 85 percent of calories from fat, the trained cyclists rode 152 minutes (to exhaustion) compared with 147 minutes following an average or moderate carbohydrate diet (50 percent of calories from carbohydrate). Critics point out, however, that during the test, the cyclists rode to exhaustion at an intensity low enough (63 percent of $\dot{V}O_2max$) to be fueled primarily by fat oxidation, not limited by glycogen depletion. In reality, most athletes train and certainly race at an intensity of 70 percent of their $\dot{V}O_2$max or above, levels at which glycogen depletion is an increasingly limiting factor. Thus, the attributed positive effect of fat loading as reported in the study isn't applicable for most endurance athletes.

On the other hand, ultraendurance athletes who perform at a relatively lower or submaximal intensity for long periods (greater than 4 hours) could possibly experience a greater benefit from fat loading. Enhanced ability to use fat as fuel would serve to spare the body's limited carbohydrate stores. Researchers continue to refine and test healthier and more realistic fat-loading protocols (e.g., 6 days followed by one day of restoring carbohydrate stores, with carbohydrate feedings during exercise). To date, studies have not shown statistically significant improvements in performance.

In general, though, fat loading, or following a high-fat diet that weighs in much above the recommended maximum of 30 percent of total daily calories, doesn't make sense for most endurance athletes. Such a diet squeezes carbohydrate out of the mix and lowers muscle glycogen stores, which reduces endurance and the ability to perform at high intensity. In the long term, eating a fat-rich diet could also increase the risk for heart disease and certain cancers. (Despite training heavily, the earlier mentioned competitive road cyclists saw their cholesterol levels rise while on the high-fat diet.) Don't forget that even lean athletes have more than enough body fat stored to fuel their endurance endeavors. If you want to improve your performance, focus on manipulating the way that you exercise or train, not the fat content of your diet. Aerobic or endurance exercise stimulates the body to use fat as an energy source. Highly trained endurance athletes are able to use more fat and less glycogen at the same absolute level of exercise, compared with less-fit athletes.

The news that merely eating more fat won't improve your performance in endurance events doesn't mean that you should shun all higher-fat foods, such as salad dressing, cheese, or an occasional bowl of ice cream. To perform at your best, you need muscles that have adapted to using both fat and carbohydrate as fuel. The metabolism of fat and carbohydrate requires different sets of enzymes. By training hard and long, you train your muscles to burn fat and spare glycogen during exercise. By eating a diet that contains adequate fat (approximately one-half gram per pound, or 1 to 1.2 grams per kilogram, of body weight), you also stimulate your muscles to make more of the enzymes necessary for fat metabolism. In other words, you support the efforts of your muscles to build extra cellular machinery for metabolizing fat.

Fat also provides more energy per pound of food. Eating an adequate amount of fat helps athletes obtain enough calories to fuel high-volume training, such as running 10 or more miles (16 km or more) per day or participating in multiple training sessions throughout the day. Athletes who eat most of their calories from carbohydrate-rich foods (about 60 percent) still have plenty of leeway for some fat and, of course, protein. Besides, how much fun is a diet without some fat in it? Keep in mind, though, that even athletes need to watch their intake of unhealthy fats, such as saturated fat and trans fats. (See the section in chapter 1 titled Choose Healthy Fats (Oils) Over Unhealthy Fats.)

Athletes with high calorie needs often train quite successfully by consuming an adequate amount of carbohydrate (for example, 450 to 600 grams a day) and a relatively high percentage of fat calories (up to 35 percent of total calories). For example, an athlete who consumes 4,000 calories a day (50 percent derived from carbohydrate, 15 percent from protein, and 35 percent from fat) still receives a substantial amount of carbohydrate (500 grams). The calories provided by fat add up quickly and allow the athlete to do something other than train and eat all day. Downing a stack of 5 pancakes with margarine and syrup, for instance, is easier than eating 10 plain pancakes, and it provides the same amount of calories.

As for trying to improve your performance by supplementing with fat before or during exercise, little evidence exists for doing so. The fat in the foods that you eat (long-chain triglycerides) takes too long to be digested and absorbed to provide readily available energy during exercise, unless you're planning to be on the move all day. Dietary fat empties slowly from the stomach, and the fatty acids it provides typically don't appear in the bloodstream (as available energy for active muscles) until 3 or 4 hours after ingestion.

Medium-chain triglycerides (MCTs) represent another type of fat that could possibly enhance performance during endurance exercise. Unlike long-chain triglycerides, MCTs are rapidly broken down to fatty acids and directly absorbed into the bloodstream and liver. Theoretically, they could be delivered to muscles quickly enough to provide energy, thereby sparing muscle glycogen. MCTs are available as MCT oil, and some energy bars, sports drinks, and meal-replacement beverages contain modest amounts of MCTs.

When it comes to supplementing with MCTs during exercise, the research is inconclusive. Of studies looking at the effect of using a carbohydrate–MCT mixture (delivered by a sports drink) on time-trial performance, one has shown a positive benefit. After a long, low-intensity warm-up (2 hours at 60 percent of $\dot{V}O_2$max), six endurance-trained cyclists immediately rode a simulated 25-mile (40 km) cycling time trial. During the rides, the athletes consumed either a carbohydrate drink, an MCT solution, or a combined MCT–carbohydrate drink. The times recorded in the time trials in which the athletes consumed the MCT–carbohydrate drink were significantly faster (by 2.5 percent) than those turned in when they used carbohydrate alone. The riders turned in their worst performances when they drank the MCT (no-carbohydrate) beverage.

Other studies, however, have not been able to duplicate the positive effect of ingesting MCTs in conjunction with carbohydrate. In addition, some people will not be able to tolerate a large enough amount of MCTs (the riders in the study ingested 86 grams) to see a benefit. MCTs can cause cramping and diarrhea when consumed in amounts greater than 30 grams. (To learn more about MCT oil, see chapter 5.)

Protein Intake

As much as you might like cereal, bread, and pasta, you can't live on carbohydrate alone if you are involved in endurance activities. Endurance exercise increases our need for protein. In fact, your daily protein requirement may be higher than that of strength and power athletes.

Endurance athletes need protein to shore up the loss of amino acids oxidized during exercise and to repair exercise-induced muscle damage, especially the trauma that occurs during eccentric muscle work, such as downhill running. Protein typically supplies 5 percent or less of daily energy needs. During extreme bouts of prolonged exercise when glycogen stores run low, however, protein is used as fuel and may contribute as much as 15 percent of the energy needed. Failing to eat enough calories from day to day to match those burned during exercise, such as when dieting to lose weight or during periods of high-volume training, also raises daily protein needs.

Endurance athletes require .55 to .75 grams of protein per pound (1.2 to 1.7 grams of protein per kilogram). For example, a 120-pound (54 kg) athlete needs around 75 grams a day. A 150-pound (68 kg) athlete should get about 95 grams, and a 180-pound (82 kg) athlete needs about 115 grams. Competitive athletes involved in extremely intense training, such as Ironman triathletes, and growing teenage athletes may need as much as .8 to .9 grams of protein per pound (1.8 to 2.0 grams of protein per kilogram).

These quantities may sound like a lot, but most well-nourished athletes easily meet their protein needs. Consider this: If you eat two eggs and cereal with milk for breakfast, a tuna sandwich and yogurt for lunch,

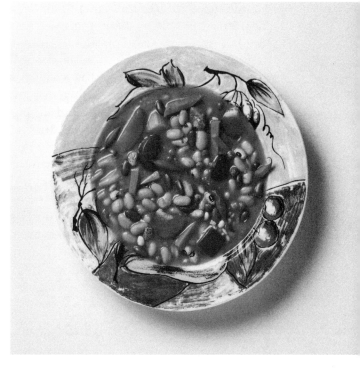

Bean-based dishes can help meet the increased protein needs of endurance athletes.
© PhotoDisc

and grilled chicken with baked beans for dinner, you've devoured almost 100 grams of protein. Between-meal snacks can also provide protein, and vegetables, whole grains, nuts, and tofu and other soy products supply varying amounts as well. Another bonus of including some protein at every meal (and for snacks, too) is that doing so helps stabilize blood sugar so that you feel full longer.

Branched-chain amino acids (BCAAs) are of particular interest to endurance athletes because of their potential role in enhancing mental strength and delaying fatigue during prolonged exercise. BCAAs, stored in muscle, can be converted into glucose and used as fuel during prolonged exercise. Normally, high levels of BCAAs help block the entry of tryptophan (another amino acid) into the brain, but during the latter stages of prolonged endurance exercise, BCAA levels may fall if they are used as energy to compensate for depleted glycogen stores. Consequently, tryptophan may have an easier time gaining entry to the brain, where it's converted into serotonin, a brain chemical that can induce sleepiness and fatigue.

Although supplementing with BCAAs during exercise to improve performance is sound in theory, the studies to date are limited. Adding BCAAs to sports drinks and other products doesn't appear to provide any additional benefits, nor does it appear to be detrimental, although large doses (most studies use 7 to 20 grams) can impair the absorption of water and contribute to stomach problems. Eating protein-rich foods, such as milk, yogurt, meat, poultry, and fish easily supplies the recommended daily dose (about 3 grams a day) of BCAAs. (To learn more about BCAAs, see chapter 5.)

Keep in mind that the goal as we train is to maintain (or build) lean muscle tissue—not break it down during workouts for fuel! Beginning all workouts with adequate glycogen stores and supplementing with carbohydrate (sports drinks, energy gels, and so forth) during long-duration efforts remain your best defense against fatigue and the breakdown of muscle tissue. A small amount of protein consumed shortly after intense or prolonged exercise (along with consuming carbohydrate during the carbohydrate window or including protein-rich foods at the following meal) will jump-start the rebuilding process of muscle protein. The carbohydrate–protein combo also helps the body replenish its glycogen stores more quickly than by ingesting carbohydrate alone.

Optimal Intake of Energy Nutrients for Peak Performance

Relying on a balanced plate (refer back to chapter 1) and your common sense may be all you need to do to keep your eating habits on track most of the time. Sometimes, however, you might wonder if you're consuming the optimal mix of energy-supplying nutrients (carbohydrate, fat, and protein) to enable you to perform at your best. Use the following guidelines to estimate your daily caloric needs, but keep in mind that the food you eat serves three basic needs: it supplies energy (measured in calories), helps regulate the body's metabolism, and supports the growth, maintenance, and repair of tissues.

Carbohydrate (about 60 percent of total calories)

Training 1 hour per day—3 grams of carbohydrate per pound of body weight (6 to 7 grams per kilogram)

Training 2 hours per day—4 grams of carbohydrate per pound of body weight (8 to 9 grams per kilogram)

Training 3 hours per day—5 grams of carbohydrate per pound of body weight (10 to 11 grams per kilogram)

Protein (about 15 to 20 percent of total calories)

.55 to .75 grams of protein per pound of body weight (1.2 to 1.7 grams per kilogram)

Fat (at least 20 percent of total calories)

Approximately .5 grams of fat per pound of body weight (1 gram per kilogram)

Use the numbers you just calculated to estimate your optimal daily caloric intake: (grams of carbohydrate $\times$ 4 calories/gram) + (grams of protein $\times$ 4 calories/gram) + (grams of fat $\times$ 9 calories/gram) = estimated total daily calories

High-Protein, Reduced-Carbohydrate Diets

Popular diet plans that restrict carbohydrate and tout more protein (and fat), such as the Atkins and South Beach diets, continue to appeal to fitness buffs as well as athletes seeking quick weight loss to hopefully boost their performance. Proponents of the 40-30-30 plan (40 percent carbohydrate, 30 percent protein, and 30 percent fat), for instance, shove carbohydrate aside and claim protein to be the most coveted nutrient for athletes. Carbohydrate is blamed for everything from unwanted pounds to low energy levels. How can this be true if glycogen (stored carbohydrate) is the body's preferred fuel during exercise, especially as intensity increases and you pick up the pace?

Take a closer look at this popular, but not necessarily beneficial, diet. The 40-30-30 balance of nutrients supposedly keeps the correct balance between two hormones that the body produces, insulin and glucagon. Advocates reason that limiting the intake of carbohydrate keeps the body from producing too much insulin and that consuming protein boosts glucagon (a hormone that counteracts the effects of insulin) levels. This optimal insulin–glucagon balance supposedly maintains blood sugar levels better, improves endurance by increasing the use of fatty acids for fuel, and reduces body fat by increasing the use of stored fat. Incidentally, all the scientific jargon referred to in these diets about good and bad eicosanoids (hormonelike substances that regulate a variety of body functions) as being the key to all health and disease is unfounded and unproven by any sound scientific research.

High-protein diets hinge on the theory that carbohydrate, not excess calories, does the damage. It begins with eating carbohydrate-rich foods, like rice and potatoes, which cause the body's insulin level to rise. High insulin levels signal the body to store excess carbohydrate as fat instead of burning it for energy. The result is a feeling of lethargy and fatigue as your blood sugar level dips (as insulin moves glucose out of the bloodstream). You're also prone to weight gain, since high insulin levels inhibit the body's ability to access its fat stores. Eating protein, on the other hand, supposedly increases the level of glucagon, which directs the liver to release glucose, thereby replenishing the body's blood sugar supply. Lower insulin levels also promote the release of fatty acids from fat cells for use as energy.

Here is the flip side of high-protein, low-carbohydrate diets. First, those who go too low in carbohydrate pay the price. Sports scientists have long established (since the 1930s) that consuming a high-carbohydrate diet enhances endurance during strenuous athletic events. As you've read in this chapter, consuming carbohydrate before, and especially during, exercise is crucial for endurance athletes. Eating carbohydrate-rich foods (for instance, an hour before exercise) does raise insulin levels and lower blood sugar levels to some degree; however, this normal physiologic response is temporary. Most healthy, active people experience no negative effects on performance. In addition, consuming ample carbohydrate after workouts to refill depleted glycogen stores is also smart science. Fail to do so consistently, and you'll find yourself recovering more slowly, and thus training less effectively.

Second, fat is an important energy source, particularly at rest and during low-intensity exercise. In fact, training (becoming fitter) promotes the increased use of fat as a fuel source. Nevertheless, it's our low glycogen (stored carbohydrate) reserves that are the limiting fuel source during endurance exercise, even in marathons and ultraendurance events. As exercise becomes more intense (you respond to a surge or turn the corner and head up a steep hill), the body shifts to burning more carbohydrate, not fat. And, for your body to function optimally, your brain needs a steady supply of carbohydrate, too. Seriously, who performs at their best when experiencing a headache and feeling grumpy and irritable? So, as terribly old-fashioned (and definitely unhip among those trying to sell you the latest discovery) as it may sound, carbohydrate is still king.

Human sports physiology hasn't changed in the last 75 years. Its principles still apply to all endurance athletes, from fast to slow. Furthermore, weight-loss or fad diets aimed at average people rarely work for active people, especially those who are serious about their athletic goals. Remember, you're eating to work out or to train, not to sit in a rocking chair. The ability to train smart and consistently leads to being fit. Fitness leads to leanness (a healthy weight that you can maintain without heroics), not the other way around.

Third, losing weight is about expending more calories than you consume. The total amount of calories burned during the day is what counts—not whether you burn fat or carbohydrate. (Otherwise, to lose weight, you could simply sleep more, an activity that burns few total calories, but a high percentage of fat calories.) Your body can pull from its fat stores at any time of day or night to compensate for the calories burned during exercise. Besides, if you consume too many calories from any source—carbohydrate, protein, or fat—your body will store the excess calories as body fat. As for high insulin levels causing people to become overweight, the reverse is more likely to be true. Being overweight drives insulin levels up. People have trouble regulating their blood sugar level and consequently feel hungrier, and thus are more likely to overeat. Losing weight through a sound exercise program almost always brings insulin levels back down within the normal range.

By the way, it's not surprising that people can lose weight quickly on high-protein, low-carbohydrate diets because most provide too few calories for active people. Besides, ketosis (when the body turns to burning fat when insufficient carbohydrate is eaten) promotes water loss and curbs appetite. (Every gram of glycogen is stored with almost 3 grams of water, so as you deplete your glycogen stores, you lose a great deal of water.) Besides dehydration, ketosis also causes bad breath, light-headedness, dizziness, and fainting, and it can be dangerous in the long run.

Why do some athletes claim that they feel, and perform, better on a high-protein, low-carbohydrate diet? Obviously, we don't all have the same nutrition needs, and not everyone is an elite athlete who trains for hours every day. Some active people, especially those who have been on carbohydrate overload (eating, for example, fruit, salad, energy bars, bagels, pasta, and more bagels), may lose weight or perform better on high-protein diets simply because they're eating a more balanced diet. Getting enough high-quality protein, iron, zinc, calcium, and a little more fat can make quite a difference. Perhaps you've been fat-phobic, eliminating most protein-rich foods, such as meat and dairy products, because they also contain fat. Adding some protein and fat back to a very low-fat diet means that you may eat less because you feel more satisfied and can resist those urges to plow through a box of fat-free cookies in one sitting.

Keep in mind that deciphering complicated formulas and eating specific percentages of nutrients at every meal and snack most likely have little to do with feeling healthier and performing better. The key lies in eating a balanced diet that tastes good, meets your energy needs, and mixes carbohydrate, protein, and fat at every meal. Eating plenty of carbohydrate, without going overboard, makes sense. Otherwise, someone should tell some of the world's fastest runners, the Kenyans, that they're doing it all wrong by eating a diet high in ugali, a starchy corn-based mash that's rich in carbohydrate.

The Body's Response to Training

Athletes of all ages and abilities frequently get caught up in manipulating what they eat in hopes of performing better, rather than choosing foods to support their training efforts. When you boil it down, the connection between your diet and your training program is simple. Food is fuel. To succeed, you must train. To have enough energy to train consistently, you must meet your energy needs on a day-to-day basis.

Sure, it's important to be knowledgeable about recommended nutrition guidelines, but those recommendations are just that—guidelines. We all know that simply eating properly doesn't guarantee a PR or put you on the winner's podium. You have to do the work. Your daily food choices or diet plays a key role in your success by affecting your ability to train consistently and recover quickly. Healthy eating habits also help you avoid losing days to injuries and upper respiratory infections, such as colds.

Endurance training offers many benefits. Keep the following in mind when you're having a hard time riding one more mile, completing one more set of swimming intervals, or running along one more trail in cold rain. Endurance training helps you in the following ways:

- It increases cardiac output (the maximum amount of blood that the heart can pump every minute), which means that you supply your exercising muscles with more oxygen.
- It increases the capacity of muscles to store more glycogen—the fuel that your body heavily relies on during prolonged exercise of moderate to high intensity (50 to 90 percent of $\dot{V}O_2$max).
- It increases muscles' capacity to store fat (triglycerides) and increases the rate at which it is released (as free fatty acids), thereby making free fatty acids more readily available for your muscles to use as fuel during exercise.
- It improves the aerobic energy system of muscles by increasing the size and number of mitochondria (site of ATP production) in skeletal muscles, as well as the activity of oxidative enzymes needed for

breaking down carbohydrate and fat to produce ATP. Consequently, a trained athlete has greater capacity to burn carbohydrate for fuel during intense endurance exercise and relies less on limited muscle glycogen and blood glucose as fuel during prolonged submaximal exercise.

- It raises lactate threshold (the pace or intensity you can maintain without causing lactic acid to accumulate significantly in the blood and contribute to fatigue) through certain types of training, such as fartlek, intervals, circuit training, and sustained tempo exercise, thereby helping to minimize anaerobic metabolism. A unit of glycogen burned aerobically (with oxygen) generates nearly 20 times the ATP that it could through anaerobic (without oxygen) metabolism. In practical terms, a higher lactate threshold means that your oxygen-dependent energy systems have improved and that your muscles are better able to clear lactic acid from the blood. You can, in other words, exercise more intensely without accumulating lactic acid—an obvious benefit because the presence of lactic acid contributes to fatigue and inhibits the ability of the body to burn fat as fuel, which increases the rate at which glycogen is broken down.

All these adaptations help you become more efficient at using fat as a fuel source during exercise. Fats are mobilized and made available to working muscles more rapidly. Training also stimulates your muscles to store more carbohydrate in the form of muscle glycogen. The benefits are twofold: Muscles start out with larger glycogen reserves, and you use it at a slower rate. You can therefore exercise at a higher absolute level (for example, maintain your pace for longer) before experiencing the fatiguing effects of glycogen depletion.

Eating balanced meals and snacks daily is the easiest way to get the necessary calories and key nutrients needed for consistently training at a high level. Athletes who accomplish their training goals arrive at the starting line more confident and better prepared to handle the rigors associated with endurance sports. By coupling the benefits of smart endurance training with nutrition strategies that target the key time periods before, during, and after exercise (see chapter 4), you'll be able to succeed at whatever endurance endeavor you choose.

3

Weighty Matters: Losing, Gaining, and Maintaining

Which weighs more, a pound of feathers or a pound of bricks? The answer: A pound is a pound!

Common sense tells us a pound of muscle and a pound of fat have to weigh the same; however, they do differ in density. Place 5 pounds of muscle and 5 pounds of fat side by side, and you will see that the muscle takes up less volume, or space, than the fat.

Are you training more than ever, but you still can't seem to lose weight? Or do you need to get stronger this season in order to get faster? Athletes participating in endurance sports typically fall into one of two categories regarding body weight: those who want to lose weight or body fat so they have less to carry around and those who want to add muscle or gain weight to boost their strength-to-weight ratio. In either case, the smart athlete will focus on establishing a solid training program, supportive eating habits, and a positive body image. These components are essential if you are to reach and maintain the leanest, healthiest weight you are genetically preprogrammed to be. If your quest becomes an obsession, however, especially if you try to live at a weight that's too low for you, you will perform poorly. You can also cause serious harm to your health and well-being.

Body-Weight Basics

Like most of the recreational athletes and elite competitors I work with, you've probably tried to lose or gain a few pounds at one time or another. You most likely set out to reshape your body in hopes of performing better.

Although most of us readily accept our height, we often invest a great deal of time and energy trying to manipulate what we weigh. An important concept to accept is that body weight is influenced by more than simply what we eat and how much we exercise. Gender, age, and height, as well as the thickness (density) of bones and our ratio of lean muscle mass to fat all influence how much we weigh at any given point in life. Obviously, most of these factors are genetically predetermined and out of your control, as is your inherited body type.

If you use a typical bathroom or locker-room scale to monitor your weight, accept its limitations. A scale cannot differentiate between fat weight and muscle weight. In other words, it can't tell you about body composition—how much of you is muscle and how much is body fat. Furthermore, when you step on the scale and it registers a number higher or lower than your last, you can't tell whether you've gained or lost muscle or body fat. Additionally, body weight is not static. It doesn't remain exact or constant from day to day or even throughout a single day. Treat body weight as a vital sign, similar to blood pressure or body temperature, that varies throughout the day.

To gain useful information from the scale, limit outside variables. In other words, don't compare readings from different scales or make drastic changes in your food choices or training program based on a single or random weight check. Rather, weigh yourself nude in the morning, once a week at most (if at all), after emptying your bladder and before you exercise or eat breakfast. Monitoring body weight over time (during a specific phase of training, for example) can be valuable. An otherwise unexplained drop in weight over a few weeks or a competitive season, combined with less-than-satisfactory performances, for instance, can signal an overtraining scenario precipitated by underfueling. Daily weigh-ins, on the other hand, provide information only on body fluid shifts.

Many variables affect your weight at any particular time. Sweat losses due to exercise or illness-induced vomiting or diarrhea will temporarily decrease your weight, whereas the scale may register a gain (sometimes literally overnight) due to water retention related to monthly hormonal changes or a carbohydrate-packed meal eaten the night before. If you're compelled to weigh yourself daily, use your time and energy productively. Weigh yourself before and after you exercise to monitor fluid losses and to assess how well your hydration plan worked. To rehydrate following exercise, drink at least 2.5 cups of fluid for every pound (1.3 L for every kg) that you're down on the scale.

As a serious athlete, don't put too much stock into standard height–weight tables or even the weight guidelines from the National Institutes of Health based on body mass index (BMI). Calculated with a formula that considers body weight relative to height, BMI can be used by health professionals to help find people at risk for obesity-related diseases, such as diabetes, coronary heart disease, and some cancers. BMI was developed, however, to be used in population studies. On an individual level, it's an inaccurate and poor predictor of fatness and health.

Many athletes and even regular exercisers, for example, often will show up on the charts as overweight (BMI of 25.0 to 29.9) or possibly obese (BMI of 30.0 or above) even when they're not. Blame your lean body mass, or muscles, which are denser and thus heavier than fat, as well as (hopefully) denser bones, too. If you work out consistently and your heart and lungs are fit (and you pass your annual medical checkup), don't be overly concerned about your BMI. Healthy bodies come in all shapes and sizes. What's important is your fitness level, not your weight.

Body Composition and Performance

Rather than relying only on the scale to evaluate the effectiveness of your diet and training program, consider your body composition, too. Simply put, our bodies are composed of two compartments, fat mass and fat-free or lean body mass (bones, muscles, organs, and connective tissue). By using one of the various body-composition analysis techniques available, you can determine, and monitor over time, how much of your body weight is fat (expressed as percent body fat) and how much is lean body mass.

Generally, leaner athletes, or those with lower percentages of body fat, perform better on tests of speed, endurance, balance, agility, and jumping ability. Excessive body fat would be detrimental for a serious-minded endurance athlete. It translates into extra weight that the athlete must transport for extended periods. The ideal body composition varies from sport to sport. In general, body-fat levels of elite endurance athletes (marathoners and triathletes) range from 5 to 9 percent in men and 8 to 15 percent in women. Keep in mind that these levels are simply what researchers have observed, not what all endurance athletes should strive for or attain.

Be careful not to confuse *correlation* with *causation*. As athletes attained an elite ranking in their sport, measurements were taken and their body-fat levels were observed to fall into (or correlate with) a particular percent body-fat range. These measurements, however, cannot prove (because observations simply don't have the scientific power to do so) that body-fat percentage is the reason (or cause) of these individuals obtaining elite status (effect). In other words, taking drastic steps to whittle your body fat down into the previously mentioned ranges doesn't guarantee that you'll enter the elite ranks. In fact, despite what athletes and those around them believe (or want to believe), rarely is an athlete's relative fatness the definitive limiting factor in his or her sport performance.

Taking your body-fat level too low, in fact, is unhealthy, and it is likely to be detrimental to your performance. Your body needs some essential fat to function. The American College of Sports Medicine estimates that men need a minimum level of 5 percent and women need at least 12 percent (higher body-fat levels are needed to protect menstrual and child-bearing functions). If you choose to monitor your body-fat percentage, be realistic. The goal is to achieve an appropriate body-fat level that allows you to perform at your best without harming your current or long-term health. As with weight, the top performers in any sport will always vary in body-fat percentage. When I was running my fastest, for example, I was involved in a comprehensive study of elite female distance runners. Most were running well at body-fat percentages between 10 and 12 percent. But the most accomplished women at that time—the top collegiate 10K runner and the world's leading female marathoner—were both significantly above that range.

Methods of Assessing Body Composition

Several techniques exist to assess body composition. The following section describes the advantages and drawbacks of the methods most commonly available to endurance athletes. In living humans, body fat cannot be measured directly, only estimated. The only way to directly measure body fat is to analyze a human cadaver—obviously an impractical approach! Keep in mind that even the best methods have an error of 2 to 3 percent. For example, if your body-fat level is given as 12 percent and the measurement technique carries a 3 percent error rate, your estimated body-fat percentage is actually anywhere from 9 to 15 percent.

Underwater (Hydrostatic) Weighing

This method requires repeated tests conducted in a special water-filled tank. You will be instructed to blow all the air out of your lungs and then asked to sit perfectly still for about 10 seconds while fully immersed underwater. The difference between our weight on land and our weight in the water is used to estimate body density. From that, body-fat percentage is extrapolated. It's desirable to be considered dense during this test, because denser bodies have less fat. If you're interested in underwater weighing, check with a local sports medicine center, a hospital with a wellness department, or a university with a physical education or exercise physiology program.

Underwater weighing has traditionally been the gold standard or technique of choice among researchers when it comes to assessing body composition. Much of the success, however, depends on the person's ability to tolerate being underwater while expelling as much air as possible. Depending on where you live and the resources available to you, underwater weighing can be expensive (US$10 to US$75), and it's more time consuming than other methods. The formulas used also may be less appropriate for some populations (such as older and non-Caucasian athletes).

Air Displacement (Bod Pod)

This technique relies on the same whole-body measurement principle as underwater weighing does; the overall density of the body is used to determine the percentage of fat and lean tissue. You sit in an enclosed egg-shaped capsule (the Bod Pod) for about 1 minute as computer sensors determine the amount of air displaced by your body. The Bod Pod quickly generates estimates of body-fat percentage, does not require the subject to get wet, and produces estimates that correlate closely with those produced by hydrostatic weighing for physically active people. Unfortunately, few facilities can afford the research-oriented version of the Bod Pod (which has the ability to measure actual lung volume), so this option can be expensive, and it may not be available in your area. Check university research laboratories and athletic facilities that serve professional and collegiate athletes. The Bod Pod version typically available in health clubs uses predicted lung volumes; thus, athletes engaged in serious training may be led awry by skewed results. With either version, it's advised you wait at least 2 hours following exercise before being tested.

Dual-Energy X-Ray Absorptiometry (DEXA)

DEXA has rapidly become the new gold standard due to its precision, accuracy, and reliability. It looks at the body using a three-compartment model: lean muscle mass, fat, and bone. As you lie quietly for 10 to 20 minutes, a whole-body scanner that emits two types of low-dose X-rays (one for bone, one for soft tissue) passes across your body. Developed to measure bone density, DEXA assumes that the amount of photon energy being absorbed is directly proportional to the mineral content of the bones. Besides letting you know what shape your bones are in (compared with predetermined standards for people of the same sex and age group), DEXA provides relative measurements of fat and lean tissue. Furthermore, DEXA shows exactly where the fat (as well as the muscle) is distributed throughout your body.

Noninvasive and easy, DEXA does expose you to low amounts of radiation (as all X-rays do), and it can be relatively pricey because the equipment is expensive, and trained professionals are required to operate it. Check universities, hospitals, and other research-based facilities.

Bioelectrical Impedance Analysis

Bioelectrical impedance analysis (BIA) involves having a low-voltage (undetectable) electric current passed through your body via electrodes attached to your hand and ankle. Lean body tissue (primarily muscle) contains most of the body's water and electrolytes; thus, it conducts the current faster and more easily than adipose or fat tissue. The faster the current travels through your body, the less body fat you have.

Although quick and noninvasive, BIA has a higher error rate (3 to 5 percent), and it can be particularly inaccurate when used with athletes. BIA tends to overestimate body-fat percentages in lean individuals, and fluid shifts in the body caused by dehydration from exercising or fluid retention due to a menstrual cycle can easily sway the results. To increase the probability of getting meaningful measurements, you must be well hydrated (although you should avoid eating and drinking for 4 hours before the test) and should avoid exercising for 12 hours before the test.

The same advice applies if you purchase a scalelike device based on BIA designed for home use (such as the Tanita body-fat scale). You need to take readings at the same time of day, when you are in a hydrated state (with an empty bladder). Avoid getting on the scale when you are most likely to be dehydrated—early in the morning or late at night, following exercise, after a sauna, or within 24 hours of consuming large amounts of caffeine or alcohol.

Skinfold Caliper Test

A skinfold caliper test involves using handheld calipers to pinch and measure the thickness of fat located right under the skin. Typically, three to seven sites are measured, for example, the abdomen, back of the arm, thigh, hip, and back of the shoulder. These measurements are plugged into a formula to estimate percent body fat. This simple, noninvasive, inexpensive technique can provide accurate and reliable readings, but only if the measurement taker is skilled and has had lots of practice. Skinfold measurements are not the most valid predictor of body fat (3 to 5 percent error). Nevertheless, they can be very useful to athletes and coaches in monitoring changes in body composition over time.

Tape Measure

You can essentially accomplish what skinfold tests do by using a tape measure. This method requires no fancy scientific formulas, just precise measurements. Simply measure selected points on your upper arm, chest, waist, hips, thighs, and calves to the nearest eighth of an inch (3 mm) with a tape measure and record those readings. You won't be calculating a specific body-fat percentage. Over time, though, as you repeat the measurements, you will be able to see your body respond as you adopt healthier eating habits or undertake a new training program.

If weight loss is your goal, for example, it can be gratifying and reassuring to use a tape measure to document your progress (i.e., to see measurements decrease over time) versus relying solely on the scale. Female athletes who intensify their training or begin a strength-training program often struggle to make sense of the scale, too. A pound of muscle (think of a brick) takes up less space than a pound of fat (think of cotton balls), so a tape measure will more accurately reflect body composition changes than will a scale.

Determining Optimal Body Composition

Many athletes I counsel want to know what they should weigh, especially those who are new to a sport or embarking on a challenging endurance endeavor for the first time. I remind them that determining an exact weight or body-fat percentage isn't necessary or even desirable. Strive to keep your weight within an optimal range, within a few pounds, for example, during a competitive season. Living on salad and rice cakes while training twice a day to reach or maintain a specific weight is a red flag that your weight goal is unrealistic.

Remember that your weight and body-fat percentage will vary some throughout the year depending on the amount and type of exercise that you are engaged in. Measuring your body-fat percentage is better than knowing only your weight; however, it's still just an estimated number. The most common mistake that I see athletes make is engaging in harmful behaviors, like crash dieting or overloading on caffeine or other stimulants to "burn fat," based on a single body-fat measurement. A second common mistake made is comparing measurements compiled from different testing methods. Science tells us that if we want to track body composition, we must use the same method each time and follow the person over time. This approach allows us to monitor changes in body composition that truly occur in response to changes in training or eating habits. Because gaining muscle or losing body fat requires time and a lot of effort, most people won't benefit from having their body-fat percentage estimated more than once or twice a year (if at all). To make such measurements worthwhile, you also need to note the type and volume of training that you were involved in at the time the measurement was taken.

Rather than focus on, or worse, obsess over your weight (which is merely an outcome of what you do), switch your focus and concentrate on your behaviors. What do you need to be doing daily to reach your desired outcome? You'll make faster progress by putting your energy into setting up and sticking to a sound training program and establishing smart eating habits. These two factors are what will carry you over the long haul. Following this approach leads you to your optimal weight range—you can realistically achieve and maintain this weight, perform well at it without compromising your physical or mental health, and fully enjoy life, too. You may not like what this optimum weight range turns out to be; however, that's another book!

What's a healthy body-fat percentage to strive for? Check out the most current research-based standards, which take in account age and sex, presented in table 3.1.

TABLE 3.1 Body-Fat Basics

Health standards:
Body-fat levels considered healthy because they do not independently increase the risk for health problems, such as high blood pressure, diabetes, or heart disease.

Men < 55 yr: 8%–22%	Women < 55 yr: 20%–35%
Men > 55 yr: 10%–25%	Women > 55 yr: 25%–38%

Fitness and physical activity standards:
Body-fat levels that reflect greater physical training. No additional benefits to sports performance occur when body fat drops below 5% (<55 yr) and 7% (>55 yr) for men and below 16% (<55 yr) and 20% (>55 yr) for women; however, health risks increase when body fat drops below those levels.

Men < 55 yr: 5%–15%	Women < 55 yr: 16%–28%
Men > 55 yr: 7%–18%	Women > 55 yr: 20%–33%

Athletes:
No body-fat standards have been established for athletes in specific sports. Body-fat values for athletes vary widely depending on gender and the sport itself.
All athletes need a certain amount of body fat, at least 5% for men and 16% for women, to insulate vital organs, regulate body temperature, and ensure adequate production of sex hormones.
The optimal body-fat percentage for an individual athlete may be much higher than these minimums and should always be determined on an individual basis because of genetic differences in body type.
In either sex, a too-low body-fat level (less than 5% for male athletes, less than 12% for female athletes) jeopardizes performance and increases the risk for serious health problems.
Athletes who strive to maintain inappropriate body weight or body-fat levels, or who have body-fat percentages below the estimated minimal safe levels, may be at risk for an eating disorder or other health problems related to poor energy and nutrient intakes.

Sources: V.H. Heyward and D.R. Wagner, 2004, *Applied body composition assessment*, 2nd ed. (Champaign, IL: Human Kinetics), and "Position of the American Dietetic Association, Dietitians of Canada, and the American College of Sports Medicine: Nutrition and athletic performance," *Journal of the American Dietetic Association* 100(2), December 2000: 1543-1556.

Altering Body Composition

In the endurance-sports world, many athletes struggle to maintain a healthy weight. Most at risk are those who need to lose weight (body fat) for medical reasons, as well as those athletes who need to gain weight (or restore weight they've lost) in order to live within their body's preprogrammed healthy or optimal weight range. Whether you maintain, lose, or gain weight is primarily a matter of energy balance. You'll maintain your weight if you consume roughly the same amount of energy, or calories, that you expend.

To gain weight, you need to consume more calories than you burn off. To lose weight, you must expend more calories than you take in—that is, you must eat less or exercise more, or ideally, do some of both. In theory, weight loss is simple and straightforward. In real life, however, it's more complex. After all, you're dealing with the human body, not a machine. And as you're probably aware, athletes, too, often eat for reasons other than physical hunger.

Strategies for Losing Weight

Before you embark on a plan to lose weight, be certain that you really need to. Don't assume that your performance will definitely improve if you lose weight or that you've automatically gained fat every time the scale registers an increase. Before attempting weight loss—or if you're a coach, before implying an athlete needs to or should lose weight—it may be helpful to determine percent body fat or to reassess skinfold measurements, especially for endurance athletes with stocky, muscular builds and for female athletes who may appear heavier because they carry their weight on their lower body (hips and thighs). Whatever the case, if your body-fat percentage is reasonable from a physiological standpoint, you won't gain anything from dieting or excessively exercising to reach a new low on the scale.

You may need to instead concentrate on accepting your inherited body type or, if you're a coach or trainer, on accepting the body types of the athletes you work with. One of my collegiate teammates, the best female cross-country runner in her state as a high school senior, is a perfect example. Tall with a lean upper body, she carried all her weight on the lower half of her body. Despite completing a successful high school career at a certain weight, our coach decided that she would perform better in college if she lost 5 pounds (2.3 kg). Living on salad, air-popped popcorn, and a small dinner (accompanied by a scoop of ice cream as a reward for making it through the day), she did lose the weight. However, she constantly battled an upper respiratory infection and even pulled some intercostal (between the ribs) muscles from coughing so hard. She ran poorly all year and never fully recuperated.

If weight loss is in order, rapid weight loss isn't an option for physically active people—especially if you're serious about competing. A loss of more than 1 pound (.5 kg) a week for female athletes or 2 pounds (1 kg) for male athletes means you're losing more than just body fat. Along with initial losses of water and muscle glycogen is a significant loss of protein from the breakdown of lean tissue (muscles and internal organs). Your competitors are the only ones who benefit from this type of weight loss. Athletes who are chronically dehydrated and operating with too-low glycogen stores will find it increasingly difficult to maintain their usual training pace, will fatigue earlier in workouts and competitions, and will be more likely to get injured. It's also harder to be confident, focused, and positive when you're anxious about your weight and preoccupied with thoughts of food and the scale.

The longer-term consequences of losing weight rapidly can be particularly costly: loss of muscular strength and power, electrolyte disturbances due to dehydration, increased susceptibility to colds and other respiratory illnesses, iron deficiency anemia, amenorrhea (loss of menstrual periods) for women or suppressed testosterone levels for men, low bone density as a result of hormonal disturbances and lack of dietary calcium, ketosis (an undesirable state that the body enters when it must use its fat to fuel the brain), and potential kidney problems. Ultimately, you may lose valuable training time or, worse, be forced to miss a competition or planned adventure altogether.

The bottom line: Attempting to lose weight during the competitive season or at a time when you need to deliver a peak performance makes no sense. Weight loss is best undertaken during early preseason, when you're ramping up your base or aerobic training, but not yet doing faster-paced or intense workouts.

Repeated attempts to manipulate body weight or body fat below a level that is normal for you are counterproductive. Significant metabolic changes result from chronic dieting and the loss of critical fat stores. If you restrict your caloric intake too drastically, your body immediately resists by dropping its resting metabolic rate—that is, your body uses fewer calories to carry on essential vital functions. This means future calories are more likely to be stored as body fat. Because your body has no way of knowing how long it must tolerate being underfueled, it will attempt to protect itself by immediately adapting to a lower calorie intake.

For most people, this reduction in resting metabolic rate doesn't appear to be permanent; however, those who lose and gain weight repeatedly may experience some long-term effects. The body apparently receives messages through brain signals and hormones that help it become more efficient at extracting energy from food and storing it as body fat. Consequently, perpetual dieters often find it progressively harder to lose weight. In the future, they must eat even fewer calories to induce further weight loss.

Keep in mind that a pound of muscle burns 7 to 10 calories per day, which is far more than the 2 to 3 calories burned to maintain a pound of body fat. When you lose weight, you are destined to lose some of it as muscle or lean body mass (research has shown it to be about 25 percent, even more if you diet and drop weight quickly). And anytime you decrease or lose muscle mass, your body will require fewer calories to remain at the same weight. By the way, it is impossible to build muscle and lose body fat simultaneously. Weight loss requires that you take in fewer calories than your body needs every day, whereas muscle building requires that you take in more calories than you need daily.

Work with a qualified expert, such as a sports dietitian, if you need help in this area. Be realistic. You can't lose body fat overnight. Focus on behaviors, such as eating less, moving more, and better managing stress or anxiety that leads you to overeat. A realistic and healthy weight is a weight that you can reach and maintain, without heroic measures, at this point in your life. Perhaps you've added children to your family or picked up additional hours at work that cut into your training time. If this is the case, don't assume that you can weigh what you did in college or even what you weighed last year.

Finally, how you eat is just as important as what you eat. Assuming that you have weight to lose, and that you want to keep it off permanently, estimate your current calorie needs (see chapter 1) and put the following strategies into action.

Keep a Food Journal

If you bite it, write it! A food journal serves the same purpose as a training log. A record of what you eat can help you or someone with a trained eye (like a sports dietitian) decipher your current eating patterns—what works for you and what doesn't. If you're serious about eating better or losing weight, this is your number one tool. As with the 1-day or 24-hour food recall exercise in chapter 1, record everything that you eat or drink from the time you get up in the morning until bedtime. Be sure to write down the time of day or night, too. Measure portion sizes at home so that you can more accurately estimate how much you're eating when you're away from home. Capturing the reason that you are eating is also enlightening. For example, are you eating because you are physically hungry? Or because you're bored? Or nervous about an upcoming race? If you overindulge on weekends, a practice that can quickly erase the healthy choices that you've made all week, start by tracking those days.

Writing it all down has been shown repeatedly to help people remain committed to a long-term goal. One study followed 38 dieters who had been on a weight-loss program for a year through the dreaded danger zone, the period from 2 weeks before Thanksgiving (at the end of November) until 2 weeks after New Year's Day. The 25 percent of participants who consistently recorded all the foods that they ate during this period managed to lose 7 pounds (3 kg)! The other 75 percent who weren't as vigilant gained an average of 3 pounds (1.4 kg).

It's the writing down or recording, not precisely what you ate, that matters. Self-monitoring forces us to be accountable for our daily actions. Like the jar of peanuts you nibbled through while working late one night. You can't as easily forget about it when it's in black and white for you to see. You also can refer to your food journal to make certain that you're eating enough of the nutrient-rich foods that you need. For best results, leave your food journal in a visible place as a visual reminder (for example, on your desk or kitchen counter) or use your favorite electronic device to keep daily records. (See the Selected Resources section at the back of the book for the best apps to use.)

Reduce What You Eat by No More Than 300 Calories a Day

Take the long road: It's true that losing 1 pound (.5 kg) a week requires that you create a deficit of 3,500 calories. The traditional golden rule of weight loss tells you how: Consume 500 fewer calories a day. If you're physically active, however, drastically reducing the amount that you eat is unrealistic and certainly not sustainable. Popular ploys, such as starving yourself while working out as hard as you can or swearing off all fun foods until you reach some ideal weight, have little to no chance of being successful. Unfortunately, the most common weight-loss strategy that athletes employ is one that actually promotes weight gain. They diet all day by skipping breakfast and skimping on lunch, become progressively hungrier as the day goes along, and then load in the calories by beating a path to the refrigerator from late afternoon until bedtime.

Trimming the amount of calories that you currently consume by small increments (200 to 300 calories a day rather than 500) shouldn't suppress your metabolism, and this approach helps limit the loss of lean muscle tissue. You also are more likely to have enough energy (and desire) to keep exercising, which is essential if you want to keep the weight off permanently.

Keep in mind that regardless of age or ability, athletes do best with weight loss that is accomplished in stages. After you lose a few pounds, let your body become accustomed to your new weight, and then decide whether you're feeling weaker or stronger before trying to lose more. Cementing even small changes into new habits takes time and effort. Stop and assess how you are doing at maintaining the healthy changes that got you to a lower weight. Can you realistically continue them? Will you be able to do more? You may find that you would be better off directing your efforts elsewhere, into strengthening your mental skills or accepting your body type, rather than continuing to try to lose more weight.

Sit Down and Eat Real Food

Don't throw nutrition guidelines out the window just because you're trying to lose weight. You still need to consume foods from all five food groups, plus a modest amount of fat daily, just like everyone else. Many female athletes I know wouldn't dream of sitting down to eat a real lunch—a sandwich and a glass of milk, for example. Instead, they nibble their way through the day, racking up calories from small chocolate treats, sports or energy bars, caffeinated beverages, and oversize muffins and fruit smoothies.

If you constantly eat out of a box, in your car, or while standing up, consider that these unfulfilling actions typically undermine weight-loss efforts. You're more likely to feel satisfied and experience less guilt or denial if you simply plan to eat three meals (of at least three food groups) and two snacks (aim for one or two food groups) daily. You'll likely eat fewer calories, too.

You may lack skills in the cooking and domestic department. I met one college athlete who lived off campus and was responsible for his own meals.

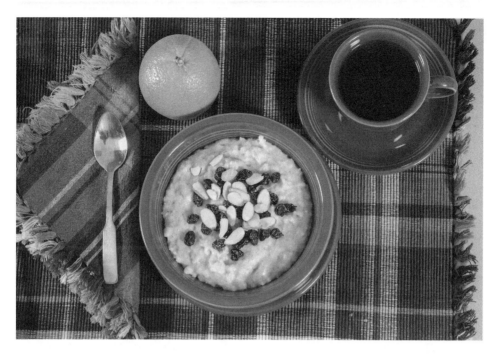

Eating breakfast fills you up and encourages you to eat healthfully all day long.

He routinely boiled four hot dogs for lunch and followed that up with four more for dinner. If you're like me and can't afford to hire a personal chef, invest some time and energy into learning basic cooking and meal-planning skills. Alternatively, invest in cost-effective dinners offered by companies that provide preassembled meals that you cook or reheat at home. Because we eat what is available and convenient, your job is to always keep a variety of nutritious and tasty foods on hand that you can assemble into a meal quickly. This "skill power" is what keeps people from racking up excess calories from takeout and fast foods—not willpower.

Eat Breakfast

Start the day out right. Eating breakfast is a habit. If you're not a regular breakfast eater, start retraining yourself now. Why? One of the crucial habits of successful weight losers, as tracked by the National Weight Control Registry (adults who have lost at least 30 pounds, or 14 kilograms, and kept it off for more than a year), is eating breakfast every day. By eating breakfast (within an hour of waking up), you jump-start your metabolism and set the stage for the rest of the day. For physically active people, eating breakfast is particularly important because we tend to get hungry more often and more quickly. If you want to end the struggle with your body, don't allow yourself to become too hungry during the day. Remember, the less you eat in the morning, the more likely you are to overeat later in the day.

Be a Portion Master

Be aware of portion distortion, especially when you dine away from home. Because of the supersizing of food portions, an average bakery bagel now provides 320 calories—the equivalent of eating three to four slices of bread! Paying attention to serving sizes can be an easy way to reel in your calorie intake, and practice brings progress. Megasized cookies, muffins, sodas, and coffee drinks may appear to be a good buy, but can you afford the 500 to 800 calories that they provide? The bottom line: Supersized portions lead to supersized people, including overweight athletes.

Even if you're training for your first marathon or century ride, you cannot afford to eat whatever foods you want in unlimited amounts. I constantly hear from disappointed recreational athletes who had assumed that they would lose weight easily while training for a new endurance challenge. If you snooze around food, however, you don't lose. You will also need to change the way that you eat (being mindful is required; being obsessed just backfires). Use a kitchen scale and measuring cups and spoons periodically at home so that you can estimate portion sizes when you dine out.

Look for easy ways to trim empty calories. If you eat out frequently, limit your intake of high-fat foods, such as salad dressings, mayonnaise, cheese, fatty meats like hot dogs and sausage, and fried items. Inquire about how foods are prepared before you order them to detect hidden fats, such as cream sauces, olive oil, and cheese. Watch out for carbohydrate overloading, too. Seriously, how often do you begin meals at home by eating a whole basket of bread?

Keeping It Off During the Off-Season

If you're like most competitive athletes, you're ready for the off-season when it arrives. This recovery period provides the body and mind with a well-deserved break from physical and mental stressors associated with strenuous training and competing. Whether you totally kick back, engage in active rest (this is a perfect time to try new activities), or enter a period of easy, light training, a decrease in exercise volume and intensity means you require fewer calories. So, you need to eat less—unless you want to pile on the pounds. I see it go best when athletes choose to enjoy some initial period of time completely off—that is, free of working on any goals. The next phase, early preseason, is when the successful ones gear it up again. This is the time to reexamine your eating habits as well as any weight-related concerns and goals you might have. If you need to lose weight (or increase muscle mass), early preseason is the time to work on it. Not later in the season when you don't want anything to interfere with or compromise important training sessions, and certainly not right before or during competition.

1. Skip the sports foods. Use energy drinks, bars, and gels strictly for their intended purposes—before, during, and after strenuous or prolonged exercise. When you're not moving continuously at a moderate-to-vigorous pace for at least 75 minutes, you don't need them. Arrange early preseason getting-back-in-shape or base-building training so that you can sit down to eat a normally scheduled, balanced meal within 60 minutes of walking in the door. This helps you avoid eating a special postworkout or recovery meal followed by your regular meal.

2. Keep moving. Besides workouts and races, many athletes are quite sedentary, especially those tied to a desk all day. With fewer planned exercise sessions, you may need to remind yourself to get up and get moving. To hold yourself accountable, buy a simple step counter. Aim to walk at least 10,000 steps a day, approximately 5 miles (8 km), by taking the stairs, running errands on foot, and pacing back and forth while on the phone. To keep your weight within a healthy range (3 to 6 pounds, or 1.4 to 2.8 kg), establish your baseline (average steps walked weekly) and then increase your weekly step goal as needed.

3. Weigh yourself weekly—on the same scale, at the same time of day, and under the same conditions. Modest weight gains are acceptable and expected. Be alert to an unexplained rapid or large gain in weight (for example, not associated with a strength-training program or the restoration of weight lost during the competitive season). Take responsibility for your body and take action before small gains add up to an unreasonable number of extra pounds.

4. Eat a fruit or vegetable at every meal and snack. Fill up without filling out. What's a good habit at any time becomes essential during the off-season. Commit to filling half your plate at lunch and dinner with fruits and vegetables—and French fries don't count! For snacks, start with a fruit or vegetable (carrot cake, strawberry Pop-Tarts, corn chips, and the like do not qualify) and then decide whether you're still hungry.

5. Eat your calories; don't drink them. It's easy to overload calories by guzzling down coffee drinks and other caffeinated beverages, like soda and energy drinks, especially if you're doing so in order to avoid eating. Bursts of caffeine and sugar will temporarily dull cravings, but hunger always comes roaring back. When awake, plan to eat every 3 to 4 hours (never go longer than 5 hours without eating). Commit to eating three balanced meals (each containing at least three food groups) daily, with one or two snacks as needed.

At mealtime, create a plate that mirrors My Plate (see chapter 1)—make half your plate or bowl fruits and vegetables. Limit grain-based foods, like potatoes, rice, pasta, and bread, to one-quarter of the plate. Fill the other quarter with lean protein–rich foods. Get a handle on how many calories you drink throughout the day, too. Cutting back on liquid calories from soda, alcohol, health shakes, energy drinks, and even juice may be all you need to do.

Include Lean Protein at Every Meal

It's no secret that people lose weight on the popular carbohydrate-controlled (higher-protein, lower-carbohydrate) diets. It's also not a mystery why: They consume fewer total calories. People report feeling fuller longer when they eat ample amount of protein, and that appears to translate into feeling less deprived and more motivated to stick with a lower calorie intake. Researchers are eagerly seeking the underlying mechanism to explain how protein works to increase the feeling of fullness. Beef up your diet by including a source of lean, quality protein, such as fish (not fried), chicken or turkey (no skin), lean red meat, low-fat dairy, eggs, soy products, or beans of any kind (pinto, black, kidney, and so on) at every meal. Stick to reasonable-size portions, such as 3 ounces (90 g) of meat, at any one time. Unlike carbohydrate and fat, protein cannot be stored by your body. If you eat protein beyond your needs, your body breaks it down and converts the excess calories into body fat.

Take Your Eating Cues From the Sun

Have you worked out today? Have you eaten today? Because most of us perform the bulk of our training, our work, and our family obligations between nine o'clock and six o'clock (even earlier if you train first thing in the morning), why do most of us insist on eating the majority of our calories after six o'clock? Concentrate on eating your calories when you need them most, which is during the day, and practicing moderation at night. Our muscles and our brains thrive on having a steady, constant supply of fuel available. To avoid becoming too hungry and devouring everything in sight, stagger your calories throughout the day. Plan to eat a meal or wholesome snack every 3 to 4 hours so that your blood sugar doesn't dip too low. Otherwise, you'll be racing for the nearest vending machine or fast-food outlet.

Be creative with your eating schedule. Even if you're trying to lose weight, you still need to be well fueled before you head out the door, and you still need to replenish your glycogen stores following strenuous exercise. If you train after work, for instance, eat less at lunchtime and save some calories for an afternoon snack closer to your workout time. A sports drink or energy bar after you finish takes the place of that second helping or extra dessert at dinner. You can control your overall intake by eating reasonable portions (a good reality check is the serving size listed on the label), by selecting lower-fat items, and by eating fewer calories at night when you don't really need them.

Marathon Training and Weight Changes

People training for marathons, ultra runs, and Ironman triathlons often become bewildered and frustrated (even panicked) if they discover that they've gained weight. You're supposed to lose weight when you train for endurance sports, right? Although this is a popular sentiment, it simply isn't true.

In reality, getting involved in endurance sports with the primary goal of losing weight is likely to lead to disappointment. A study presented at the 2011 American College of Sports Medicine's annual conference, for example, looked at the different motivations between first-time marathoners and dropouts. Those running to lose weight (or gain recognition) were more likely to drop out of marathon training. In another study, researchers put 64 people on a 3-month marathon training program. The end result: 78 percent experienced no change in body weight, 11 percent lost weight, and 11 percent gained weight. Of the 7 who gained weight, 6 were women.

What's going on here? First, an increase on the scale doesn't automatically mean you've gained body fat. As an endurance athlete, some weight gain can be expected due to physiological changes induced by training, such as an increase in blood volume, larger glycogen stores (which also means more water is held in the body), and increases in connective tissue, as well as possible gains in muscle mass. Second, while the study does not tell us why some women gained weight during the rigorous endurance training program, three-quarters of the women in the study did report eating more as they trained more, as compared to only 48 percent of the men. An increase in appetite is one of many proposed theories why women, in particular, often struggle to lose weight when engaged in endurance-type training. Other theories include muscle-efficiency differences that result in women's bodies burning fewer calories, hormonal differences affecting how women process carbohydrates, and women's increased likelihood of falling victim to reward syndrome. The latter involves mind games based on wishful or erroneous thinking, such as "I'm training for a marathon, so I can eat whatever I want, when I want," or "I just ran 18 miles (30 km), so I deserve another slice of pie."

The bottom line: Train to improve your performance, not to lose weight. Listen to and respect your body. Fuel up before you go (and during training sessions as recommended) and promptly refuel after prolonged or intense efforts. Lastly, don't use food rewards as a motivator to get you through the training you've elected to do.

Make Friends With Fat

Good fats aren't bad. The fat that you eat in foods doesn't inevitably reappear as body fat. You can still obtain a desirable level of body fat if you snack on half a bagel spread with peanut butter or a salad with dressing drizzled over it. Be sure to keep enough fat in your diet. Besides supplying energy and essential fatty acids, fat allows your body to absorb and use fat-soluble vitamins.

Fat also heightens the flavors of food, curbs cravings, and helps you feel satisfied. Without enough fat in your diet, you will feel unsatisfied and will be more likely to overeat, especially in the carbohydrate department. How many times have you passed on eating a burger or a piece of pizza because you tell yourself that it's too fattening, only to end up an hour later reaching for another sugary, caffeinated drink (or two) or answering an out-of-control chocolate craving? The fact remains that we do not gain weight simply from eating foods or meals that contain fat. Excess calories, whether they come from fat, carbohydrate, protein, or alcohol, are the culprit.

Eating a diet that contains an appropriate amount of fat, at least 20 percent of total calories or one-half gram per pound (1 gram per kilogram) of body weight, is not overdoing it. The key is to concentrate on eating the better kind of fat. Nuts and nut butters, seeds, avocados, and oils such as olive, canola, and flaxseed are rich in heart-healthy monounsaturated fat. Of course, even these heart-healthy fats supply concentrated calories (9 calories per gram), so use modest amounts spaced throughout the day.

Fats that we all need to limit in our daily diet are saturated fats and partially hydrogenated fats, or trans fats. To reduce the saturated fat in your diet, choose low-fat dairy products and lean cuts of meat. Limiting traditional fatty foods—fried food, fast food, and processed foods containing partially hydrogenated vegetable oils, such as stick margarine, snack foods, and bakery goods—will help keep the amount of trans fat that you consume under control.

Complement Your Aerobic Training With Anaerobic or Strength Training

Ignore misguided advice that you must train long and slow in order to burn fat and lose weight. Exercise performed at lower intensities (aerobic exercise) does use a higher percentage of fat than high-intensity exercise (anaerobic activities, such as interval or speed work). Exercise, however, does more than just help you burn fat. Exercise helps create a calorie deficit in the body; in other words, exercising helps you expend more calories than you consume. Remember, you need to create a deficit of 3,500 calories (by eating less, exercising more, or some combination of the two) to lose 1 pound (.5 kg). No matter which fuel source is burned during exercise, the body can pull from its fat stores later to make up for the calories expended during exercise.

The amount of calories that you burn during exercise depends on many factors—your body weight, the type of exercise, the intensity and duration, and whether you are a novice or a trained athlete. As an endurance athlete, you're most likely focusing on putting in the distance. But strength or resistance training and higher-intensity exercise, such as intervals, tempo workouts, and fartlek training (you break up your normal pace with fast bursts), can help you lose weight as well as boost performance. Don't forget that during exercise, a combination of fat and carbohydrate are burned for energy. Given the same time period, lower-intensity exercise uses a greater percentage of fat than higher-intensity exercise; however, it burns fewer calories overall. During faster-paced activities, a greater percentage of calories from carbohydrate are burned than from fat; however, the total calories burned is much higher. What matters most is the total number of calories used, not the percentage of fat to carbohydrate. Higher-intensity exercise helps you lose weight because it uses more calories per minute.

Think about it this way: A large percentage of a small number can be smaller than a small percentage of a large number. For example, a 150-pound (68 kg) cyclist averaging a leisurely 12 miles (19 km) per hour may burn 380 calories an hour, and about 70 percent of the energy is derived from fat. The same cyclist may burn approximately 780 calories per hour riding at 18 miles (29 km) per hour, and fat provides about 50 percent of the necessary fuel. But 70 percent of 380 is 266, and 50 percent of 780 is 390, so the more intense ride burns over 100 more fat calories. More important, because few people have unlimited time to exercise, riding more intensely burns 400 more calories in the same period (780 versus 380).

Trained athletes burn more fat as fuel for two reasons. First, they use fat sooner during exercise (training helps you store more fat within muscles for easy access). Second, they have the ability to work at higher intensities (thanks in part to an elevated lactate threshold) than recreational athletes do, so they burn more overall calories as well as proportionally higher amounts of fat. Of course, you can't just go flying out the door and start training fast and furiously in an attempt to lose weight. You won't burn many calories sitting on the couch if you injure yourself.

Lower-intensity or slower-paced workouts are necessary for preparing your body for the future stresses that come with more intense or strenuous activity. In the meantime, as you're working up to handling higher-intensity workouts, the duration or length of time you spend exercising becomes a greater factor. To succeed at weight loss, you'll need to exercise longer to make up for the lower number of calories used per minute. Consider increasing your training volume by adding more distance to your weekly training program. And become more active outside of planned workouts. Throughout the day, look for opportunities to move more. Take the stairs instead of the elevator and walk instead of drive to complete errands.

Make visiting the weight room a priority, too. Strength training helps to preserve muscle mass, a major determinant of resting metabolic rate. The more muscular you are, the more calories you burn—even at rest. Weight training also makes it more likely that any weight you do lose is primarily body fat, not muscle.

Strategies for Gaining Weight

Gaining weight can be an advantage if speed, power, leverage, or mass comes into play in your sport or activity. Of course, you most likely want to gain lean muscle tissue, not fat. Adding muscle mass can increase your strength-to-weight ratio, which ultimately increases your strength and power, enabling you to perform at a higher level. Depositing extra body fat does little to enhance power or strength. On the other hand, some endurance athletes find that carrying a little extra padding may help them fend off illness and better weather the rigors of hard training.

Like athletes who are trying to lose weight, you need to be realistic about the amount of weight or lean body mass that you can gain. Adding a few pounds before you head off to an ultra run or adventure race is one thing, but expecting to transform your physique is a completely different ball game. Your genes, gender, diet, training program (including the amount of strength training that you're willing to do), and motivation all count. Look at the other members of your family, especially your parents, to get a clear picture of your potential. If you're a well-trained athlete or simply a hard gainer, you may find it difficult, if not impossible, to gain weight without substantially increasing the amount of calories that you eat or cutting back on your training.

The bottom line, of course, is that to gain or build muscle, you must consume more calories than you expend. In general, you'll need to eat an extra 400 to 500 calories a day to gain about 1 pound (.5 kg) of lean muscle in a week. Don't look to supplements as a substitute for hard work and good nutrition. No magic nutrients exist that promote substantial gains in strength and muscle mass. (See chapter 5 for a complete review of creatine and other supplements touted for their potential to enhance muscle mass in athletes.) Keep the following guidelines in mind as you attempt to add lean muscle mass.

Up Your Calorie Intake and Do More Strength Training

Contrary to popular opinion, total calorie intake, not protein, is the determining nutrition factor when it comes to gaining muscle. Building new muscle, or adding mass, requires that you consume enough calories to meet normal daily energy demands, as well as support new tissue growth. If you fail to take in enough calories, protein that you consume will be used to help satisfy energy needs rather than to build new muscle tissue. You must also commit to a well-designed strength- or weight-training program. Eating extra calories or protein, or ingesting vitamins, amino acids, or other supplements, won't magically do the trick. Strength training helps muscle cells become more efficient at using available protein to synthesize new cells.

If you're training and eating appropriately, the majority of any weight gained will be muscle. Of course, if you simply overeat (literally consume more calories than you burn off), then extra calories from any source—carbohydrate, protein, or fat—will result in weight gain, primarily from an increase in body fat.

Make Eating a Priority

Many athletes need to make eating a high priority to ensure that they get enough calories. Eat frequently throughout the day (starting within an hour of when you arise) and eat well at meals, even if you don't feel hungry. Don't let mealtimes slip away on weekends, business trips, or during busy times, like the holidays. Also, consciously plan to eat mini meals (snacks) two or three times a day. Be smart and plan ahead by buying and keeping healthy snacks on hand at home, at the office, and in your car (see Performance-Enhancing Snacks in chapter 8). Refuel promptly after all training bouts—don't wait until your hunger returns.

Choose Higher-Calorie, Healthy Foods

You can easily boost your calories by choosing heartier versions of various foods, such as granola over cornflakes and split-pea soup instead of chicken noodle soup. Eating larger than normal portions of healthy foods, such as another helping of baked beans or an extra sandwich, will also add calories. If you're crunched for time or planning to exercise soon, drink your calories. Liquid-meal products, homemade liquid meals such as milk shakes and fruit smoothies, and even 100 percent fruit juice (cranberry juice has more calories than orange juice, for example) can be easy ways to down additional calories.

Eat Carbohydrate and Protein With Each Meal and Snack

Special protein powders or weight-gainer supplements aren't essential when you're trying to put on muscle or gain weight. Eating more protein, such as meat or eggs, won't translate automatically into more muscle, either. Athletes who struggle to gain weight typically fail because they don't consume enough calories or enough carbohydrate in their day-to-day diet, not because they lack protein. Although protein requirements do increase, most athletes naturally fulfill their quota from the additional food that they eat to boost their calories. Carbohydrate-rich foods still need to supply most of these calories. Your body relies on carbohydrate to fuel weight-training sessions as well as the endurance activities that you participate in. Consuming adequate carbohydrate also replenishes muscle glycogen stores so that you can continue to train effectively day after day.

To meet your protein and carbohydrate needs simultaneously, eat a variety of foods. Meat, poultry, fish, eggs, cheese, and tofu all supply quality protein (as well as fat, obviously), but virtually no carbohydrate. Few foods, though, are composed of one nutrient. Milk (regular and soy), yogurt, cottage cheese, and beans and lentils are good sources of both protein and carbohydrate. Vegetables and other carbohydrate-rich foods like pasta, rice, bread, and cereal supply relatively small amounts of protein, but small amounts add up when eating large portions.

Remind yourself of the importance of eating enough carbohydrate and protein by including a protein-rich food (from the protein foods or dairy group) with your carbohydrate-based meals and snacks. For example, melt cheese on a whole wheat bagel; add tuna, chicken, or a hard-boiled egg to a salad; top pasta with a meat sauce; and serve baked beans over rice or on top of a baked potato. Pay particular attention to your food choices when you first hit the weight room. When you add a strength-training program to an already ambitious training schedule, your body's need for protein rapidly increases.

If you're still concerned that you're not getting enough protein, consider sports shakes or complete meal-replacement powders. These products offer a more complete nutrition package than straight protein powders or supplements. They're relatively expensive, so you might consider saving them for travel or for days when a busy schedule would otherwise result in missed meals. If you're not lactose intolerant, you can add nonfat dried milk powder to just about anything, such as homemade shakes or smoothies, or stir it into oatmeal, soup, or cooked rice. Nonfat dried milk is a high-quality, inexpensive protein supplement (a quarter-cup provides about 11 grams of protein) without the unproven additives that many other supplements provide.

Fuel Up Before and After Workouts

Time your nutrition right. Feed your muscles at two key times—before and after exercise. During exercise, muscle fibers are ripped apart and broken down. Repair of damaged muscle fibers and formation of new muscle tissue happen only postexercise, when you allow your body to rest and recover. To optimize gains of lean muscle and strength, eat a small amount of protein (along with carbohydrate, of course) just before and after you strength train. Take advantage of the situation—your muscles are primed at these times, so give them what they need. Scientists at the University of Texas, for example, found that drinking a protein-fortified sports drink (containing only 6 grams of protein—slightly less than the amount of protein contained in 1 ounce, or 30 grams, of meat or a cup of yogurt) before a weight-training workout resulted in greater gains in lean body mass than drinking it afterward. Researchers theorize that a ready supply of essential amino acids (the building blocks of protein) in the bloodstream combined with the increased blood flow to muscles during exercise translated into the amino acids being ready and waiting in the muscle for postexercise repair.

It's well known that consuming a carbohydrate-rich sports drink or meal immediately after exercise (during the carbohydrate window) helps the body refill its glycogen stores more quickly. Adding protein to the mix jump-starts muscle repair and growth. The carbohydrate (which is broken down into glucose) stimulates the release of insulin, a powerful hormone that directs glucose out of your bloodstream and into your cells where it can be used as fuel, or into muscle and liver cells, where it is stored as glycogen. Insulin also decreases the rate at which body proteins are broken down and, simultaneously, the rate at which they are rebuilt—a perfect scenario for an athlete seeking to gain lean muscle mass. Researchers still don't agree on the ideal ratio of carbohydrate to protein (3:1 to 7:1 have been used in studies) to produce a significant effect, although a small amount of protein (about 10 grams) appears to be sufficient. Opt for lean, animal-based protein sources because they provide ample amounts of the essential amino acids that our bodies cannot make.

Three Dangerous Ds: Body Dissatisfaction, Dieting, and Disordered Eating

A chapter about athletes and weight would not be complete without a discussion about disordered eating. That's right—*disordered eating*, not *eating disorders*. (For more on eating disorders, such as anorexia and bulimia nervosa, see chapter 6.) The National Eating Disorders Association defines disordered eating as "attitudes about weight, food, and body size and shape that cause a person to have very strict or rigid eating and exercise habits that jeopardize their health, happiness and safety." Sports-minded people who are constantly at war with food, dissatisfied with their body size or shape, and obsessed with controlling their weight (which usually means trying to lose weight) are often trapped in disordered eating.

Disordered eating involves trying to consciously control what, when, and how much you eat, not by tuning into your body's signals of hunger or fullness (as normal, healthy eaters do) but by tuning them out. Adhering to external rules and guidelines (like diets, prepackaged drinks and meals, and self-imposed rules about good and bad foods) takes precedence over listening to what your body needs. As a result, disordered eaters become overly preoccupied with eating a certain way, such as avoiding all sugar and white flour or eating as little fat as possible. They may obsessively count calories or fat grams, or eat in irregular and chaotic ways, such as skipping meals, fasting, or bingeing. Dieting or restrained eating—eating less than the body needs at a given time or actively resisting the intake of specific foods or entire food groups—also fits the definition of disordered eating. In fact, many experts who specialize in food, body image, and weight issues believe that dieting itself is the chief cause of most disordered eating.

According to nutrition and body image experts, two main styles of disordered eaters exist: deprivation eaters and emotional eaters. I routinely see both in the clients with whom I work. Deprivation eaters have a history of dieting (usually with accompanying "fat" and "thin" weights), of disliking their bodies and trying to change them with exercise or by restricting the foods that they eat. They divide foods into good and bad categories and then attempt to eat only the good or "legal" foods. They spend a great deal of time worrying about whether the foods that they eat are going to make or keep them fat, or berating themselves from not being able to stay away from their forbidden foods.

Of course, you can't stay on a diet or avoid all your favorite foods forever, especially when you expect your body to perform physically. Nor can you drastically alter your inherited body type. The natural response to deprivation or restrained eating is bingeing or overcompensating, particularly on all the foods that you've deprived yourself of. Deprivation eaters, however, use this as further evidence that they are controlled by food or out of control when it comes to food. They thus believe that they need a diet or meal plan to follow. Their own body signals of hunger and fullness certainly can't be trusted when it comes to figuring out what, when, and how much to eat. Deprivation eaters can also engage in emotional eating. For example, feeling guilty about eating a food that they think they shouldn't eat drives them to eat even more. As long as they hold on to the diet mentality, deprivation eaters tend to be miserable around food and on a constant quest to change their bodies.

Emotional eaters, both undereaters and overeaters, eat either less or more than their bodies need in response to intense or uncomfortable emotions. Emotional overeaters attempt to numb distressing thoughts and feelings by distracting or comforting themselves with food. Because food is a temporary solution at best, and it doesn't resolve the true issues (the feelings come back and the problems remain), eating continues. Those who frequently overeat to cope with emotional distress eat past feeling full and sabotage their struggle to lose weight and keep it off.

Emotional undereaters also numb themselves. They are trying to stay away from feelings altogether—which includes feeling hungry. Emotional undereaters do this by finding ways to ignore their hunger, such as staying busy and "forgetting to eat," using caffeine, and going places where food isn't allowed or available, like the gym. Although emotional undereaters may lose weight, they don't do it in a healthy, sustainable manner.

Why do some fitness enthusiasts and competitive athletes become trapped for years in the world of disordered eating? As an athlete or person interested in fitness, you can easily hide or rationalize disordered eating behaviors under the guise of improving health or as a means of boosting your performance or fitness level. Furthermore, the culture surrounding many endurance sports emphasizes, even worships and rewards, lean physiques and low body weights, helping to fuel disordered eating. Sadly, so many sports- and fitness-minded people are currently engaged in disordered eating that you may believe that these disordered beliefs, attitudes, and behaviors

Recognizing Disordered Eating

Do you, or does someone you know, struggle with disordered eating? You don't have to suffer from a full-blown eating disorder, such as anorexia or bulimia nervosa, to do yourself harm. Abnormal eating habits alone can impair your health, performance, and enjoyment of life. To get a handle on your beliefs and attitudes about food and your body, answer the following questions honestly.

Do you eat when you're not hungry or wait until you're extremely hungry to eat?

Do you frequently diet or avoid certain foods or food groups?

Are you aware of the calorie content of the foods that you eat?

Do you eat until you are physically uncomfortable?

Do you find yourself excessively preoccupied with food, dieting, your appearance, or your weight, shape, or size?

Are you terrified about being overweight or gaining fat?

Do you feel guilty, disgusted with yourself, or out of control when you eat?

Do you avoid social situations because you fear food or your eating behaviors?

Are you uncomfortable eating in front of others?

Do you think about burning up calories when you exercise?

Do you feel that food controls your life?

The more yes answers that you gave to the preceding questions, the more you will benefit from seeking help from a qualified professional, such as a mental health expert or a sports dietitian, to deal with your restrictive eating attitudes and behaviors.

---

are normal or essential to performing at your best. The oft-promoted tagline that the thinner you are, the faster you'll run (bike, swim, climb, or whatever) is difficult to ignore, especially for adolescent girls and anyone else for whom weight and self-esteem are closely linked.

Although disordered eating does not meet the strict diagnostic criteria of a full-blown eating disorder, it has its own very real and serious consequences, including the increased risk of spiraling out of control and escalating into an actual disorder. According to the NCAA's *Sports Medicine Handbook*, disordered eating can lead to semistarvation and dehydration, resulting in loss of muscle strength and endurance, decreased aerobic and anaerobic power, loss of coordination, impaired judgment, and other complications (like iron-deficiency anemia, menstrual irregularities, and stress fractures) that decrease performance and impair health. Obviously, this is a poor approach for anyone whose happiness or job performance (such as a student–athlete) depends on his or her body.

Compulsive exercise is another complicating factor typically intertwined with disordered eating habits. Are you dedicated and training hard, or are you training beyond your coach's knowledge or more intensely than athletes of similar fitness levels? People who struggle with compulsive exercise and underfueling may look fit and healthy. However, they typically present with one or more of the following symptoms:

- They have passed out during a workout or race
- They have a history of stress fractures
- They have exercise-induced amenorrhea if they are female (loss of three or more consecutive menstrual cycles or failure to start menstruating by age 15) or a low or suppressed testosterone level if they are male
- They face a perpetual struggle with poor body image and low self-esteem
- They are primarily drawn to endurance activities as a way to burn calories and control their body weight

For example, I've counseled numerous pregnant women who, even before they deliver, commit to endurance-type races that will take place just 2 to 3 months after their expected due date. With a history of not trusting themselves around food and of feeling anxious about their weight, they view enforced exercise and an eating plan from a sports nutritionist as the best way to get their bodies (and life) back under control. Many experts in the field of preventing and treating eating disorders believe that one way to uncover disordered eating is to determine whether the person is exercising compulsively. Although not all compulsive exercisers are disordered eaters (some middle-aged men, for example), experts think that most (particularly girls and women) are.

As a sports dietitian, I look for other disordered-eating patterns besides compulsive exercise among endurance athletes. These include an unbalanced vegetarian eating style, multiple self-diagnosed food allergies, numerous or chronic stomach problems that interfere with preexercise fueling, undertaking prolonged training efforts and races (marathons and century rides) on water alone because of being unable to tolerate sports drinks, being excessively critical about their own body (characterized by lots of negative body talk), weighing themselves more than once a week, and avoiding food-related social situations, such as family gatherings, team outings, or eating at restaurants.

Disordered eaters are not simply misinformed eaters (those concerned about nutrition and their eating habits who may have dieted on and off, but who simply operate with a great deal of misinformation). Misinformed eaters, when sufficiently self-motivated, are generally capable of improving their daily eating habits by using basic nutrition information and following appropriate guidance. For those struggling with disordered eating, however, more rules, plans, diets, and nutrition information aren't helpful and may do more harm than good. If you fit this profile, seek guidance from a credible health professional, such as a sports dietitian or therapist, so you can learn how to invest your time and energy into something other than trying to control your weight (see Selected Resources).

4

Timing Fuel and Fluids for Optimal Results

For endurance exercise lasting 30 minutes or more, the most likely contributors to fatigue are dehydration and carbohydrate depletion, whereas gastrointestinal problems, hyperthermia, and hyponatraemia can reduce endurance exercise performance and are potentially health threatening, especially in longer events (> 4 hours).

Source: A.E. Jeukendrup, 2011, "Nutrition for endurance sports: Marathon, triathlon, and road cycling," *Journal of Sports Sciences* 29(S1): S91-S99.

You've logged the miles and set your sights on completing an endurance-focused challenge. It may be scaling a 14,000-foot (4,200 m) peak, finishing your first century ride, or surviving an open water swim. Or, if you've been bitten by the competitive bug, the possibilities are endless. Choose your weapon—racing flats, a bike helmet, swim goggles, oars, snowshoes, skis, or trekking poles.

Before packing the necessary gear, however, be certain that you aren't leaving home without your most important piece of equipment—a properly hydrated and well-fueled body. Also make sure that you have a solid fluid and fuel plan in place for what lies ahead. Otherwise, you won't be going anywhere very far or very fast. Dehydration and glycogen depletion are two relentless foes that all endurance athletes battle as they push their bodies to perform. Just remember, fancy and expensive equipment may get you to the starting line, but what propels you across the finish line is adequate fluid and fuel.

Timing Is Everything

Nutrition plays a crucial role, especially on race day, as the following account about a world-class athlete who was at the top of her game clearly illustrates.

Colleen De Reuck, a former three-time Olympian for South Africa, quickly became one of America's top marathoners when she became a U.S. citizen. When she was just 10 days shy of her 40th birthday, De Reuck was the surprise champion of the U.S. Olympic Marathon trials ahead of overwhelming favorite Deena Kastor, the American record-holder who came into the race with a PR 7 minutes faster than her nearest competitor. Blowing past Kastor at mile 24, De Reuck ran to a stellar Olympic trials course record of 2:28:25. This performance demonstrates that a lot can change in a year. Just 1 year earlier, on the same course, De Reuck had been the U.S. Women's Marathon Championship prerace favorite. Instead, passed at mile 25, she struggled to hold on to finish second in 2:37:41.

What had De Reuck learned from her struggle-to-the-finish experience? What did she plan to do differently the following year at the trials race? Her answer speaks volumes on the importance of timing your nutrition: "I'm going to make sure I get all my fluids, and I'm going to start taking my Clif Shots earlier in the race. I'm going to try some glucose tabs also."

This real-life account illustrates several key points about hydrating and refueling for peak performance. First, even top-level athletes don't always get it right. De Reuck was able to pull herself through the U.S. Championships race by relying on her superb fitness level and honed mental skills, as well as her considerable experience as a long-time marathoner. If you are less gifted genetically, less fit, or have less racing experience, the need to follow nutrition recommendations is even greater. You simply don't have the knowledge or the experience to fall back on.

Second, there's almost always more than one way to get the task done. Your job is to start with the science and apply it to yourself. No one else can do the work for you. At least once a week, I meet with an endurance athlete who is in denial—who is convinced that the basic laws of physiology and nutrition science simply do not apply to him or her. In reality, of course, this isn't true. Hydration and refueling need always to be at the top of the list. After all, your success on the big (in this case, long) day hinges on your ability to train consistently. It's during weekly workouts and training sessions that nutrition strategies must be practiced and honed. This chapter provides a general foundation for how to best address three key nutrition periods for endurance athletes—before, during, and immediately after exercise. The second half of the book (chapters 9 through 16) delivers detailed nutrition tips, as well as tried-and-true strategies from well-known and successful athletes and coaches on how to successfully navigate the varying distances and conditions that you will undoubtedly find yourself in.

Timing is everything, especially for endurance athletes who must squeeze meals and snacks in among work, family obligations, social commitments, and lengthy workouts (sometimes more than once a day) that can involve multiple sports or activities. The fueling cycle (see figure 4.1) depicts an easy way to remember the key time periods to be nutritionally prepared—before, during, and immediately following exercise. During sports nutrition checkups, most people I counsel can readily tell me their plan for any given day (work or school schedule, for example) as well as specifics about their intended workout (for example, masters swim workout at 6 a.m. or weekly group hill ride at noon.). Few, however, can state what their nutrition game plan is for the day.

Nutritionally challenged athletes tend to fall into one of two camps. Some say, "I eat when I can. I try to fit it in (for example, a midafternoon prework-out snack), but it doesn't always happen." Others say, "When I'm hungry, I grab whatever I can find." No wonder so many athletes come to view food as problematic, responsible for everything undesirable and disastrous—from indigestion to dropping out of a race.

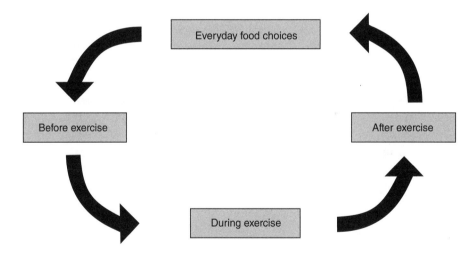

FIGURE 4.1 The fueling cycle highlights key times for active people and competitive athletes to pay attention to their body's need for fluid and fuel.

Glycemic Index and Glycemic Load

Some people appear to be extremely sensitive to the initial drop or lowering of blood sugar (in response to an increase in the hormone insulin) that naturally occurs after we eat. For these people, eating within a half hour to even a few hours before exercise can produce sugar lows (hypoglycemic reactions), with symptoms such as sweating and feeling light-headed, shaky, or lethargic as they begin to exercise. Besides the timing, the type of carbohydrate eaten preexercise may also play a role. A numerical system that ranks carbohydrate-containing foods based on their effect on blood sugar has been developed. Based on the glycemic index (GI), along with glycemic load (GL), this system may help sensitive athletes meet their nutrition needs and avoid or limit negative reactions.

Carbohydrate-rich foods and beverages that are quickly broken down or digested in the small intestine trigger a rapid rise in circulating blood sugar. The greater the blood sugar response, the higher the GI number. Low-GI foods, in contrast, are digested more slowly. They enter the bloodstream more slowly and produce a small rise in blood sugar. Don't be fooled into thinking, however, that this system neatly divides carbohydrate-containing foods into simple and complex categories. Don't assume, for instance, that less-healthy simple carbohydrate (sugar in a candy bar) raises blood glucose rapidly and, consequently, insulin, leading to the rebound lowering of blood sugar that some people are sensitive to. Don't assume that foods with wholesome complex carbohydrate (starch in whole wheat bread) produce the desired slow release of glucose and insulin. On the contrary, whole wheat bread (high-GI food) triggers a rapid blood glucose response, and chocolate (low-GI food) induces a slow rise in blood glucose.

The glycemic index, however, is no longer the only factor you need to consider. The GI system tells only part of the story, that is, how rapidly a particular carbohydrate turns into sugar (a quality issue). The GI doesn't tell you how much of that carbohydrate is in a serving of a particular food (a quantity issue). Scientists now feel that glycemic load (GL), which takes into account the quantity of available carbohydrate, is just as important as the GI. You need to know both the GI and the GL to understand a food's effect on blood sugar.

The GL is the food's GI divided by 100 and multiplied by its available carbohydrate content (carbohydrate minus fiber) in grams. GL rankings are as follows: high (20 or more), medium (11 to 19), and low (10 or less). Foods that have a low GL almost always have a low GI, too. Foods with medium or high glycemic load, however, can range from a very low GI to a very high GI. The glycemic index, for example, of one-half cup of carrots and an 8-ounce (240 ml) Coca Cola are similar (47 and 58), but the GL of the soda (15) is five times that of the carrots (3). For a list of some common foods with their corresponding GIs and GLs, see table 4.1. (You can find the definitive table for both the glycemic index and the glycemic load of more than 2,480 individual foods at www.mendosa.com/gilists.htm.)

If you're sugar sensitive, think low before you go. Experiment with preexercise meals based on low-GI foods, especially before prolonged efforts. You may benefit from the more sustained release of glucose that these foods promote. Conversely, moderate- to high-GI foods and beverages make glucose available more quickly; thus, they are best consumed during exercise.

TABLE 4.1   Glycemic Index by Glycemic Load of Various Foods

	Low GI (1–55)	Medium GI (56–69)	High GI (70–100)
Low GL (1–10)	All-bran cereal 8/38 Apple 6/38 Carrots 2/39 Chickpeas 8/28 Lentils 5/29 Grapes 8/46 Kidney beans 6/22 Orange 4/40 Pinto beans 8/33 Strawberries 1/40 Sweet corn 9/52 Peanuts 1/14 Milk, skim 5/37 Milk, full fat 5/41 Oatmeal cookies 10/55 Peanut M&M's 5/33 Honey 10/55	Pineapple 7/59 Cantaloupe 4/65 Popcorn 7/65 Wheat crackers 9/67 Yogurt, sweetened 3/66 Ice cream, regular 8/61 Couscous 9/65	Waffle 10/76 Watermelon 4/72 White or wheat bread 10/70 Whole wheat bread 9/71
Medium GL (11–19)	Apple juice 11/40 Orange juice 12/50 Milk, chocolate 12/43 Banana 11/47 Spaghetti, whole wheat 15/37 Fettuccine 18/40 Rice, white 14/38 Rice, brown 16/50 Sourdough wheat bread 15/54 Chocolate 12/43 Banana cake 18/47 Ensure 16/48 Frozen yogurt 11/51 Potato chips 11/54	Raisin Bran 12/61 Oatmeal, instant 17/66 Corn chips 17/63 Angel food cake 19/67 Cola soft drinks 16/63 Bran muffin 14/60 Honey 12/61	Cheerios 15/74 Grape Nut Flakes 17/80 Shredded Wheat 15/75 Potatoes, mashed 14/74 Potatoes, instant 17/85 Gatorade 12/78 Rice cakes 17/82 Graham crackers 14/74 Pretzels 16/83 Vitasoy rice milk 17/79
High GL (20+)	Long-grain wild rice 21/49 Vanilla cake with vanilla frosting 24/42 Chocolate cake with chocolate frosting 20/38	Raisins 28/64 Bagel, white 24/69 PowerBar 24/58 Clif Bar 22/57 Mixed fruit, dried 24/60 Rice, instant 28/69 Spaghetti, white 27/61 Pancakes 38/67 French fries 21/64	Potatoes, baked 26/85 Sweet potato 22/70 Cornflakes 20/81 Rice Krispies 21/82 French fries 22/75 Fig fruit bars 21/70 Pop-Tarts 25/70 Jelly beans 22/78

The first number listed is glycemic load (GL); the second number is glycemic index (GI).

GL: low = 10 or less; medium = 11–19; high = 20+

GI: low = 55 or less; medium = 56–69; high = 70+

Foods with higher glycemic values produce a faster rise in blood sugar (glucose) than do foods with lower values. Nothing produces a faster rise in blood glucose than pure glucose, which has a glycemic index of 100. A slow, steady rise in blood glucose is generally better tolerated than a sudden rise in blood glucose. Foods with a glycemic index below 70, therefore, are preferable for usual consumption.

Eating high-GI foods following exercise also may help your body replenish more quickly the glycogen used during exercise.

As easy as this method may sound, it doesn't necessarily work for all athletes in all cases, so don't rely on GI/GL as your only criterion when selecting what to eat. Combining foods at meals introduces other nutrients (such as fat, protein, and fiber) which tend to slow digestion and cause blood sugar to rise more slowly. Even the way a carbohydrate-rich food is prepared will affect the GI of that meal. You need also to consider practical concerns when choosing what to eat before (as well as during and following) exercise, such as taste, how well you tolerate the item, and how easily it can be prepared and toted around.

Experiment during training to determine which options and combinations work best for you. Besides, you really need to pay attention only to the major carbohydrate players in your daily diet, that is, foods that provide the most carbohydrate. If you're like most active people I meet, that means choosing breakfast cereals, breads, crackers, potatoes, pasta, rice, energy bars, and soft drinks, versus high-GI foods like watermelon, carrots, honey, or overripe bananas.

Strategies Before Workouts

Many athletes I know would rather not eat than risk being stuck in the bathroom before a workout. Obviously, no one wants to start out with a stomachache, cramps, or diarrhea from eating the wrong thing or eating too much of the right thing too close to heading out the door. Studies repeatedly show, however, that athletes who consume carbohydrate up to 1 hour before exercise improve their performance in endurance events. Why does this work? It's simple. This extra dose of carbohydrate helps maintain blood sugar levels and tops off glycogen stores.

As expected, eating a carbohydrate-rich food before you exercise, such as cereal, yogurt, an energy bar, or a glass of juice, raises your blood sugar (glucose) level. In response, your body releases insulin (a hormone produced by the pancreas). Insulin's job is to rapidly move glucose out of the bloodstream and into cells, where it's typically used right away for energy. In the case of the liver and muscle cells, excess glucose can be stowed away as glycogen for later use. Back in the 1970s, people thought that athletes should avoid eating before exercise because a high insulin level would be responsible for lowering their blood glucose level (bringing it perhaps too low) as well as suppressing the body's ability to access its fat stores. This was bad news for endurance athletes, who need to use fatty acids for fuel to spare limited glycogen stores. Numerous studies since then have revealed that this isn't the case. Although blood glucose levels may be lowered and insulin levels may be high following a preexercise meal, the condition is only temporary. Within 15 minutes after the start of exercise, insulin levels fall and glucose levels rise to normal. In most cases, the person exercising doesn't feel a thing, and performance is not negatively affected.

Keep these general guidelines in mind when deciding what to eat before you exercise: The longer you have before working out, the more you can (and often need to) eat; the closer you are to the start of the workout, the more important it is to choose carbohydrate. Eat at least 1 hour before exercise to allow glucose and insulin levels to normalize before you head out the door. If you don't have that much time, say, before an early morning ride, run, or swim workout, try to eat or drink something containing readily digestible carbohydrate as close to the start of exercise as possible. Good options include fruit juice or a sports drink, an energy gel, or even a banana or piece of toast with jam. See table 4.2 for more preworkout guidelines.

This preexercise carbohydrate may be just the fuel you'll need to finish strong, because depending on when you last ate, your liver glycogen stores can be cut in half by the time morning rolls around. Remember, your body breaks down liver glycogen to keep your blood sugar level constant—during the day, while you're sleeping, and during exercise. Liver glycogen can also supplement muscle glycogen as fuel for working muscles. Lastly, being well fueled during exercise will keep your brain happier. The pool won't feel quite as cold; the wind won't feel quite as strong.

Eating before exercise: The longer you have, the more you can (and often need to) eat; the closer you are to working out, the more you should reach for some carbohydrate.

You will also benefit from staying adequately hydrated. Many athletes walk around slightly dehydrated, especially those who train in the heat (especially if more than once a day) or complete long exercise bouts on successive days. However, being in an air-conditioned environment all day doesn't let you off the hook, because that comfortable environment may make it more difficult for you to acclimatize to the heat. A simple method for monitoring how well you're keeping up with or matching any fluid losses is to weigh yourself before and immediately after exercise (especially during warm weather). Any weight loss following exercise represents fluid lost as sweat or urine. If you progressively lose weight over the course of a few days, you're most likely dehydrated. Replace every pound lost during daily exercise bouts by consuming at least 2.5 cups (replace every kilogram lost with at least 1.3

TABLE 4.2   Preworkout Fuel Guidelines

If you have:	Choose:	Containing:
3 hr–4 hr	Meal	Carbohydrate + prot
2 hr	Mini meal/snack	Carbohydrate + p
1 hr	Fluids	Carbohydrate
5 min–10 min	Fluids or energy gel	Carbohydr

liters) of fluid as soon as possible. Better yet, try to consume that amount of fluid while you exercise. Incidentally, you should be able to urinate before and after you exercise. If you're unable to do so or your urine is dark yellow, work on drinking more throughout the day and while you exercise.

Strategies During Workouts

Don't be anxious about consuming carbohydrate *during* exercise. Other hormones are released during exercise to suppress insulin production and to single out muscles as the main recipient of glucose. This way, any carbohydrate-rich sports drinks and foods that you consume during exercise will be used to help stabilize blood sugar and to provide additional fuel to working muscles, extending your body's limited glycogen stores. You definitely need to plan to consume carbohydrate if you will be engaged in continuous exercise lasting 60 to 90 minutes or longer, especially if you'll be pushing the pace or really exerting yourself.

Avoid Hitting the Wall and Bonking

Eating a balanced sports diet (about 60 percent of calories from carbohydrate) enables you to store 1,400 to 1,800 calories worth of muscle glycogen on any given day. An athlete can burn through that in 1 to 3 hours of continuous moderate- to high-intensity exercise. When muscle glycogen stores become depleted during exercise, an experience often referred to as hitting the wall, muscle fibers lack the fuel needed for contraction and fatigue takes over. Depleted muscle glycogen stores force you to reduce your pace drastically, and they may even prevent you from finishing what you set out to do. Sure, your body continues to burn fat, but it can't turn it into usable energy quickly enough. If you've ever watched or run a marathon yourself, you may have witnessed even top athletes shutting down and basically shuffling to the finish, running on almost-empty muscle glycogen reserves.

blood sugar level during exercise depends on a balance between the liver and the uptake of glucose by the muscles. source of energy for the brain and ner- the point that the liver can no longer he brain and working muscles, you're ne carbohydrate to burn as a pilot light What happens if no carbohydrate exists is system shuts down, making exercise what it means to bonk. ing enough energy to function properly, find it difficult to concentrate. You may may experience tunnel vision and find it your balance. Essentially, when you bonk, ble mountains. Feeling miserable, you can

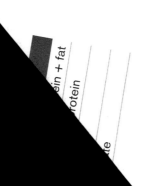

87

easily make a costly or dangerous error, such as taking a wrong turn or riding your bike right off the road, or find yourself forced to stop altogether to avoid more severe health consequences.

The length and intensity of your chosen activity or sport will dictate which foods and fluids you need to consume during exercise. Stopping to eat a sports bar during a 45-minute run doesn't make much sense, but having a bunch on hand for a daylong ski fest does. Dehydration, hitting the wall, and bonking don't happen only during prolonged races and adventures. Every time you head out the door, you need to be prepared to battle these two relentless foes: dehydration and glycogen depletion.

Meeting Fluid Needs During Workouts

The loss of body fluids, typically referred to as dehydration, can stop you in your tracks long before your fuel reserves run low. If you exercise, you'll sweat, especially on a warm day, which can mean a loss of as much as 4 pounds (1.8 kg) of water per hour. As the water content of the body drops, blood volume drops, which means that the heart pumps less blood with every beat and that less blood is delivered to exercising muscles and the skin. Muscles receive less oxygen, and waste products, such as lactic acid, build up. The core temperature of the body rises because less heat is being carried (in the blood) to the skin where it can evaporate as sweat. Your body attempts to compensate by working harder. Your heart rate increases as much as seven extra beats per minute for each 1 percent loss in body weight due to dehydration.

Athletes of all abilities battle the fatigue associated with dehydration as an elevated body temperature and increased heart rate take their toll. Studies have shown that athletes slow down by about 2 percent for each 1 percent loss in body weight. For example, a 150-pound (68 kg) runner would slow down by 4 percent after sweating off only 3 pounds (1.4 kg) of water (2 percent loss in body weight). At a pace of 8 minutes per mile (5 minutes per kilometer), slowing down by 4 percent means an additional 20 seconds per mile (12.4 seconds per kilometer). Greater losses, in the range of 6 to 10 percent of body weight, can lead to life-threatening conditions such as heat exhaustion and heat stroke (see chapter 14).

Even being mildly dehydrated can affect your ability to make decisions and perform complex skills. Keep that in mind the next time you head out on your bike to bomb down a route with hairpin curves at 45 miles (72 km) per hour, or negotiate a trail in the dark, or need to get yourself to safety under whiteout conditions. Dehydration also increases the risk of stomach problems, including vomiting, because it slows the rate at which fluids leave the stomach and move to the small intestines to be absorbed.

Although the risk for dehydration increases the longer you push your body to perform, you'll benefit from staying on top of your fluid needs every time you exercise. The closer your fluid intake comes to matching your sweat losses, the better you will feel and perform. Unfortunately, left to their own devices, most athletes don't do a very good job, ingesting only one-half to two-thirds of the fluid that they need. The following general recommendations for drinking during exercise apply to all endurance athletes. Be prepared, however, to experiment to find the best program that meets your individual needs and suits the specific needs of your sport. The bottom line: No one-size-fits-all formula exists. For additional condition-specific recommendations, see chapters 9 through 16.

Three Reasons to Put In the Effort to Stay Hydrated

1. Keeping your body hydrated proves that you really do respect it and want to treat it well.

2. You drink while on the move because you want to enjoy your workout and get the most out of it.

3. You accept the responsibility to drink during workouts because you understand the need to practice fluid-replacement strategies that you intend to rely on during upcoming events and races.

What to Drink

Water is acceptable for workouts lasting 30 to 60 minutes. Ingesting a flavored beverage, such as a sports drink, however, isn't likely to do any harm, and it can be a plus if it leads you to consume more fluid. It takes time, however, for ingested carbohydrate to be absorbed, transported to, and actually used by the muscles as fuel. Traditional thought has been that the percentage of any carbohydrate ingested during shorter-duration exercise (30 to 60 minutes) would be too small to provide additional fuel, and thus wouldn't result in any tangible performance benefit. Recent research, in fact, suggests otherwise. Merely rinsing your mouth with a carbohydrate-containing beverage during shorter-duration exercise can delay fatigue and boost performance. One study, for example, documented a 1-minute improvement for male cyclists in a 40K cycling time trial. Furthermore, the performance boost, surprisingly, appeared to be as great as if the carbohydrate-supplying beverage was actually ingested.

Since hypoglycemia (low blood sugar) doesn't develop when exercising for 60 minutes or less, some other mechanism must be at work. Even though none of the carbohydrate actually enters the body with carbohydrate-rinsing (no carbohydrate is absorbed in the mouth), it seems that the carbohydrate, nevertheless, has a positive effect on the brain. Researchers believe that mouth receptors for carbohydrate signal the brain that food is on the way, and this reduces the perception of effort, making the exercise task easier. To date, the most effective approach used during exercise lasting 30 to 60 minutes is to rinse the mouth about every 10 minutes, using a more concentrated carbohydrate solution (10 to 20 percent or 10 to 20 grams per ml) than a traditional sports drink (6 to 8 percent).

If your plan includes being on the move at a moderate to fast pace for 60 minutes or longer, use a sports drink. Sports drinks designed for use during exercise provide modest amounts of carbohydrate (6 to 8 percent) and electrolytes (for example, sodium). The carbohydrate extends your limited glycogen stores and may be just what you need to finish workouts strongly. Sodium helps you absorb and retain water and stimulates you to drink more.

Drinking carbohydrate-containing beverages during intense exercise or competitions (as well as before and after) also appears to lessen the effect of stress hormones on your immune system, which may help protect you against colds and other upper respiratory infections.

Although dehydration remains the most common foe, hyponatremia (low blood sodium) is a real possibility for endurance athletes who exercise continuously for 3 hours or longer, especially in hot, humid weather. This condition, which causes you to become bloated, weak, confused, and disoriented, arises if you rely only on water or other low-sodium drinks to replace fluid losses during prolonged exercise bouts. Because the body can lose substantial amounts of both sodium and fluid through sweating, drinking too much plain water can dilute the remaining sodium in the blood to a dangerously low level.

The sodium supplied by sports drinks (and foods eaten before or during exercise) is usually enough to protect most athletes from hyponatremia during prolonged endurance exercise. If you sweat excessively, have problems in the heat, or have access only to plain water, you need to have a plan to replace sodium losses, which may include taking salt or electrolyte tablets. (For more information on preventing hyponatremia and taking salt tablets, see chapters 5 and 14.)

Drinking fruit juice and defizzed soft drinks during exercise may increase your risk for nausea, cramps, or diarrhea because of their high sugar content (10 to 12 percent carbohydrate). Some athletes dilute them to half strength with water or ice. If you can tolerate it, however, fruit juice or a defizzed soft drink could provide a welcome change from sports drinks during long workouts and races. Be aware that these beverages contain minimal sodium and that cola drinks may contain more caffeine than you may want.

If you will be traveling into the backcountry (ski trips, hikes, trail runs, adventure race practices), check beforehand into the quality and availability of water along the way. No matter how clean the water looks, you need to protect yourself from microorganisms that can cause significant gastrointestinal problems. Educate yourself on how to use a water-filtration device and iodine and neutralizing tablets (in case your filter breaks) to purify backcountry water sources. Water filters and iodine treatment kits are available at stores that sell camping or outdoor adventure gear. Water bottles that contain small filters are also available; however, they weigh considerably more than a standard water bottle. Be prepared to lug at least 2 quarts (~2 L) of water per person per day if no water is available.

When to Drink

As a general rule, aim to drink at least every 15 to 20 minutes from the start of your workout. Follow a predetermined drinking schedule instead of relying solely on thirst. If you wait until you feel thirsty, you've waited too long. The goal is to minimize the effects of dehydration instead of trying to reverse them later. Athletes often falsely blame their sports drink for causing stomach upset or diarrhea when dehydration may be the real culprit. Dehydration slows the movement of fluids out of the stomach and their subsequent absorption from the intestinal tract. You can get caught in a self-perpetuating cycle in which you become increasingly dehydrated because you avoid drinking something that you believe is causing the discomfort. If need be, set an alarm on your watch as a reminder to drink frequently.

Be especially diligent when exercising in warm weather and during activities that jostle the stomach, such as running. Cold-weather events and sports during which you maintain a relatively stable or horizontal position, such as swimming or cycling, tend to present less risk for developing abdominal pain and diarrhea.

Our thirst sensation always lags behind our body's need for fluid. Cold weather further depresses thirst, so adhere to a predetermined drinking schedule when exercising in cold conditions. You lose a substantial amount of fluid on cold, dry days through rapid breathing (expired air contains water) and sweating, especially if you're working intensely and wearing the proper amount of clothing for the cold. Other confounding factors include exercising at altitude and on windy days, when sweat evaporates so quickly that you may not realize how much fluid you are losing.

When exercising in warm weather, keep in mind that pouring water over your head or body or using sponges can help you feel cooler and can provide a psychological boost, but it doesn't help you stay hydrated. When given the option of drinking or pouring fluid over your head, drink it.

How Much to Drink

As a general rule, drink 2 to 8 ounces (60 to 250 ml) at a time. Think in terms of gulps instead of ounces. For most adults, one gulp equals roughly 1 ounce (30 ml). For younger athletes, two gulps equal roughly 1 ounce (30 ml). Most standard water bottles hold 20 ounces (600 ml). The amount that you will need to drink during exercise is highly individual. We all sweat at different rates, and the rate at which fluids (and food) empty the stomach also varies widely. Your fluid requirements also depend on the weather and how fit you are to deal with it. The goal is to match your fluid intake to what you are losing via sweat (and urine) on that particular day. Don't wait until you are outright thirsty; however, monitor how much (or little) you are sweating and drink to thirst.

Begin exercise having drunk the largest volume that you can comfortably tolerate, and continually refill your stomach as a portion of this empties.

Larger volumes of fluid (for example, 8 ounces) tend to empty from the stomach faster, as do colder fluids.

To determine whether you are drinking the right amount, weigh yourself before and after exercise. Fluid losses should be modest, a few pounds (1 kg) at most. If you lose more than that, you need to do a better job of rehydrating while you are exercising. To determine whether you're drinking enough during exercise bouts lasting several hours, monitor your ability to urinate, as well as its color. Your urine should be pale yellow, not as clear as water and not dark yellow like straw. If your weight is up after you exercise or you feel increasingly bloated during exercise (your rings and watch get tighter, for example), it indicates that you are consuming too much fluid. This greatly increases the risk that you'll develop hyponatremia. If you're struggling in this area, or simply want to improve, make time now to determine your individual sweat rate so you can minimize fluid loss during exercise without overdrinking (for details, see How to Estimate Average Hourly Sweat Rate).

How to Estimate Average Hourly Sweat Rate

Preexercise weight – postexercise weight (in pounds or kilograms) + fluid intake during the activity (in ounces or liters) = individual hourly sweat rate

Notes

- Body weight pre- and postexercise is taken in the nude.
- Every pound lost equals 16 ounces (480 ml) of fluid; every kilogram lost equates to approximately 1 liter of fluid.
- This formula assumes no urine output during this period.

Example One

Preexercise weight: 60 kilograms

Postexercise weight: 58.5 kilograms

Volume of fluid consumed during exercise: 1 liter (1 kilogram)

Exercise duration: 2 hours

1. Fluid deficit in the body: 60 kilograms – 58.5 kilograms = 1.5 kilograms or 1.5 liters
2. Total sweat loss: 1.5 liters + 1 liter (fluid consumed during exercise) = 2.5 liters
3. Sweat rate (liter/hour) = 2.5 liters/2 hours = 1.25 liter/hour
4. Drink to match sweat losses = .31 liters (310 milliliters) every 15 minutes

> continued

> continued

Example Two

Preexercise weight: 140 pounds

Postexercise weight: 139.5 pounds

Volume of fluid consumed during exercise: 24 ounces

Exercise duration: 1 hour

1. Fluid deficit in the body: 140 pounds – 139.5 pounds = .5 pounds or ~ 8 ounces
2. Total sweat loss: 8 ounces + 24 ounces (fluid consumed during exercise) = 32 ounces
3. Sweat rate (ounces/hour) = 32 ounces/1 hour
4. Drink to match sweat losses = ~8 ounces every 15 minutes

How to Drink While on the Move

Because going without fluid isn't an option for an endurance athlete, you need to become proficient at meeting your fluid needs without expending a lot of energy. Practice simple techniques, such as drinking on the run. Grab a paper cup and pinch it slightly on the sides to create a funnel from which to drink, or add handles to your water bottles. On a bike, grip the handlebar next to the stem when reaching for your water bottle to avoid veering or swerving as you ride one-handed. Endurance swimmers must master drinking while doing a resting backstroke.

Whatever your preferred endurance sport or activity, the ability to drink on the move, without spilling or losing your focus, is an essential technique to master.

Adventure racers can conserve energy by sharing water bottles when traveling in single file while walking or running. Reach forward to grab the water bottle from the carrier worn by the person in front of you, instead of struggling to reach around your back. (Obviously, the first person in line must drink from his or her own bottle, but you should be swapping the lead anyway!)

Situations in which you need to carry your own fluid (such as long rides and runs and backcountry travel) present an additional challenge. Fortunately, a host of hydration systems exist. Experiment with waist (hip-mounted) belts, big bottle waist packs, fluid belts, sports vests, or fluid-toting over-the-shoulder packs with bladders to determine what works and what doesn't.

Meeting Fuel Needs During Workouts

If you eat every 3 to 4 hours throughout the day, timing meals and snacks around workouts (for example, eating within a reasonable time frame before and after you exercise), you should have plenty of muscle and liver glycogen to handle workouts lasting an hour or less. Sports drinks, traditionally, haven't been promoted as necessary or useful in improving performances in shorter exercise bouts (60 minutes or less) because adequate body stores of glycogen can readily fuel 90 to 120 minutes of hard exercise.

Researchers have found otherwise, however. Taking in carbohydrate and water during shorter exercise bouts appears to be more beneficial than ingesting water alone. One study looked at cyclists who pedaled intensely (80 percent of maximal effort) for 50 minutes and then tried to kick the last several minutes. Cyclists who consumed 6 ounces (175 ml) of a sports beverage were 6 percent faster than cyclists who consumed 6 ounces of water. Cyclists who consumed 32 ounces (1 L) of the sports beverage were an additional 6 percent faster, or 12 percent faster than those who only drank water. Try drinking a sports beverage in prerace situations, such as interval workouts or other short, intense efforts, to see whether it works for you. If your performance improves, consider whether the improvement is enough to offset the time that it takes to drink and the extra weight if you must carry the beverage.

Since the time that you will be on the move at a moderate to faster pace exceeds 60 continuous minutes, be prepared to monitor your need for extra fuel (beyond the body's glycogen stores) in addition to your fluid needs. Consuming an exogenous or outside source of carbohydrate during prolonged exercise is crucial on two accounts: to maintain an adequate blood sugar level and to serve as an extra source of fuel for working muscles. Mastering an effective refueling routine in training is the key to being successful during the race.

Consuming enough carbohydrate during exercise is especially vital in certain situations. Relatively speaking, supplemental carbohydrate appears to be more critical during prolonged cycling (2 hours or longer) than during prolonged running or walking. Athletes may have a harder time maintaining a steady blood sugar level when cycling due to a smaller active muscle mass using glucose at a faster rate, so the key is to eat often, rather than loading up every few hours or only at the half-way point. Eat by your watch during ultralong efforts to counter an increasing lack of appetite caused by fatigue or sleep deprivation. Snack every 20 to 30 minutes, for example, aiming for 125 to 200 calories each time (e.g., a large banana, or three or four fig bars).

A properly formulated sports drink (6 to 8 percent carbohydrate plus at least 110 milligrams of sodium per 8 ounces) should be part of any refueling plan for longer events and competitions, so now is the time to practice with one. Sports drinks are the most practical way to get the carbohydrate and fluid that the body needs during exercise lasting 60 minutes or longer. High-carbohydrate beverages, such as Ultra Fuel (21 percent carbohydrate), and liquid food supplements, such as Ultramet and a CytoSport Muscle Milk nutritional shake, however, are generally best tolerated before and after, but not during, vigorous exercise.

The high carbohydrate concentration of these beverages (along with any fat or protein) means that they empty from the stomach more slowly, increasing the risk of dehydration, nausea, cramps, and diarrhea. Ultraendurance athletes often include them, however, during long-duration events when the need for calories is almost as high as the need for fluid.

Following exercise, the research supports consuming a sports drink or other recovery beverage with a carbohydrate–protein combo; however, the evidence remains far less compelling for including protein during exercise. If the sports drink you favor during exercise includes protein, and it's well tolerated when you're pushing the pace, go with it. The protein may help slightly to protect muscles and decrease muscle soreness. If not, don't worry that you're missing out. As long as you're taking in carbohydrate at the higher end of the recommended range during exercise, adding protein isn't likely to give you any performance boost.

Sodium is the most important electrolyte for endurance athletes to monitor. Sodium supplied by the foods that we eat daily, as well as sports drinks and sports foods consumed during exercise, satisfies the needs of most athletes. If, however, you sweat heavily, have had problems dealing with heat in the past, or engage in outings that last 4 hours or longer, be prepared to experiment with consuming extra sodium. Your options include ingesting actual table salt; salty foods like soup, tomato juice, pickles, and pretzels; or electrolyte tablets. (See chapter 5 for more information on electrolyte tablets.)

Carbohydrate-rich solid foods, such as energy gels and bars, fruit, candy, low-fat cookies, bagels, and potatoes, can be equally effective at supplying carbohydrate (as well as various amounts of sodium) during extended exercise bouts. Plus, eating solid food can help you feel more satisfied than consuming fluids alone. Foods with low water content, such as cookies and energy bars, are compact and easy to carry; however, they can be difficult to chew when you're working hard. On top of that, solids take longer to empty from the stomach, which could lead to greater intestinal problems, especially if you're running. Remember, the most important nutrient needed during exercise is water. Solid foods (including semiliquid energy gels) don't help in that regard, so you will have to drink plenty of fluid along with these items.

The following guidelines for refueling during workouts apply to all endurance athletes. All athletes, however, should be prepared to develop (and practice) their own unique refueling plan for undertaking endurance events and competing in endurance races. Read chapters 9 through 16 for additional condition-specific recommendations.

Five Reasons to Put In the Effort to Stay Well Fueled During Workouts

1. You work diligently to refuel because it enables you to complete and to enjoy (as much as possible) what you set out to do.

2. You want to decrease your chances of getting injured or coming down with an upper respiratory infection afterwards. You understand that your best defense, in that regard, is to avoid prolonged periods of low blood sugar while exercising.

3. You accept that you must experiment with or test your intended nutrition plan during training efforts so that you can rely on it when you compete. Training your stomach, (just as you do your mind and muscles) is necessary for developing a personal cache of tried-and-true foods that are familiar and tolerable (having passed the test in training) to eat during competitions.

4. For workouts that include teammates or partners, you realize that others are depending on you and you want to send a strong message that you're committed to doing your part.

5. Last but not least, getting yourself (and others) home or back to the car safely can literally be a matter of life and death. A well-fueled brain and the ability to think clearly and solve problems while on the move could be the definitive factors during an endurance outing.

When to Refuel

To delay fatigue, you need to replace carbohydrate throughout exercise and definitely before muscle glycogen reserves are depleted. In other words, don't wait until you are feeling poorly or you can no longer maintain your pace. Begin to supplement with carbohydrate immediately (within the first 30 minutes) when you know that you will be moving (at a moderate to fast pace) for 60 to 90 minutes or longer. Because it takes some time for its rate of uptake to reach maximum, you benefit the most when you start taking in carbohydrate during the very first hour of exercise. Otherwise, you experience an even longer delay before your body can fully utilize, and benefit from, any carbohydrate you do consume.

Have a long chat with yourself if you have any doubt about the value of drinking and eating during endurance events and races. Be prepared, especially in the early stages when you feel good and things are going well, to hear a little voice in your head that squawks, "You're wasting time," when you think about slowing down or stopping to drink or eat something. Switch over to a new mental tape, the one that says, "Food is fuel, and I'm increasing my chances of going faster or farther or both."

Always do what you can to protect what most serious-minded endurance athletes bemoan, at some point, as their weakest link—the stomach. Drink frequently and try to eat (if applicable) small amounts continually, rather than large amounts sporadically, which causes blood (carrying oxygen and nutrients) to be diverted away from working muscles to the digestive tract.

Learn to quickly recognize the signs of bonking or hypoglycemia (low blood sugar). If you or a teammate (or an athlete whom you coach) is acting exceptionally irritable, combative, disoriented, indecisive, or lethargic, suspect hypoglycemia. For the quickest relief, immediately stop and ingest rapidly absorbable carbohydrate, such as a sports drink, non-diet soft drink or juice, a packet of energy gel, glucose tablets, sugar cubes, or even sugary candy (gumdrops, jelly beans, and so on). If energy bars or other solid foods are your only available option, eat those. From this point on, pay extra attention to your food and fluid intake (or keep an eye on susceptible individuals in your group), since you're likely operating on borrowed time. Finally, keep in mind that hypoglycemia impairs shivering during cold-weather exercise, thereby increasing the risk of hypothermia (dangerously low body temperature).

How Much to Take In

Stick with the science and apply this well-established basic guideline—consume 30 to 60 grams of carbohydrate each hour of exercise. Remember, sports drinks supply fluid and carbohydrate simultaneously. Most supply 14 to 20 grams of readily absorbed and easily digested carbohydrate (50 to 80 calories) per 1-cup serving or 35 to 50 grams per one standard 20-ounce (590 ml) water bottle (140 to 200 calories). The longer you'll be on the move, the more your body needs a readily available supply of fuel of at least 200 carbohydrate calories per hour. Consider the total duration of your race or adventure, work out how much carbohydrate you want to take in, and then divide that amount as evenly as possible throughout the event or race. This approach is far easier on your stomach, too.

For ultraendurance athletes, emerging research confirms what many have been demonstrating in real life—the ability to absorb and utilize more than 60 grams of carbohydrate per hour during extended exercise. Up to now, it has been widely accepted among sports scientists that humans generally couldn't process more than 1 gram of carbohydrate (glucose) per minute, so 60 grams of carbohydrate (glucose) per hour was the absolute maximum—hence the preceding guideline. The bottleneck or rate-limiting step in trying to get carbohydrate to our muscles is getting it absorbed or across the intestinal wall in the first place (which, incidentally, doesn't depend on your size or weight). Over the past few years, however, as more sports drinks have included multiple carbohydrate blends, that threshold has been pushed up to 90 grams of carbohydrate per hour.

Asker Jeukendrup, professor of exercise metabolism in the school of sports and exercise sciences at the University of Birmingham, England, has documented that sports drinks containing multiple sources of carbohydrate, such as glucose and fructose, increase the total amount of carbohydrate the body can absorb. How is this possible? The sources are being absorbed across the intestinal wall by different mechanisms. In other words, both glucose and fructose (which is absorbed more slowly than glucose) are being absorbed at the same time. Added together, it reaches about 1.7 grams of carbohydrate per minute that the body actually uses. Ultraendurance athletes training 3 hours or more can benefit from choosing a drink containing multiple sources of carbohydrate and ingesting it at higher rates. Aim to ingest 90 grams of carbohydrate per hour. Don't, however, wait until race day. You need a well-trained digestive tract in order to oxidize carbohydrate at a rate greater than 1 gram per minute.

How much and how frequently you need to eat to maintain a readily available supply of blood glucose for fuel varies widely among individuals. Table 4.3 offers some general recommendations from Jeukendrup, which you can use as a starting point as you experiment to determine what works

TABLE 4.3 Recommendations for Fueling Up With Carbohydrate While on the Go

Sports scientist and Ironman competitor Asker Jeukendrup recommends ingesting the following amounts of carbohydrate during exercise, depending on the duration of the exercise.

Less than 45 min:	No carbohydrate needed. (Note: Recent studies, however, now show that mouth rinsing with carbohydrate can have a positive effect during exercise bouts as short as 30 min.)
45-75 min:	Mouth rinsing, with any type of carbohydrate
1-2 hr:	Up to 30 g/hr; any type of carbohydrate
2-3 hr:	Up to 60 g/hr, with carbohydrate that is oxidized rapidly like glucose or maltodextrin
More than 2.5 hrs:	Up to 90g/hr; must be a combination of carbohydrate that is absorbed via different mechanisms (e.g., glucose or maltodextrin combined with fructose in a 2:1 ratio)

Adapted from A.E. Jeukendrup, 2011, "Nutrition for endurance sports: Marathon, triathlon, and road cycling," *Journal of Sports Sciences* 29(S1): S91-S99.

best for you. Getting a handle on how to best meet carbohydrate and calorie needs while avoiding or minimizing intestinal problems requires that you experiment in training, ideally under conditions similar to what will be expected during the upcoming race or event. This is a trial-and-error endeavor. If you participate in several sports (for example, a triathlon), you'll need to develop and practice strategies for each activity.

Exercising under extreme conditions, such as heat and humidity, cold, or while at altitude, boosts the body's need for carbohydrate and calories. At altitude (especially extended stays), extra calories are needed for countering an increased metabolic rate. The emphasis is on ingesting more carbohydrate as skeletal muscles shift to relying more on carbohydrate than fat for fuel. In cold weather, muscle glycogen, supplemented with carbohydrate-rich foods and fluids, remains the most important fuel. Exercising in the heat (especially if you're not acclimated) also accelerates the rate at which muscle glycogen is burned for fuel. (For specific strategies for exercising in extreme environmental conditions, see chapters 14 through 16.)

Remember to pay particular attention to your fluid needs early on. Dehydration wreaks havoc with the digestive tract and isn't immediately reversible. Practice drinking ample amounts of your chosen sports drink and then supplement with solid foods (if applicable) as the duration of your workout increases. If you've got a hypersensitive stomach, be wary of caffeine and fructose, a sugar found in fruit, honey, and products made with high-fructose corn syrup (including some energy bars). Even small amounts can cause some athletes to struggle with abdominal distress and diarrhea.

Options for Refueling While on the Move

Sports drinks and sports foods such as energy gels (25 grams of carbohydrate per packet), blocks, chews, and chomps (25 to 30 grams), and bars (20 to 50 grams) are the easiest and most convenient way to refuel while on the move. Many exercisers and athletes find that sports drinks made with maltodextrin (small glucose chains) are more palatable because they taste less sweet. Depending on your activity, however, any familiar and well-tolerated carbohydrate-rich solid or liquid food can supply needed fuel. Try a banana (30 grams of carbohydrate), for example, or one-quarter cup of raisins (30 grams), or a meal-replacement beverage (20 to 50 grams per 8 ounces). Other options, especially to temporarily boost a too-low blood sugar level, include hard candy, glucose tablets, Jelly Belly Sport Beans, fruit juice, and non-diet soda.

As you go longer, listen to your body and eat what you crave or can keep down. Many athletes perform perfectly well while eating foods and drinking beverages that fall outside the established guidelines. Getting down some type of nourishment is better than consuming nothing during endurance exercise.

The most successful competitors have a defined eating and drinking game plan in place; however, they are also flexible and keep an open mind. It's normal for tastes to change during hours of exercise, particularly in warm-weather conditions or at altitude. You may need to abandon, for example, your intention to eat only fruit and wholesome sports bars, and instead try M&M's and potato chips. Forcing the same routine or giving up on eating altogether almost always spells disaster.

Develop a taste for a liquid meal-replacement product, especially if you're training for a single-day ultraendurance event, such as a 100-mile (160 km) running race, or a multiday or multistage event, such as a hut-to-hut ski trip or the Race Across America (RAAM) individual and team cycling race. Liquid meals are easier to consume than solid foods, especially when you're exhausted or you have no appetite. They also make good prerace meals, since they reduce the need to defecate. Foods containing moderate amounts of fat and protein also help satisfy cravings, and they can provide a much needed psychological boost during ultraendurance outings. Use long training efforts to become accustomed to drinking a meal-replacement beverage during exercise.

Ironman Triathlon: Going the Distance

To finish an Ironman, you've got to survive the run. And the best nutrition plan for the run is a smartly executed bike nutrition plan. Pace yourself appropriately on the bike and fuel up with rapidly absorbed and digested carbohydrate (at least 30 grams an hour). Hopefully, this two-pronged approach will set you up to start the run with a full tank of glycogen. A full tank of glycogen helps reduce problems that triathletes often struggle with, like stomach shutdown. It allows you to consume fewer calories when running while your body relies on some of its stored glycogen.

Each of the following provides about 50 grams of carbohydrate, or the amount you want to eat during a 1-hour bike segment of an Ironman race:

- 26 oz (800 ml) sports drink
- 2 energy gels
- 2 packets Jelly Belly Sport Beans
- 6 Clif Shot Bloks chews

Solid Foods

- 2 or 3 medium-sized bananas
- Jam sandwich (2 slices white bread with 4 teaspoons jam)
- Muesli/cereal bar (1.5 or 2 bars)—lower-fat variety
- Energy bar (1 or 1.5 bars)—lower-fat variety
- 2 oz (60 g) pretzels
- Milk chocolate candies (1.5 oz or 45 g) are higher in fat; however, they can help to relieve hunger and boredom.

Take energy gels with adequate fluid; otherwise, they can end up as a thick syrup sitting in your stomach. Ideally, to recreate an absorbable sports drink that falls into the optimal 6 to 8 percent carbohydrate range, drink 6 to 8 ounces (180 to 240 ml) of water with every packet of energy gel consumed. To carry the contents of three to five gel packets, use a small, closeable plastic container that clips onto your shorts or can be stashed in a jersey pocket until needed. For backcountry adventures, get a refillable tube (like a toothpaste tube) from a camping supply store that you can fill yourself.

Other sports foods options for long outings are blocks, chews, and chomps, such as Shot Bloks by Clif Bar. These simple-to-handle, easy-to-chew jelly-like blocks provide similar nutrition to a gel (three blocks provide 24 grams of carbohydrate and 100 calories) and can make tracking the day's caloric intake easier and more enjoyable.

Recovering After Workouts

Your job, unfortunately, isn't done when you finish your workout and stagger back to your car or flop down on the sofa. You need to make an immediate effort to rehydrate and refuel if you want to recover quickly from the workout you just completed and reap large dividends later. Keep in mind that the effects of dehydration and muscle glycogen depletion are cumulative. If you want to head back out in several hours, hit the road or trail again the next day, or just rejoin the land of the living as soon as possible, you will have to pay attention to your fluid and fuel needs when you least feel like it. You increase your risk of soft-tissue injuries every time you head out with even partially dehydrated or glycogen-depleted muscles, and you are more likely to make poor decisions when you try to function in a depleted state.

Replacing lost fluids and refilling glycogen stores are the immediate priorities as you begin to recover and prepare for tomorrow. (Yes, there is a tomorrow.) Your muscles are most receptive to reloading glycogen in the 15- to 30-minute window immediately following exercise. The blood flow to muscles is enhanced immediately following exercise. Muscle cells can pick up more glucose and are more sensitive to the effects of insulin, a hormone that promotes the synthesis of glycogen (by moving glucose out of the bloodstream and into cells).

In addition to boosting the rate at which muscles restore glycogen, you can also speed up recovery and repair of muscle fibers by ingesting protein in combination with carbohydrate at this time. The carbohydrate–protein combo appears to produce a greater secretion of insulin than eating either carbohydrate or protein alone. Along with glucose, insulin also stimulates greater uptake of protein into muscle cells. Eating an exact or specific balance of protein and carbohydrate isn't necessary (even scientists haven't definitively figured out the optimal recipe). A good rule of thumb is to consume 1 gram of protein per 4 grams of carbohydrate. You don't need to purchase specialty products, though; chocolate milk fits the bill perfectly!

Replacing Muscle Glycogen

Because it takes at least 20 hours of refueling with carbohydrate-rich foods to replenish muscle glycogen stores fully, you need to start as soon as possible. Whether you eat or drink your carbohydrate after vigorous or prolonged bouts of exercise doesn't matter, as long as you do it quickly. Aim to consume .5 to .75 grams of carbohydrate per pound (1.1 to 1.65 grams per kilogram) of body weight within the carbohydrate window, particularly the first 15 to 30 minutes (of the first 2 hours) immediately after you finish. This equates to 50 to 100 grams of carbohydrate for most athletes.

Sports drinks are probably the most efficient and convenient way to meet your needs, since they provide both fluid and carbohydrate. Because most popular brands intended for use during exercise contain only 14 to 20 grams per cup, make sure that you drink enough of them or choose a high-carbohydrate sports drink (50 grams per cup), fruit juice (25 to 40 grams per cup), or, in a pinch, a non-diet soft drink (40 or more grams in a typical 12-ounce, or 360-milliliter, can). Low-fat milk shakes and smoothies will also do the trick.

Just as you can't rely solely on thirst to tell you when you need to drink, don't wait until you feel hungry or until your appetite returns to start the refueling process. The longer you wait to eat, the less glycogen you store and the longer it takes to recover. Intense or exhaustive exercise, especially in warm weather, depresses appetite. Anticipate and prepare for this by stocking foods that you like and can tolerate. A good rule to follow is to drink or eat at least 50 grams of carbohydrate as soon as possible after exercise, and then follow up by eating a well-balanced meal within 2 hours.

The best recovery plan also includes well-tolerated carbohydrate-rich foods. As soon as you can, ease in common postrecovery favorites, such as yogurt, pudding, fresh fruit, a milk shake, an energy or breakfast bar, or a bagel. Aim to consume an additional 50 to 100 grams of carbohydrate every 2 hours until your next full meal. Some wholesome examples include a bagel with jam (about 50 grams), a banana with four fig bars (about 70 grams), a cup of yogurt with cereal stirred in (about 60 grams), or a baked potato (about 50 grams).

Carbohydrate-rich foods with moderate or high glycemic index ratings (absorbed and digested quickly so that they elevate blood sugar quickly) should, at least in theory, enhance glycogen storage after exercise. Examples of moderate and high glycemic index foods include ripe bananas, mangoes, orange juice, sports drinks, cornflakes and muesli cereals, rice, instant oatmeal, baked and instant mashed potatoes, cooked carrots, white or wheat bread, jelly beans, and ice cream. (Refer to table 4.1 for more options.)

Go ahead and satisfy a craving for salt, especially if you've lost substantial weight during exercise or if you sweat heavily. The salt will help your body hold on to fluid and stimulate you to drink more. Use the saltshaker at meals and include salty foods, such as soup, vegetable or tomato juice, salted pretzels and popcorn, pickles, low-fat crackers, baked goods, spaghetti sauce, and pizza. (If you have high blood pressure, check with your physician about consuming some salt following prolonged bouts of exercise or during periods of hot weather.)

Replacing Fluids

Be sure to address your fluid needs soon after your workout as well. Even when you do a good job consuming fluids during exercise, you can only hope to match 80 percent of what you lose by sweating. You can suffer from headaches and nausea for hours after you finish simply because you're still dehydrated.

Drink at least 2.5 cups (600 ml) of fluid for every pound you lose during exercise. Weighing yourself periodically in training (before and after exercise) can help you estimate how much fluid you typically sweat off. If you haven't urinated within a few hours after an endurance activity or if you feel headachy or nauseated, you most likely need to concentrate on taking in more fluid.

Be careful not to consume copious amounts of plain water, however, because you also need to replenish electrolytes lost in sweat, particularly sodium. Again, fluid-replacement drinks containing sodium are a convenient option. Alcoholic beverages are a poor choice, particularly if you're dehydrated, so if you consume them, do so only after you've filled up with adequate amounts of nonalcoholic beverages.

Replacing Protein and Other Nutrients

Plenty of recovery drinks with protein are now available; however, you can get the job done just as easily by drinking a glass of chocolate milk or eating a cup of yogurt. Including modest portions of meat, poultry, or fish at your next meal (3 ounces, or 85 grams, the size of a deck of cards, provides 20 to 25 grams of protein) can also do the trick. A postrace meal of rice, chicken, and vegetables, for example, or a bowl of whole-grain cereal with milk, a bagel with a thick slice of cheese and a piece of fruit, or a tuna sandwich with a piece of fruit provides the optimal combination of carbohydrate and protein.

Complete meal-replacement products such as Ensure and Boost and other liquid food supplements such as Endurox R4 and Gatorade Recover protein shake are other convenient options. These products provide a balance of energy nutrients, with approximately 40 to 70 percent carbohydrate, 15 to 30 percent protein, and 5 to 25 percent fat. Choose one with a taste you enjoy.

Four Reasons to Make the Effort to Begin Your Recovery Immediately After Your Workout

1. Replenishing your fuel stores after workouts signifies that you respect your body and that you understand the value of training consistently.

2. By refueling promptly, you acknowledge that smart day-to-day nutrition recovery habits lessen the risk of catching a cold or of getting injured.

3. You also want the energy to do something other than lie around on the couch for the rest of the day (or significant others want this for you).

4. Basically, you refuel after a workout because you're committed to doing whatever it takes to be ready to get out there again tomorrow.

Take Note

Even if you want to forget the whole experience, quickly jot down some notes immediately following your workout or race. This will help you prepare for and succeed in future endurance endeavors. As soon as you can, record fluid and fueling strategies that worked well (for example, one bottle of sports drink and one energy gel per hour) and those that didn't (cookies were too dry or the cold made the candy bars too hard to eat). Note how your tastes and cravings changed as the time that you exercised progressed. Write down any intestinal problems that you incurred during or after your outing, note your ability to handle the elements, and list the drinks or foods that you want to have available next time.

Strategies Before Long Events and Races

Congratulations! After months of deliberation, you finally registered for that killer century ride, mountain run, or your first triathlon. With the entry fee paid, it's now time to start eating smarter. The following prerace nutrition countdown will get you to the starting line a step ahead of the competition.

Well In Advance (a Few Weeks to Months Out)

The smartest way to prepare for an upcoming endurance event or race is to plan backwards. You can't get the job done by stuffing in pasta the night before or waiting until the race is underway to experiment with a new food or sports drink. Make the most of daily food choices and workouts. Just as you experiment with and develop new mental and motor skills in training, experiment with sports foods (such as sports drinks, bars, and gels) to establish the types and amounts that you will tolerate in competition or under stressful conditions. Do you really want to lug a hip pouch or bum bag full of your favorite sports bars only to find that they're rock hard and inedible because of the cold? Or that after being on the road for 3 hours you can no longer tolerate your favorite candy?

Learn what you can before you head out for your long-anticipated adventure or you toe the starting line. Talk to other participants and visit websites to read race instructions closely. Find out what will be provided at aid stations and what you will be expected or allowed to provide for yourself. Adventure races, for example, provide no outside assistance, whereas standard road-running races and cycling events typically supply fluids and foods along the way. If you don't currently use the sports drink that the organizers will provide, get used to it during your training. Familiarize yourself with the ever-expanding options for toting fluid and food, such as bladder systems, multiple-bottle waist belts, flask belts, and fluid reservoirs that affix directly to a bike. Rehearse drinking out of a bottle or grabbing cups and swallowing liquid on the move without choking. Your main job is to test in training what you plan to do during the race.

Travel, particularly to another time zone or country, can interfere with your preparations and routines. Gather information about restaurants, food stores, and other resources near your lodging and talk to athletes and coaches who have previously been to the area. If you're traveling into the backcountry, be sure that your water filtration device is in working order or have a supply of iodine and neutralizing tablets on hand. Scan outdoor and adventure travel magazines and cookbooks or visit your favorite camping store to research the latest options for lightweight, portable meals.

It may be advantageous, in some cases, to gain a few extra pounds before participating in an endurance activity. An extended stay at high altitude or a prolonged backcountry trekking or skiing trip can lead to extensive weight loss if you're burning extreme amounts of calories with limited or inadequate options for adequate refueling. An experienced mountaineering friend often reminisces about eating a stick of butter every couple of days during his final preparations for expeditions to Everest and other Himalayan adventures.

To put on weight before you depart, you must increase the amount of calories that you consume or reduce the amount that you burn through physical activity. If you desire to gain lean weight (muscle mass), you must increase your calories and, at the same time, engage in a substantial strength- or weight-training program. Otherwise, most people can expect to gain a few pounds by eating larger portions of foods than they currently consume, adding more snacks or mini meals throughout the day and before bedtime, and supplementing with high-calorie foods such as commercial or homemade liquid meals or shakes. Tapering your training will also help you create and store excess calories.

One Week in Advance

The goal the week before endurance adventures and races lasting longer than 90 continuous minutes is to carbohydrate-load—a process of loading muscles with the glycogen (stored carbohydrate) that will be used to fuel the activity and help delay the onset of fatigue. The greater your preexercise muscle glycogen stores, the greater your potential to perform well. What you may not know about smart carbohydrate loading is that it involves more than just eating some extra pasta and garlic bread.

Traditionally, endurance athletes prepared for long races by doing a long, hard effort 7 days before their event. The scientific rationale behind this exhaustive bout of exercise was to reduce muscle glycogen stores intentionally because endurance training itself is known to provide a powerful stimulus for the resynthesis and storage of muscle glycogen. After following a high-protein, high-fat, low-carbohydrate diet for the next few days (the depletion phase) while continuing to exercise (or at least trying to), endurance athletes then fed their by-now totally starved muscles a high-carbohydrate diet for the remaining 3 days before the race (loading phase). The muscles would rebound by stocking up on every gram of carbohydrate that they could get. Although this approach worked well for some athletes, timing it just right was challenging. Feeling poorly (which occurs during the low-carbohydrate depletion phase) so close to an important event or race is mentally taxing, and some athletes couldn't tolerate the growing stiffness and muscular discomfort associated with superpacked glycogen stores.

Today, it is clear that a modified carbohydrate-loading regimen is the way to go. This method has proved to be just as effective at maximizing muscle glycogen stores before a long or ultralong competition, and you're more likely to get it right. Skip the last strenuous exercise bout (unless it's part of your typical preparation routine) and the depletion phase. Instead, with a week to go, gradually taper your training while continuing to eat as you normally would. (Female athletes need to keep reading!) For the last few days of the week, further reduce your training, perhaps even resting completely for 1 to 3 days. During this time, consume a high-carbohydrate diet, which is generally defined as up to 5 grams of carbohydrate per pound of body weight (or 8 to10 grams per kilogram body weight). This approach helps to superload muscles with glycogen, and it can boost endurance by about 20 percent.

Sex differences for carbohydrate metabolism do exist, however, so the recommendations for intake are different for men and women.

Male endurance athletes benefit from consuming the recommended amount (8 to 10 grams per kilogram of body weight). Female endurance athletes benefit by taking a slightly different approach. Early studies on carbohydrate loading were conducted using only male athletes, and they typically concluded that women required less carbohydrate (6.4 g/kg body weight) when compared to their male counterparts (8.2 g/kg body weight). Unfortunately, women experienced a significantly lower performance benefit (as low as 5 percent) while some men enjoyed improvements in excess of 40 percent when following this guideline.

Subsequent studies established that a carbohydrate-loading threshold of 8 to 10 grams per kilogram is necessary for achieving the performance-enhancing benefits attributed to carbohydrate loading, hence the updated genderless recommendation. Researchers, nevertheless, continued to see female endurance athletes lag behind males in their capacity to superload muscles with glycogen. The women, not surprisingly, also failed to derive the same boost in performance as their male counterparts. Several theories abounded as to why; however, it now appears that a female athlete's lower caloric intake may best explain her reportedly lower capacity to glycogen load as compared with male counterparts.

The most recent studies reveal that women, in fact, are able to increase their muscle glycogen stores by a magnitude that's similar to that seen for men in response to a higher energy and carbohydrate intake. In other words, to supercompensate glycogen stores and gain the full advantage from carbohydrate loading, women need to consume carbohydrate at a level of around 12 grams per kilogram. From a practical standpoint, however, the only way to do this is to consume extra calories (about 700 calories/day) in the 3 to 4 days preceding the endurance endeavor, rather than to simply increase the proportion of carbohydrate consumed. Otherwise, a female athlete would be able to eat nothing other than carbohydrate during those 3 to 4 days. Even then, depending on how much muscle mass she has, she still might not achieve a high enough carbohydrate intake.

Remember—if you don't simultaneously cut back on training, you run the risk of simply using the extra carbohydrate to fuel your last training sessions rather than stockpiling it for race day. If your competitive season involves several races longer than 90 minutes and you cannot reduce your training each time for the full week, try to back off for the 3 days right before the event and concentrate on eating more carbohydrate than usual. It takes at least 3 full days of eating a high-carbohydrate diet to achieve maximum glycogen stores.

Many athletes I meet, however, are hesitant to cut back their exercise and eat more carbohydrate-rich foods during the week leading up to an important event or race. The fear of gaining weight (or fat) or even just feeling heavy increases their anxiety. Endurance-focused athletes need to realize that a temporary increase in weight means the carbohydrate-loading process is going properly. It's due to every gram of glycogen being stored with almost 3 grams of water, which can result in a temporary gain of up to 5 pounds (2.5 kilograms).

The stiffness and heavy legs felt by some athletes as they glycogen-load dissipates with exercise. If the stiffness or heavy feeling is worrisome to you, remind yourself of the benefits of carbohydrate-loading. You will arrive at the starting line well fueled and you will be able to maintain your pace for longer. The extra fluid on board helps to delay dehydration. You can also take a rest day 2 days before your event or race (rather than the day before), and exercise lightly the day before.

Carbohydrate loading is not about sitting around and eating boxes of bonbons for 3 days either. Use your common sense. Male athletes don't need to consume piles of extra food because cutting back on training means they will expend fewer calories than normal. What does need to increase, however, is the proportion of calories that come from carbohydrate. Although bonbons and other chocolate-covered treats do provide carbohydrate (in the form of sugar), they also contain a lot of fat and little else in the way of useful nutrition. You don't have to stop eating these familiar foods, but save the extra helpings of high-fat candies, cookies, muffins, pastries, doughnuts, chips, and ice cream for after your event or race.

If you typically consume 3,000 calories a day, for example, with 60 percent of your calories coming from carbohydrate, you consume about 450 grams of carbohydrate a day. (Here's the math: .6 × 3,000 = 1,800 carbohydrate calories. 1,800 carbohydrate calories / 4 calories per gram = 450 grams of carbohydrate.) To boost your carbohydrate intake to 70 percent of your total calories, you would need to eat about 525 grams of carbohydrate. What are the smartest options for boosting carbohydrate intake? Concentrate on consuming ample servings of complex carbohydrate. Starchy foods, such as bread, cereal, rice, pasta, beans, and potatoes, and all types of fruit deliver plenty of carbohydrate (15 grams or more) in a relatively small amount of food—an additional slice of bread or one-half cup of fruit, for example. (See chapter 1 for more information about serving sizes.) Milk and yogurt weigh in next at 12 grams of carbohydrate per cup. If you're having trouble consuming enough carbohydrate from food group sources, add an energy bar or supplement what you eat with liquid carbohydrate, such as 100 percent fruit juice, sports drinks, high-carbohydrate recovery drinks, or a meal-replacement beverage.

The key is to load up on carbohydrate, not fat (see table 4.4). For instance, opt for low-fat frozen yogurt over premium high-fat ice cream, pasta with marinara sauce rather than Alfredo sauce, and thick-crust pizza topped with vegetables instead of fatty meats. Check the Nutrition Facts label of your favorite snack foods, too. As a rule, snacks that supply at least 4 grams of carbohydrate for every gram of fat can be considered low-fat, high-carbo-hydrate foods. A chocolate-covered doughnut, for example, doesn't fill the bill. It supplies only 21 grams of carbohydrate (40 percent carbohydrate) for 13 grams of fat (59 percent fat). A cup of instant pudding made with low-fat milk is a better choice, offering 56 grams of carbohydrate (75 percent carbohydrate) and 5 grams of fat (15 percent fat).

Carbohydrate-loading will not help you run faster, but it can help you maintain your pace longer before tiring. If your race or event will last less than 90 continuous minutes, a 10K road race or one leg of a relay race, for example, you won't gain any advantage from carbohydrate-loading. Eating normally, including a substantial prerace meal, will ensure that you have enough glycogen on board to complete short-duration events and races.

If you will be on the move or engaged in low- to moderate-intensity endur-ance exercise for several hours, your fat stores provide most of the energy that you need to perform. You still, however, must have enough carbohydrate on board to oxidize the fat. Fat-loading with a week to go will not enable you to burn more fat, instead of glycogen, during endurance activities. In fact,

TABLE 4.4 High-Carbohydrate, Low-Fat Meals

Waffles with fruit and syrup	Chili with beans
Bagel (half or whole) with peanut butter	Rice
Low-fat milk or hot cocoa	100% fruit juice
	Low-fat frozen yogurt
Whole-grain cereal with banana and low-fat milk	Grilled chicken sandwich
Whole wheat toast with jam	Baked potato
Orange juice	Low-fat chocolate milk
	Frozen fruit bar
Roast beef sandwich on whole-grain roll with tomato and lettuce	Pizza with veggies
Applesauce or small box of raisins	Salad (leafy greens and veggies) with low-fat dressing
100% fruit juice	Breadsticks
Low-fat milk shake	Water or 100% fruit juice
Spaghetti with tomato and meat sauce	Chicken on romaine salad with sliced apples and low-fat dressing
Garlic bread	Oatmeal raisin cookies
Salad (leafy greens and veggies) with low-fat dressing	Low-fat breakfast yogurt
Low-fat milk	100% fruit juice or lemonade
Low-fat frozen yogurt	
Bean burrito	Turkey sub
Baked tortilla chips with salsa	Baked chips
Lemonade or 100% fruit juice	Apple
	Sports drink
Pasta with tomato sauce and vegetables	Rice with vegetables and black beans
Italian roll	Salad (leafy greens and veggies) with low-fat dressing
Strawberries	Fresh fruit cup
Iced tea or lemonade	Low-fat milk

Source: S. Nelson Steen, 1998, "Eating on the road: Where are the carbohydrates?" *Sports Science Exchange* #71, 11(4): 1-5.

eating too much fat makes it more difficult to load up on the carbohydrate that you definitely need. Aerobic training, of course, teaches your body to prefer fat and spare your limited glycogen reserves, but you can't influence that factor with only a week to go.

Be alert to situations or factors that can put you at additional risk for dehydration during the week leading into your long event or race. A low-grade fever, nausea and vomiting, menstruation, or sunburn can promote fluid loss. Other situations that increase your risk for dehydration include traveling by airplane, acclimating to altitude, and working out in hot and humid weather, especially if that isn't your normal training environment. Carry bottled water or a personal water bottle with you throughout the day to remind yourself to drink.

Keep an eye out for the early warning signs of dehydration: flushed skin, trouble tolerating the heat, feeling light-headed or unusually fatigued, loss of appetite, or production of only small amounts of dark yellow urine. You want to be well hydrated without being overhydrated. Drink healthy beverages with your meals and snacks because the fluid will stay in your body longer rather than run right through you. Be sure to drink before you head out to exercise (1 to 2 cups, or 250 to 500 milliliters, of fluid 15 to 30 minutes beforehand), during exercise if need be (a couple gulps every 15 to 20 minutes), and enough afterwards to replace 150 percent of body weight lost during exercise (this translates into at least 2.5 cups for every lost pound, or about 1.5 liters for every kilogram). You should be able to urinate before and after exercise. If you're properly hydrated, your urine will be pale yellow. Alcoholic drinks, as well as caffeinated beverages for those who don't typically imbibe, promote loss of body fluids, setting the stage for dehydration and early fatigue. Alcohol negatively affects how the liver metabolizes carbohydrate as well.

Consider how travel will affect your nutrition game plan. Most airlines can accommodate special requests if you notify them at least 48 hours in advance (even better, reserve a special meal when you make your airline reservation). Of course, your flight may not include a meal. Make visiting airport concession stands worthwhile by choosing healthy low-fat, high-carbohydrate snacks, such as frozen yogurt, unbuttered popcorn, bean burritos, baked potatoes, soft pretzels, bagels, fruit juices, low-fat milk and smoothies, and fresh or dried fruit. Another smart move is to pack your own supply of nonperishable foods. Depending on the destination and length of your trip, include such items as cold cereals, instant oatmeal, instant breakfast powders, low-fat cookies and crackers, pretzels, dried fruit, prepackaged puddings, granola, breakfast and energy bars, canned fruit or fruit juices, instant soups, a peanut butter and jelly (or honey) sandwich, bottled water, and sports drink powders, including high-carbohydrate and meal-replacement options. If you need it to perform well, bring it with you.

International travel, in particular, can cause unwanted problems. Don't test your immune system after you arrive by experimenting with local bugs.

Drink only bottled water (even for brushing teeth), avoid swallowing shower or pool water, turn down ice cubes made from the local water supply when ordering beverages, and stick to familiar foods if possible. Your best bets are foods that have been well cooked, fruits that can be peeled (bananas, grapefruit, oranges, kiwi, and mangoes), and prepackaged ready-to-eat items. Avoid salads and other uncooked foods that kitchen staff workers handle directly and abstain from milk and milk products if pasteurization and refrigeration practices are questionable.

Eating on the Trail

Stacy Allison was the first American woman to reach the summit of Mount Everest. She offers the same food advice to day hikers and expedition-bound trekkers who set out to enjoy the great outdoors:

- Bring foods that you really like. Allison, for example, never leaves home without fancy dark chocolate.
- Bring enough of your favorites to share with others. Sharing food builds trust and cements the bonds that form (we hope) between group members during a trip.
- Bring fun foods, like popcorn. There's no better way to make friends or alleviate boredom on bad-weather days that confine you to your tent than sharing a pot of freshly popped popcorn.
- Bring a variety of foods so that no one ever goes hungry. Understand that food takes on a whole different meaning on the trail. The quality and types of food on hand can boost morale or cause a whole trip to fall apart.
- Add spices to your trail cooking kit. They barely add any weight, but can quickly give new life to the same old foods you typically bring.
- Take the job of staying properly fueled and hydrated seriously. Keep foods and water accessible (not buried in the bottom of your pack), force yourself to eat when necessary (plan at least three mealtimes a day), and try drinking your calories (sports drinks and shakes) when the going gets really tough.
- On extended trips, get everyone to sign off beforehand on the types and quantities of food that the group is taking. The time to find out about likes, dislikes, and possible food allergies is before you leave home.
- Add butter to foods to boost the calorie intake and help foods go down when eating gets really tough, for example, at high altitudes. Allison maintains that this is her secret to never losing weight on an expedition.

One Day in Advance

The main goal when it comes to eating the day before your endurance adventure or race is to eat in a way that leaves you physically ready and mentally prepared. Top off your glycogen reserves and avoid any last-minute pitfalls. No experimenting! Trying new foods the day before an important race or event is risky. Jen, an avid runner I met while receiving physical therapy, learned this lesson the hard way. After diligently training for months for the Boston Marathon, including experimenting for the first time with using a sports drink, Jen was on pace to set a new PR when I left her office a few days before the marathon. When I paid her a visit the following week, I was shocked to hear that she didn't finish the race. Her enthusiastic friends and husband had taken her to a new ethnic restaurant the night before, and she awoke with stomach pains and diarrhea. She started the race but ended up dropping out at the 8-mile mark.

Keep it simple. Eat foods that you like and that you eat all the time. Eat them in normal-sized amounts. Graze or eat frequently throughout the day, so that you don't feel as if you have to stuff yourself at the evening meal. The ideal prerace dinner is carbohydrate rich and contains modest amounts of fat and protein. Pasta is a proverbial favorite, but it's not a magical meal. Choose foods that you feel comfortable with or that you believe enhance your performance. I routinely ate pizza before my races, dating back to my first year in college when my coach, Jack Bacheler, the ninth-place finisher in the 1972 Olympic Marathon, recommended it. Other elite athletes dine on baked potatoes, or fish or poultry with vegetables and rice. Choose what works best for you. You have enough on your mind at this point, so don't make your prerace meals a cause of added anxiety.

Here are some tips to keep in mind the day before the event:

- Drink a healthy beverage with every meal and snack. Don't overload with plain water. (See chapter 14 for a discussion on how overloading with water increases your risk of hyponatremia.)
- Avoid beans, broccoli, cabbage, radishes, and other gas-causing foods if you suffer from digestive problems.
- Avoid high-fiber foods such as raw fruits and vegetables with thick skins, bran cereals, nuts, and seeds.
- Avoid sugar substitutes like sorbitol and mannitol (in gums, candies, and other foods), which may cause diarrhea.
- Limit alcohol or avoid it altogether.
- Set out, prepare, and pack everything ahead of time that you need. Don't wait until the morning of the race!
- Eat or drink a bedtime snack to squeeze in a few more calories and help you sleep better.

Morning of the Event

You don't want to be stuck in the bathroom when the gun goes off, or to hold back the group because you're running on empty after only an hour. The most important action you can take is to eat a light to moderate prerace meal. If you've satisfied your carbohydrate and fluid needs throughout the week, you should be adequately hydrated, and your muscle glycogen stores should be at their peak. Your liver glycogen, however, may be substantially depleted, especially if you were tossing and turning all night. Liver glycogen is converted back to glucose to maintain normal blood sugar (the fuel used by the brain) and provide fuel for exercising muscles, especially during prolonged endurance exercise. In other words, eating a meal before you compete helps you make wise decisions while you're on the move, like staying on course or remembering to change shoes between events.

Eating a single carbohydrate-rich meal can quickly restore liver glycogen reserves to normal. Your job will be to find a happy medium in terms of the foods and the amounts that you can tolerate; you don't want to suffer from a stomachache or diarrhea, nor do you want to arrive at the starting line feeling hungry and light-headed. Choose familiar foods that you enjoy. I'll never forget my first international race, a women's 10K road race that took place in the United States. The Russian women downed a full breakfast of eggs, toast, and bacon, and they didn't seem to suffer one bit during the race. Obviously, they knew what they were doing. (Remember, you have plenty of opportunities to practice what you'll eat before an endurance event or race. They're called training days.)

Plan to eat 1 to 4 hours before start time (you can always go back to bed after you eat), and aim for 50 grams of carbohydrate for each hour before the start. For example, consume 150 grams of carbohydrate 3 hours before the race by eating a large bagel (50 to 60 grams) with jam (13 grams per tablespoon), 8 ounces of fruit yogurt (34 grams), and 16 ounces of fruit juice (50 to 60 grams). Some athletes feel satisfied longer if their prerace meal also contains higher-fat foods, such as peanut butter or cheese. Eat early, especially if you'll be exercising or competing intensely, because these meals take more time to empty the stomach. If you do well by eating closer to the starting time, make it a carbohydrate-rich snack (50 grams of carbohydrate), such as an energy bar (30 to 45 grams) or instant oatmeal (12 grams) with a medium banana (27 grams) and 8 ounces of low-fat milk (12 grams). Be sure to drink ample fluids with your meal. Aim for at least 2 cups of fluid 2 hours before exercise and another cup as close to the time of the race as practical.

If your stomach is tied in knots on race morning, or you have an ultrasensitive stomach and simply cannot eat before prolonged exercise, make an effort to eat extra food the day before, including a substantial bedtime snack. Liquid meals, such as breakfast shakes, high-carbohydrate sports drinks, or meal-replacement beverages (for example, Ensure or Boost) empty from the stomach faster than solid foods do and contain less fiber, a frequent driver of digestive discomfort during exercise. Liquid meals are usually well tolerated up to 2 hours before exercise, and are handy if you are in transit or have an early start time.

If you shy away from eating on race morning because you're sensitive to blood sugar fluctuations, consider experimenting with a prerace meal based on low-glycemic, carbohydrate-rich foods, such as milk, flavored yogurt, whole wheat bread, bran cereal, pasta, baked beans, apples, and oranges. High-glycemic, carbohydrate-rich foods eaten before exercise, such as honey, white bread, cornflakes, and sports drinks, may cause undesirable reactions for those with sensitivities. (Refer back to table 4.1 for ideas on which foods to choose.)

Using Supplements Effectively

Although energy drinks and energy shots contain a number of nutrients that are purported to affect mental or physical performance, the primary ergogenic nutrients in most of these products appear to be carbohydrate and caffeine. The ergogenic value of caffeine on mental and physical performance has been well established but the potential additive benefits of other nutrients contained in energy drinks and energy shots remains to be determined.

Source: B. Campbell, C. Wilborn, P. La Bounty, et. al., 2013, "International Society of Sports Nutrition position stand: Energy drinks," *Journal of the International Society of Sports Nutrition* 10(1): 1-16.

Taking supplements isn't a new phenomenon. Athletes, for centuries, have attempted to get the winning edge by looking to supplements for an ergogenic (performance-enhancing) boost. Endurance athletes are no exception. Unfortunately, more often than not, supplements don't deliver on their promises. The typical response that I hear from athletes is "There's no harm in trying it." Investing time, mental energy, and money on supplements that don't work, however, does come at a cost. At the very least, it's a poor use of time, mental energy, and money. Furthermore, supplements can contribute to health problems or interfere with medications you take, hurt rather than improve your performance, and, for competitive athletes, result in disqualification for ingesting a banned substance.

If you're similar to the athletes I counsel, you don't intend to harm yourself or sabotage your performance when you jump on the latest supplement-of-the-month bandwagon. You probably rationalize that taking supplements compensates for a less-than-ideal diet or inadequate training, or you believe that you have special nutrient needs resulting from strenuous exercise. If you're highly competitive, you may hope a supplement will help you avoid colds and injuries or simply give you that little extra competitive edge. Let's face it: You're not out there to lose.

This chapter features sound and credible information on popular supplements that endurance athletes frequently use—some with proven benefits and others with the potential to improve performance. The latter portion of the chapter focuses on how to determine whether a supplement is safe, legal, and effective, and it provides guidelines for evaluating supplement manufacturers' claims and promises.

Understanding the Supplement Hype

The extraordinary drive that endurance athletes possess to improve and excel (you know, the drive that keeps you going hour after hour), unfortunately, also leaves you vulnerable to the lure of dietary supplements. The supplement industry capitalizes on this weakness by spending vast sums of money to market the latest promise of the day, including vitamins, minerals, herbals, botanicals, amino acids, and other substances such as phytochemicals, extracts, and glandular concentrates and metabolites. The opinions of those who perform better than we do can also easily sway us. Advertisers recognize this and use successful athletes and coaches to represent or pitch products. To make matters worse, you probably have at least one friend or teammate who swears by how well a particular supplement works. These influences, coupled with the fact that most adults haven't had a nutrition science class since high school, make it easy to understand how misinformation and pseudoscience about sports supplements continues to thrive.

My friend Peter, an avid and dedicated trail runner, performed a ritual every morning and evening for years. He religiously swallowed a tablespoon (15 ml) of a smelly, vile-tasting concoction that he affectionately referred to as bark juice. For more than 7 years, he drank this awful-tasting stuff daily because he was convinced that it was the key to recovering from running 60 miles (100 km) and cycling 150 miles (240 km) week after week.

Whether it worked or not may be hard to prove. As with loads of supplements, the scientific evidence doesn't exist yet to rule definitively on what effect, if any, a particular substance may have on health or athletic performances. If you rely on your body to perform, I recommend that you learn a great deal about any supplement that you are considering—before you consume it. You also need a healthy dose of skepticism, and a bit of common sense, to successfully sidestep potential minefields. In the end, after all, it's Vitamin T (where *T* stands for training) that trumps them all. (See figure 5.1.)

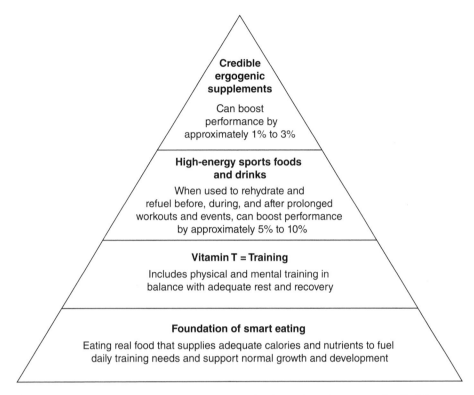

Credible ergogenic supplements

Can boost performance by approximately 1% to 3%

High-energy sports foods and drinks

When used to rehydrate and refuel before, during, and after prolonged workouts and events, can boost performance by approximately 5% to 10%

Vitamin T = Training

Includes physical and mental training in balance with adequate rest and recovery

Foundation of smart eating

Eating real food that supplies adequate calories and nutrients to fuel daily training needs and support normal growth and development

FIGURE 5.1 Think of supplements and sports foods as the icing on a cake. Build a strong food base first, since the greatest nutrition benefits come from eating in a way that leaves you physically ready and mentally prepared to train.

Adapted from Australian Sports Commission, "Supplements FAQ." [Online]. Available: www.ausport.gov.au/ais/nutrition/supplements/supplements_in_sport [August 29, 2013].

Popular Supplements for Endurance Athletes

The following section identifies supplements that may help you stay healthy and perform better while undertaking endurance activities. Before looking to supplements for a boost, make sure that you have in place a smart sports diet and a sound training program—and even then, don't expect miracles. My advice is based on the guidelines developed by the department of sports nutrition at the Australian Institute of Sport (AIS), the world leader in the sports nutrition field. AIS has an active research program that includes scientific evaluation of dietary supplements and nutrition ergogenic aids to find practical nutrition strategies that athletes and coaches can use to achieve optimum performance. Keep in mind, however, that you may fail to respond positively or to gain any performance-enhancing effect from a supplement, despite using it as recommended.

Supplements With Scientifically Proven Benefits

The following supplements are considered to be safe when used as directed. They are backed by enough science to have been proven reasonably effective. In terms of boosting athletic performance, they are legal to experiment with. One caveat, however, is that any seemingly harmless dietary supplement can still be contaminated with a banned substance. The presence of prohormones, compounds that can be converted in the body into an active hormone (testosterone, for example), continues to be a significant problem.

Sports Foods and Fluid-Replacement Drinks

The most powerful supplements that you have at your disposal are sports foods—those carbohydrate-rich beverages and food items created specifically for athletes to consume before, during, or after exercise. These include energy bars, gels, blocks, and chews, as well as sports drinks. During endurance exercise, after all, you won't get far without adequate fuel, and you can't last long without staying on top of your fluid needs.

Water is adequate for exercise bouts lasting an hour or less; however, a properly formulated sports drink (6 to 8 percent carbohydrate plus at least 110 milligrams of sodium) does triple duty by providing fluid, electrolytes, and carbohydrate. As athletic adventures and races stretch past an hour, your success (whether that means placing, setting a personal record, or just finishing) can hinge on consuming a fluid-replacement drink.

The closer you come to replacing your fluid losses during exercise, the better you'll perform, especially in hot weather. An adequate fluid intake helps your heart beat efficiently, attenuates the rise in body temperature that results from exercise, and delays the onset of dehydration. Study after study has shown that athletes offered either water or a sports drink during exercise will drink a greater amount of the sports drink.

Bars, gels, chews, blocks, and sports drinks ingested during exercise also supply carbohydrate that stabilizes blood sugar and fuels hard-working muscles. To perform at your best during events and races lasting longer than 90 minutes, you must consume a minimum of 30 grams of carbohydrate per hour of exercise. The majority of sports drinks provide 14 grams of carbohydrate per 8 ounces (240 ml); gels, blocks, and chews offer 25 grams per packet or per serving; and bars (if you can tolerate solid food during your event or race) range from 20 to 50 grams per bar. Thanks to powders and convenient packaging, you can now refuel easily during most endurance endeavors.

Fluid-replacement drinks and sports bars can also be part of a carbohydrate-loading regime before prolonged exercise, as well as a convenient source of carbohydrate and protein postexercise to jump-start glycogen replenishment and muscle repair and recovery. The research also strongly suggests that beyond boosting performance, consuming carbohydrate-containing beverages in events and races lasting longer than 90 minutes can bolster the immune system to the physiologic stress initiated by prolonged exercise.

Possible Side Effects Fluid-replacement drink and other sports foods may cause gastrointestinal distress, such as nausea and diarrhea, during exercise. Energy bars may compromise overall nutrient intake if they routinely replace meals and snacks based on real foods from the five food groups.

Advice The best fluid-replacement drink is the one that you enjoy drinking. Experiment during training sessions with different flavors and brands to find products that taste good and sit well with your stomach. Fluid-replacement drinks formulated for use during exercise (6 to 8 percent carbohydrate concentration and at least 110 milligrams of sodium), such as Gatorade, Cytomax, and Clif Shot electrolyte drink, are generally tolerated best (see table 5.1 for a comparison of some of the most popular fluid-replacement drinks on the market). Even participants and competitors in shorter-range

TABLE 5.1 Comparison of Fluid-Replacement Drinks (per 8 oz, or 240 ml, serving)

Beverage	Carbohydrate type	Calories	Carbohydrate (g)	Carbohydrate concentration	Sodium (mg)
Accelerade	Sucrose, trehalose	80	14	6%	127
Clif Shot electrolyte drink	Fructose, maltodextrins	80	19	8%	200
Cytomax	Maltodextrin, fructose, dextrose, alpha L-polylactate	72	17.6	7%	96
Enervit G Sport	Fructose, maltodextrin, glucose, sucrose	60	14	6%	112
First Endurance EFS	Complex carbohydrate, dextrose, sucrose	64	16	7%	200
Gatorade G Pro endurance formula	Sucrose, dextrose	50	14	6%	200
Gatorade G Series	Sucrose, glucose	50	14	6%	110
Gu Electrolyte Brew	Maltodextrin, fructose	50	13	5%	125

> continued

< continued, **Table 5.1**

Beverage	Carbohydrate type	Calories	Carbohydrate (g)	Carbohydrate concentration	Sodium (mg)
Hammer Heed	Maltodextrin	50	13	5.5%	31
Infinit Speed	Maltodextrin, dextrose, sucrose	115	28.5	12%	187
Maxim/Extran thirst-quench-ing powder	Fructose, maltodextrin	60	14.6	6%	81
Nuun Active Hydration (1/2 tablet)	Sorbitol	4	<1	<1%	180
Osmo Active Hydration	Sucrose, glucose	35	9.5	4%	155
Powerade Isotonic	Sucrose, maltodextrin	80	19	8%	70
PowerBar Ironman Perform	Maltodextrin, fructose, dextrose	70	17	7%	190
Red Bull	Sucrose, glucose	115	28	12%	215
Skratch Labs Exercise Hydration Mix	Sucrose, glucose	40	10	4%	155
Succeed! Ultra	Maltodextrin, sucrose	59	15	6%	75
Ultima Replenisher	Maltodextrin	10	3	1.7%	25
Vitalyte (Gookinaid)	Glucose, fructose	40	10	4%	68
Compared with:					
Coca-Cola	High-fructose corn syrup or sucrose	100	27	11%	35
Orange juice	Fructose, sucrose	120	29	12%	trace
Vita Coco coconut water	Pineapple puree, coconut puree	56	15	6%	28
Water	N/A	N/A	N/A	N/A	N/A

events lasting 30 to 60 minutes (10K road race or 40K cycling time trial, for example), have been shown to benefit from rinsing the mouth with a sports drink. Make the effort and experiment in training sessions. (For more information, review the chapter 4 section What to Drink.)

During exercise lasting 60 minutes or longer, consume a sports drink (or water and an energy gel, energy blocks, or energy chews) to prevent precipitous dips in blood sugar. A low blood sugar level causes the body to release large quantities of stress hormones, particularly cortisol. Elevated cortisol levels profoundly suppress the immune system, leaving you vulnerable to colds and other upper respiratory infections in the days following the exercise bout. Ultraendurance athletes will benefit from training with (and using on race day) a sports drink with multiple carbohydrate sources (glucose or maltodextrins and fructose, 2:1 ratio) to increase the total amount of carbohydrate the body can absorb during prolonged exercise.

Experiment with energy bars and other sports foods, too. Reduce the risk of stomach problems by taking energy gels, blocks, or chews with plenty of water, ideally 6 to 8 ounces (175 to 240 ml), rather than a sports drink. Avoid flavor fatigue during daylong or multiday events by developing beforehand a taste for more than just one flavor of your favorite brand energy bar or gel. In terms of training diet or everyday eating, energy bars make handy snacks. Use them, however, to supplement, not replace, wholesome foods.

Liquid Food Supplements

High-carbohydrate beverages, such as Ultra Fuel and Maxim/Extran, supply a concentrated dose of carbohydrate (40 to 50 grams per 8 ounces) to help build muscle glycogen stores before exercise and to replenish those stores following exercise. Low-fat chocolate milk and products, such as Ensure, Clif Shot Recovery, and Endurox R4, provide a mixture of nutrients—carbohydrate, protein, and fat, as well as various vitamins and minerals. Consume them 2 to 5 hours before exercise as a low-fiber pre-event meal or immediately afterward to enhance recovery. Liquid food supplements also can be a concentrated source of calories, carbohydrate, and other nutrients during periods of heavy training or if you need to restore or gain weight. Lastly, these products can also serve as an easy-to-ingest source of fuel during ultraendurance events (see table 5.2 for a comparison of some popular liquid food supplements on the market). Powdered varieties provide portable, convenient nutrition while traveling.

Possible Side Effects Liquid food supplements may cause gastrointestinal problems and dehydration when consumed during exercise, nutrient deficiencies or excesses if routinely used to replace wholesome foods at meals, and potential weight gain from consuming excess calories.

Advice To recover more quickly from daily training bouts and reduce your risk of injury, get in the habit of replenishing muscle glycogen stores as soon as possible. Drink either a high-carbohydrate beverage or

TABLE 5.2 Comparison of Liquid Food Supplements

Beverage	Serving size	Calories	Carbohydrate (g)	Protein (g)	Fat (g)
Boost	8 oz (240 ml) bottle	240	41 (68%)	10 (17%)	4 (15%)
Carbo-Pro	2 oz per 20–24 oz (590–710 ml)	224	56 (100%)	0	0
Champion Endurance	1 scoop per 8 oz (240 ml)	120	6 (20%)	19 (64%)	1.5 (11%)
Clif Shot Recovery	2 servings per 16 oz (480 ml)	290	62 (86%)	10 (14%)	0
CytoSport Muscle Milk nutrition shake	2 scoops per 10–12 oz (300–350 ml)	310	18 (23%)	16 (21%)	12 (35%)
EAS Recovery Protein	2 scoops per 10–12 oz (300–350 ml)	270	42 (62%)	20 (30%)	2 (6%)
Endura Optimizer	2 scoops per 12 oz (350 ml)	280	58 (83%)	11 (16%)	1 (3%)
Endurox R4	2 scoops per 12 oz (350 ml)	270	52 (77%)	13 (19%)	1 (3%)
Enervit R2 Sport	3 scoops per 16 oz (480 ml)	220	40 (73%)	2 (4%)	1 (4%)
Ensure	8 oz (240 ml) bottle	250	40 (64%)	9 (14%)	6 (22%)
First Endurance Ultragen	2 scoops per 12 oz (350 ml)	320	60 (75%)	20 (25%)	0
Fluid Recovery drink	2 scoops	128	25 (78%)	7 (22%)	0
Gatorade Post-Game Recovery beverage	8 oz	60	7 (46%)	8 (54%)	0
Gatorade Recover protein shake	1 carton	270	45 (66%)	20 (30%)	1.5 (5%)
Generation UCAN protein	1 powder packet	180	30 (66%)	13 (28%)	0
Hammer Perpetuem	2 scoops	270	54 (80%)	7 (10%)	2.5 (8%)
Hammer Recoverite	2 scoops	170	31 (73%)	10 (24%)	0

Beverage	Serving size	Calories	Carbohydrate (g)	Protein (g)	Fat (g)
Infinit Endurance	2 scoops	280	66 (95%)	4 (5%)	0
Interphase Recovery Matrix	2 scoops	194	10 (21%)	34 (70%)	1 (6%)
Kona Endurance Super Recovery	1 serving	375	70 (75%)	24 (25%)	0
Low-fat chocolate milk	8 oz	170	28 (66%)	8 (20%)	2.5 (13%)
Maxim/Extran energy drink	3 scoops	233	58 (100%)	0	0
OS Pre-Load	1 pouch per 24 oz (710 ml)	400	83 (91%)	15 (16%)	1 (2.5%)
OS Re-Load	1 pouch per 24 oz (710 ml)	370	66 (65%)	31 (33%)	2 (4%)
PowerBar Recovery sports drink mix	1 scoop	90	20 (88%)	3 (12%)	0
SiS REGO Rapid Recovery	1 sachet (50 g/500 ml)	179	29 (65%)	13 (29%)	1 (5%)
Spiz	4 scoops per 20 oz (590 ml)	517	97 (75%)	19 (15%)	5 (9%)
Succeed! Amino	1 1.3 oz pouch	150	37 (97%)	1 (3%)	0
Sustained Energy (from Hammer)	3 scoops per 8–12 oz (240–350 ml)	320	68 (85%)	10 (13%)	0
Ultramet	1 packet per 12 oz (350 ml)	280	24 (34%)	42 (60%)	2 (6%)
Ultra Fuel	4 scoops per 16 oz (480 ml)	400	100 (100%)	0	0

1 cup = 250 ml

a meal-replacement product within 30 minutes following intense or prolonged exercise, especially if you don't plan to eat a meal within an hour or two. Aim to consume at least .5 grams of carbohydrate per pound (~1.0 g per kg) of body weight and 10 to 20 grams of protein. High-carbohydrate beverages and meal-replacement products also come in handy as prerace meals and as part of a carbohydrate-loading regimen before endurance races that will last longer than 90 continuous minutes.

Liquid food supplements are also the easiest and most convenient way to meet energy needs during ultraendurance events, such as 100-mile (160 km) ultra runs or century bike rides. Experiment in training with any product that you intend to consume during an event or race so that you know what it will taste like and how it will settle in your stomach. Ingesting both carbohydrate and a small amount of protein in the latter stages of ultraendurance events may help lessen the breakdown of muscle tissue associated with those strenuous efforts.

Round out a healthy sports diet with these products if you need extra calories or are trying to restore or gain weight. Homemade milk and yogurt smoothies, beverages fortified with nonfat dried milk powder, or instant breakfast drinks can serve the same purpose. Keep in mind that you need adequate protein, carbohydrate, and calories (along with a weightlifting program, of course) to build lean muscle mass. Consuming protein beyond your needs (as supplied by high-protein drinks) will be stored as fat instead of contributing to muscle growth, and it will increase your need for fluid. If you're trying to lose weight, watch out for the calories packed into these products.

Finally, keep a supply of meal-replacement products on hand to use as backup meals while recovering from exhausting efforts or races, when traveling, or on busy days when you would otherwise skip meals or eat poorly.

Multivitamin and Multimineral Supplement

Take a multivitamin and multimineral supplement to bolster a diet that is sometimes less than adequate. Examples include if you fast, skip meals, or diet frequently; if you're lactose intolerant (possible riboflavin, calcium, and vitamin D deficiencies); or if you avoid foods because of food allergies or sensitivities. Multivitamins are also appropriate for vegetarian and vegan athletes (who run the risk of being low in iron, zinc, and other nutrients), as well as women trying to become pregnant (at least 400 milligrams of folic acid are needed daily for preventing birth defects) or who struggle with exercise-induced amenorrhea (fail to have a normal monthly cycle due to consuming too few calories).

Possible Side Effects   Some athletes may rely too heavily on a multivitamin to compensate for a poor diet. Multivitamins and multimineral supplements may supply too little or too much of key nutrients.

Advice   Along with taking a multivitamin or multimineral supplement, take a look at your everyday eating. Work on making better food choices. Vitamin and mineral supplements don't give you energy (calories), fiber, phytochemicals, or yet-to-be-discovered performance enhancers that occur naturally in foods. Eating well is still, and will always be, key. Choose a brand with 100 percent of the daily value for most nutrients and be sure that it carries the United States Pharmacopeia (USP) stamp of approval. The USP stamp guarantees that the supplement will dissolve properly in the body (although that doesn't guarantee that nutrients will be absorbed effectively). To enhance absorption, take a daily multivitamin or multimineral supplement with food (at mealtime).

Men and nonmenstruating (perimenopausal) women may need to consider a supplement with little or no iron (10 milligrams or less) to avoid iron overload. Most multivitamins also contain negligible amounts of calcium (the pill would be too big to swallow), so don't rely solely on a multivitamin or multimineral pill if you need to supplement your calcium intake, too.

Calcium

Besides building strong bones and teeth, calcium helps muscles to contract, nerves to send messages, and blood to clot properly. Consuming an adequate amount throughout life, especially during adolescence and the early adult years, reduces your risk of osteopenia (low bone mass) and osteoporosis (a condition characterized by brittle bones that break easily). Calcium may also play a role in alleviating symptoms of premenstrual syndrome and hypertension (high blood pressure).

Possible Side Effects   Calcium supplements may contribute to kidney stones in some people. Some athletes may rely too heavily on calcium supplements to compensate for poor eating habits.

Advice   Calcium can be found in foods from all the food groups, so work on including alternative sources if you don't drink milk or eat dairy products (see Power Nutrient: Calcium in chapter 1). Aim for 1,000 milligrams a day (1,300 milligrams per day for younger athletes ages 9 to 18, 1,200 milligrams for adults over age 50). People gain peak bone mass between the ages of 16 and 25. The more calcium that you deposit into your bones, the more withdrawals you can withstand (as you get older) before you get into trouble.

If you can't get all the calcium that you need from the foods you eat, take a supplement. To get the best absorption, take calcium supplements at mealtimes and divide your dose throughout the day, taking no more than 500 milligrams at a time. (Pay attention to the amount of *elemental* calcium listed per tablet.) Don't take more than you need and be careful not to treat supplements (like Tums or Viactiv soft calcium chews) as candy.

Choose a calcium supplement that also contains vitamin D (needed by the body for absorbing calcium efficiently) or, if you also take a multivitamin, check that it provides at least 600 IU of vitamin D. Calcium carbonate is generally well absorbed; however, choose calcium citrate if you tend to take supplements between meals. If you take a multivitamin containing iron as well as a calcium supplement, don't take them at the same time. High doses of calcium from the supplement can impair the body's ability to absorb iron. To experiment with alleviating mild to moderate premenstrual symptoms, take 1,200 milligrams of calcium a day for at least 2 months.

Vitamin D

Vitamin D, also known as the sunshine vitamin, is a fat-soluble vitamin that acts or functions like a hormone. It can be synthesized in the body when skin is exposed appropriately to ultraviolet (UVB) radiation. Vitamin D facilitates calcium's absorption from the digestive tract, and it's necessary throughout life for optimizing bone health. Vitamin D is also thought to play a role in maintaining a healthy immune system and to be important for optimal muscle function. Those with a vitamin D deficiency have an increased risk of bone injuries, such as stress fractures, chronic musculoskeletal pain, and susceptibility to viruses like the flu and common cold. Our principal source of vitamin D comes from exposure to UVB radiation from sunlight.

Possible Side Effects   Possible side effects are toxicity (hypercalcemia-elevated calcium in the blood) if consumed in excess, and sunburn and an increased risk of skin cancer in the event of overexposure to UVB (natural sunlight or tanning beds).

Advice   Any factor that limits the quality of exposure to the sun can compromise vitamin D status. For athletes, these factors include geographic latitude (especially northern climates), regular use of sunscreen, wearing clothing that covers most or all of the body or training indoors, training sessions during times when sun exposure is limited (e.g., early morning or late afternoon), as well as aging, dark skin pigmentation, and minimal or excessive body fat. Vitamin D is stored in subcutaneous (under the skin) body fat and is released, as needed, during the winter months or during other periods of low exposure; however, this process appears to be less effective in athletes with high or very low levels of body fat.

Small amounts of vitamin D can be found in egg yolks, fattier fish, and fortified foods like milk, orange juice, breakfast cereals, and margarine. Food alone, however, will not provide sufficient vitamin D.

No universally accepted definition of vitamin D deficiency exists; however, a vitamin D blood level (25(OH)D) of less than 20 nanograms per milliliter is frequently cited (and below 32 ng/ml as insufficiency and above 32 ng/ml as vitamin D sufficiency). A higher status may be desirable for athletes, so work closely with your health care provider.

If you're tested and found to have a low level of vitamin D, vitamin D_3 is the preferable supplement form. In 2010, the recommended dietary intake for vitamin D (assuming no sun exposure) was increased to 600 IU per day. Many experts now recommend at least 800 IU of vitamin D per day for adults (even up to 2000 IU/day as a maintenance dose once a deficiency is corrected).

Iron

Iron is an essential component of the oxygen carriers hemoglobin (found in red blood cells) and myoglobin (found in muscle cells), as well as some of the oxidative enzymes needed for converting food into fuel that working muscles require. Hemoglobin and body iron stores (ferritin) affect how the body transports and uses oxygen. An inadequate amount of either will greatly impair your ability to perform endurance activities.

Possible Side Effects   Iron supplements may cause constipation or diarrhea, or contribute to hemochromatosis (iron overload) in susceptible individuals.

Advice   Work at obtaining adequate dietary iron by eating foods rich in heme iron (meat, fish, and poultry) and nonheme iron (plant sources such as dark green leafy vegetables, tofu, dried beans, dried fruit, and fortified foods). Keep in mind that heme iron is absorbed much better than is the iron in plant foods or supplements. To increase the absorption of the nonheme iron in plant foods, consume these foods with heme-rich foods, such as three-bean chili with a small amount of meat added, or eat a vitamin C–rich food along with the item providing nonheme iron. Drink a glass of orange juice, for example, with a bowl of iron-fortified cereal.

Monitor your iron status through blood tests that measure at least hemoglobin, hematocrit, and ferritin (iron stores). Female endurance athletes and athletes training at altitude, in particular, often need to supplement with at least the recommended daily dose of iron to prevent iron depletion during training. The recommended daily amount is 18 milligrams for teenage girls and adult women, 11 milligrams for teenage boys, and 8 milligrams for adult men. Most multivitamins contain iron, so check the label before you take an additional supplement.

If your hemoglobin and ferritin levels are normal, ingesting large doses of extra iron through supplements will not provide a performance boost, and it could be harmful. Hemochromatosis, or iron overload, is a genetic disorder that affects as many as 1 in every 200 people. Hemochromatosis disrupts iron metabolism in such a way that the body absorbs too much iron. The excess iron deposits in the liver, heart, joints, and other tissues, damaging those tissues and potentially increasing the risk for heart disease and cancer. Because this disorder is not routinely screened for, take large doses of supplemental iron only if your physician has diagnosed you as iron depleted or anemic, and then only until your iron status normalizes.

Antioxidants

Antioxidants, such as vitamins C and E, protect cells and tissues by working to neutralize the damaging effects of free radicals (by-products of strenuous aerobic exercise, pollution, cigarette smoke, and so on). Consuming supplemental doses of antioxidants at key times might translate into less muscle tissue damage, speedier recoveries, and a bolstered immune system. Antioxidants have not been found, however, to directly improve athletic performance.

Possible Side Effects   Excessive vitamin C (such as 1,000 to 3,000 milligrams) can cause diarrhea and kidney stones in some people. Because vitamin C enhances iron absorption, high doses could also lead to harmful or excessive iron levels in the body (especially for those at risk for hemochromatosis). Excessive vitamin E (over 1,000 milligrams) can lead to fatigue, headaches, and diarrhea, as well as impaired immunity and excessive bleeding. Vitamin E supplements also interfere with anticlotting medications, including daily low-dose aspirin.

Advice   Antioxidants found in food cannot always be replicated in a pill. For example, not only did vitamin E supplements fail to lower the risk of chronic disease (heart disease and cancer) in a large-scale research trial involving smokers, they may actually have increased the risk by working as pro-oxidants. Nutrients tend to work in concert in the body; therefore, consuming too much of a single nutrient through a supplement might do more harm than good by creating an imbalance. Your best bet to obtain vitamin C is to eat a daily diet rich in nutrient-dense fruits and vegetables. Develop a taste for brightly colored fruits and vegetables such as papaya, cantaloupe, strawberries, apricots, oranges, grapefruit, kiwis, mangoes, sweet potatoes, carrots, spinach, collard greens, broccoli, red peppers, and kale.

Meeting the recommended daily intake for vitamin E (15 milligrams or 22 IU from natural source of vitamin E or 33 IU of the synthetic form), however, can be difficult for even nutrition-conscious athletes. Vitamin E is found primarily in vegetable oils, margarine, and nuts and seeds. Consider supplementing your diet with a small daily dose of vitamin E (if you don't take anticlotting medications or daily low-dose aspirin), especially if you eat a very low-fat diet or exercise in heavily polluted areas. To get the most from a vitamin E supplement, choose one that contains natural vitamin E (also called d-alpha tocopherol or RRR-alpha) rather than a synthetic version (dl-alpha-tocopherol or all-rac alpha).

Antioxidants work quietly behind the scenes. Don't take megadoses to try to see an effect, since excess antioxidants from supplements have the potential to behave as damaging pro-oxidants. The AIS suggests that a daily dose of 500 milligrams of vitamin C and 500 IU of vitamin E for no longer than 2 weeks may be helpful while adjusting to a new level of oxidative stress (which temporarily may overwhelm the body's antioxidant defense system). Antioxidants may be helpful, for example, when you substantially increase your training volume or intensity or you shift to training in a more stressful environment (move to a hot environment or to altitude or begin altitude house training). Taking a vitamin C supplement (about 600 milligrams) for at least 1 week before participating in an ultraendurance event may protect important immune cells and reduce the risk of an upper respiratory infections.

Supplements That Might Be Helpful

The following section profiles several popular supplements that may improve health or boost performance in endurance activities, but the research results are mixed, and athletes may find it difficult to obtain positive results. I consider these supplements reasonably safe (within limits as noted), backed by enough science to warrant a closer look, and legal for endurance athletes to experiment with (with limits as noted). Keep in mind that I'm not suggesting nor advocating the use of any particular supplement. My job is to inform, to evaluate the science, and to present the potential benefits and the risks. Your job is to make an informed decision about what, if any, supplements you will ingest. Athletes who may be tested for doping must be aware, as always, that sports supplements may be contaminated with prohibited substances. Understand the issues. Learn to reduce risk. (Visit www.usada.org/supplement411 for more information.)

Caffeine

Sound evidence, as summarized in the 2010 International Society of Sports Nutrition position stand on caffeine and sports performance, confirms that caffeine can reduce times in marathon and cycling time trials, as well as increase the duration over which trained elite and recreational athletes are able to exercise vigorously—at least in the laboratory. Small but credible performance boosts have been shown across a wide spectrum of exercise protocols of interest to endurance athletes: prolonged high-intensity events (20 to 60 minutes), endurance events (90 or more minutes of continuous exercise), and ultraendurance events (4 or more hours).

Caffeine's performance-enhancing effect was originally attributed to its ability to promote an increased reliance on fat as fuel during exercise, thereby conserving precious muscle glycogen. Exercising muscles, in other words, are able to keep working at a high level for a longer period of time. Athletes always were warned, however, that caffeine-containing drinks acted as diuretics and would lead to dehydration. Scientists now discount both of these effects of caffeine. Further research revealed that not all athletes respond to caffeine during submaximal exercise by demonstrating a glycogen-sparing effect; thus, other mechanisms must be at work. Most likely, the effect of caffeine on the central nervous system—its ability to stimulate the brain and alter our perception of fatigue—makes the exercise seem easier.

Caffeine supplementation, in addition, has been shown to directly affect skeletal muscles by enhancing strength of contractions and delaying fatigue. Furthermore, an extensive scientific literature review confirmed what loads of people repeatedly report in everyday life—caffeine-containing beverages (coffee, tea, and cola drinks) routinely supply a substantial source of fluid, with minor, if any, effect on urine losses. This effect is particularly true for die-hard habitual caffeine users.

Possible Side Effects Caffeinated beverages or supplements consumed prior to or during exercise may cause nausea and abdominal cramps, as well as increased urination in some people. Excessive caffeine, especially by novice users, can cause anxiety or jitteriness and rapid heartbeat. It also interferes with sleep. Habitual users often experience headaches and insomnia when they consume less caffeine than they do normally. Routinely consuming large amounts of caffeinated beverages can lead to poor nutrient intake (since other, more nutritious beverages and foods are consistently passed over), calcium loss from bones, impaired iron absorption, and problems trying to conceive. For collegiate athletes, high caffeine consumption can result in a failed drug test.

Advice Studies investigating the effect of caffeine on performance during real-life sports and athletic events are scarce, so solid caffeine supplementation protocols do not currently exist. You really need to experiment with caffeine as a potential performance aid. Some people feel no lift at all, and others find that the physical side effects outweigh the benefits. Try it in training first under various conditions. Don't wait until the morning of your big event. Because the caffeine content of tea and coffee, as well as herbal products and sports foods, varies widely depending on the brand, the way the beverages are prepared, and the size of the cup or mug, laboratory studies don't use caffeine in any of these forms. Studies, in general, use a low-to-moderate caffeine dose based on body weight (about 3 milligrams per pound, or ~6 milligrams per kilogram). For the typical trained athlete, this equates to 300 to 500 milligrams of caffeine taken 1 hour before exercise.

To decrease caffeine tolerance and receive the maximal performance boost, some researchers believe that habitual caffeine users may need to reduce or abstain from caffeine for 3 or 4 days before competition. Avoiding the headaches and general malaise associated with caffeine withdrawal, however, can be tricky. During exercise, don't underestimate caffeine's potential side effects (from drinking caffeinated sodas, for instance), such as nausea and abdominal cramps, because those issues already occur with high frequency during endurance events and races. More recent studies reported that athletes involved in prolonged exercise (lasting 60 minutes or longer) experienced benefits when they ingested small to moderate amounts of caffeine (70 to 150 milligrams of caffeine) at numerous times before or throughout exercise, or toward the end of exercise when they became fatigued.

For elite athletes subject to drug testing following competitions, the World Anti-Doping Association removed caffeine from its prohibited list in January 2004. The National Collegiate Athletic Association (NCAA), however, still restricts caffeine (and guarana, which has an active ingredient that is nearly identical to caffeine). A caffeine concentration in the urine that exceeds 15 micrograms per milliliter is considered positive (performance enhancing), and would result in a failed drug test. Many medications (Vivarin, and No Doz, for example), as well as supplements and energy drinks (Red Bull, for example), contain significant amounts of caffeine. Since athletes metabolize caffeine at very different rates, an unaware athlete's intake could add up quickly.

Low-to-moderate doses of caffeine can boost performance in endurance exercise, but no further enhancements in performance are seen with higher dosages (greater than 9 milligrams per kilogram). The goal is to find the lowest effective dose. Take care not to combine caffeine with other stimulants that are like or similar to ephedrine, since an irregular heartbeat can result. That combo also increases the risk of heat illness.

Don't abuse caffeine on a daily basis. No credible health experts support consuming large amounts of caffeine (more than 500 milligrams per day) long term. Water, low-fat milk, 100 percent fruit or vegetable juice, and sports drinks (used appropriately) make far healthier choices than tea, coffee, soda, and chocolate-covered espresso beans. (The average caffeine content in 8 ounces, or 240 milliliters, of brewed coffee is 80 milligrams; in 8 ounces of instant coffee, 60 milligrams; and in 8 ounces of tea, 27 milligrams.) Caffeine can leach calcium from bones, so boost your calcium intake with at least 2 extra tablespoons of milk or yogurt for every cup of coffee that you drink. If you have problems with iron-deficiency anemia, drink caffeinated beverages between meals so that the caffeine doesn't interfere with your body's ability to absorb iron. Women trying to conceive should consume as little caffeine as possible and continue to restrict themselves (to two cups or less daily) while pregnant to reduce the risk of miscarriage or giving birth to an underweight baby.

Glucosamine and Chondroitin Sulfate

Synthesized by the body, glucosamine plays a major role in building and repairing joint cartilage, as well as inhibiting the breakdown of existing cartilage. Chondroitin reportedly helps joints remain fluid and inhibits enzymes that break down cartilage. Short-term (4 to 8 weeks) controlled trials have found glucosamine sulfate as effective as ibuprofen in relieving pain and increasing range of motion in people with osteoarthritis, a degenerative joint disease.

Possible Side Effects   Glucosamine and chondroitin sulfate may cause gastrointestinal discomfort and diarrhea in some people. Some athletes may gain a false sense of security that a supplement will heal or cure an exercise-induced injury.

Advice Glucosamine appears to be safe, but no long-term studies have been done on either supplement or the combination together. Don't be fooled by claims that glucosamine or chondroitin sulfate can cure osteoarthritis. The evidence doesn't exist, especially because glucosamine apparently can't influence the repair of cartilage when little or no cartilage remains. If you decide to try these substances for relief of everyday aches and pain or a more serious injury, the commonly recommended dose is 500 milligrams three times a day. Just don't neglect or abandon well-established treatments for athletic or overuse injuries, such as stretching, massage, physical therapy, strengthening exercises, orthotics, and so forth.

Quercetin

Quercetin is a naturally occurring flavonoid found in a variety of fruits and vegetables, including red grapes (and therefore also red wine), red apples, red onions, green tea, berries (particularly blueberries and cranberries), broccoli, and other green leafy vegetables. Like vitamin C, quercetin has been shown to have antioxidant and anti-inflammatory properties. An average adult eating a normal, healthy diet consumes about 25 to 50 milligrams of quercetin daily. People with a high intake of calories (hard training athletes, for example), as well as those who eat loads of fruits and vegetables, get far greater amounts than this.

Quercetin may boost performance with its anti-inflammatory properties by preventing upper respiratory tract infections (URTIs) following intense exercise, which could interfere with optimal training and subsequent competitive performances. Another theory is that it increases the number and function of mitochondria, the energy-producing factories in muscles for aerobic endurance exercise. It also may provide a caffeinelike boost to the central nervous system.

Possible Side Effects Quercetin supplements in general seem safe, although pregnant women are advised to avoid them. Maximum doses for children and nursing women have not been established. Quercetin can interact with many drugs, including aspirin. At high doses, antioxidants can have undesirable pro-oxidant effects and can produce symptoms such as pain in small joints.

Advice Dr. David Nieman, who is a runner and a respected sports nutrition researcher at Appalachian State University in the United States, is largely responsible for the first description of the so-called "J-shape" relationship between exercise and the risk of illness and infection. That is, our immune system's ability to fight off infection appears to be enhanced when we engage in moderate levels of exercise. With very high levels of exercise stress, however, athletes seem to be more susceptible to minor illnesses and infections.

Neiman has conducted numerous important studies on this topic, including field studies on marathon and ultramarathon runners.

To date, some studies indicate quercetin supplementation may help prevent URTIs, including possibly suppressing cold viruses, in exercise-stressed athletes. Research findings as to whether quercetin supplementation increases aerobic endurance capacity, however, are less promising. Perhaps it does have this effect in untrained, nonexercising individuals, but no studies show this benefit for athletes who are already well trained.

Quercetin is currently is available in various forms (soft chews, powder, concentrate, ready to drink, and food bars) as a sports supplement. If you desire to try quercetin as a means to prevent illness following intense exercise, keep to the recommended dosage of 1,000 milligrams daily (usually taken in two 500 milligram doses) and only supplement during a 1- to 3-week recovery period. Check with your health care provider beforehand, particularly if you take other drugs.

Fish Oils (Omega-3 Fatty Acids)

Called essential fatty acids for a reason, omega-3 fats must come from foods we eat because our bodies don't make them. The major players, eicosapentaenoic acid (EPA) and docosahexaenoic acid (DHA), come directly from fish. Alpha-linolenic acid (ALA) comes from vegetarian sources such as flax seed and flax oil, nuts, and hemp and chia seeds. Most of the research on omega-3 fats focuses on the two that come from fish (EPA and DHA). It had been thought that eating ALA was sufficient, since it converted to the others; however, recent data suggest that conversion is very minimal (around 0.1 percent).

For athletes, fish oil supplements are purported to reduce inflammation, as well as the undesirable effects of oxidative stress, and to counteract the immune dysfunction associated with strenuous exercise.

Possible Side Effects   Fishy tasting burps and diarrhea can occur. High dose supplementation (beyond your physician's approval) can lead to compromised immune function.

Advice   Your best way to get EPA and DHA is to eat fish regularly, particularly fattier fish like salmon, mackerel, lake trout, and albacore tuna. The American Heart Association recommends eating at least two servings (up to 12 ounces, or 340 grams) per week. (Vegetarians can look for an algae-based supplemental source of DHA.) Consume a variety of fish to minimize any potentially adverse effects of environmental pollutants.

Keep in mind that in studies using trained athletes, omega-3 fatty acid supplements have failed to show improvements in inflammation or immune responses or performance. Athletes who may benefit the most from a protective effect of omega-3 fatty acid supplements (EPA and DHA) are those with exercise-induced asthma.

No dietary reference intake (DRI) has been established to date, so do not exceed 3 grams per day of EPA and DHA from all sources (food and supplements) and 2 grams a day from a dietary supplement. Be cautious with cod liver oil. It's not an acceptable substitute because it may cause toxicity, due to its high levels of vitamins A and D.

Branched-Chain Amino Acids (BCAAs)

BCAAs (leucine, isoleucine, and valine) are located primarily in muscle, and they can be broken down and burned for energy during prolonged exercise (e.g., over 2 hours) as muscle glycogen levels fall. Supplementing with BCAAs may improve performance by preventing muscle protein breakdown and damage or by delaying the mental fatigue that arises in the latter stages of prolonged exercise when blood levels of BCAAs fall. Findings of research studies are promising but inconclusive on the effect of BCAAs on performance.

Possible Side Effects Large doses may cause gastrointestinal distress. Routine consumption might interfere with the absorption of other amino acids into the body.

Advice Supplementing with BCAAs to alleviate mental fatigue during exercise is promising for endurance athletes. Studies to date, however, have found that carbohydrate-containing beverages are just as effective in improving performance as are drinks containing both carbohydrate and BCAAs. To capitalize on potential benefits, experiment with supplements and sports drinks that contain added BCAAs during prolonged training efforts, when blood levels of BCAAs decrease and you're most likely to be in a glycogen-depleted state. BCAA supplementation appears to be safe, but the effects of long-term use, if any, are unknown. Don't overdo it, because large doses can contribute to stomach upset.

You can maintain your muscle mass most effectively by consuming enough calories and adequate protein each day. Protein-rich foods that provide 10 to 15 grams of protein per serving (meat and milk in particular) provide ample amounts of BCAAs as well. A sound training program and a carbohydrate-rich diet will also help spare your protein stores from being converted to fuel during exercise. Ingesting large doses of individual amino acids on a daily basis could influence the absorption and metabolic balance of other amino acids, so choose supplements or powders that provide a full complement of amino acids. Don't be duped by the large numbers on labels. For example, 10,000 milligrams of amino acids may sound like a lot, but it equates to only 10 grams of protein, an amount that you can get more easily (and for a lot less money) by drinking a glass of milk.

Electrolyte (Salt) Replacement Supplements

Traditionally used to prevent muscle cramps in athletes who exercise in the heat, electrolyte (salt) tablets can aid endurance athletes in maintaining an adequate blood sodium level during prolonged exercise, like marathons, ultra runs, and triathlons. Sweating causes a loss of electrolytes, primarily sodium. Athletes can lose as many as 1,000 milligrams of sodium for every 2-pound (1 kg) sweat loss.

Electrolyte deficits (the most worrisome being sodium) can result from training repeatedly in extreme heat and humidity. They can also be caused by increased sodium losses that occur when the body begins to acclimate to a hot climate. A sodium deficit can also develop during endurance and ultraendurance events and competitions, especially in those athletes who rehydrate only or primarily with plain water. Hyponatremia (a low blood sodium concentration of 135 milliequivalents per liter or less) is a potentially dangerous condition that can arise during prolonged exercise. It results from excessive sodium losses (through sweating), excessive intake of plain water, or both.

Possible Side Effects   Salt tablets may cause nausea and vomiting and dehydration if not taken with adequate fluid.

Advice   Moderately salting your food (a half teaspoon of table salt provides 1,200 milligrams of sodium), choosing salty foods in the few days before a competition, and consuming a sports drink that contains sodium during exercise will be more than adequate most of the time. Use caution if you decide to experiment with salt tablets or other electrolyte replacement supplements or powders during exercise. Save them for intensive exercise (bouts lasting 3 hours or longer) or for when you exercise in extreme conditions (e.g., temperature above 80 degrees Fahrenheit, or 27 degrees Celsius, and 70 percent humidity or higher). If you plan to use salt tablets when you compete, try them first in similar training situations.

Most salt tablets supply 200 to 350 milligrams of sodium per tablet. Other electrolyte replacement supplements (tablets and powders) provide varying amounts of sodium (check the label) to allow you to customize the amount that you take. No definitive guidelines exist, so start with the recommended dose. Electrolyte loading typically consists of taking one or two salt tablets (300 to 600 milligrams of sodium, depending on your body's tolerance) 30 to 60 minutes before your race or workout as you sip on small amounts of fluid. From there, it's one tablet per hour depending on the weather and how heavily you sweat. Be sure to consume plenty of fluid at the same time; otherwise, the body draws water away from hard-working muscles and into the stomach to dilute the tablets, thereby negating the potential benefits of taking them. Choose a buffered variety to reduce the risk of nausea and vomiting. Salt tablets don't increase your thirst as salty foods do, so don't overdo it.

MCT Oil

Consuming high-fat foods during exercise provides inefficient fuel for working muscles because of the extended time required for digesting and absorbing regular fats. Medium-chain triglycerides (MCTs), on the other hand, a unique form of fat characterized by shorter-than-normal fatty acids, are digested and burned for fuel at a much faster rate, similar to carbohydrate. Consuming MCTs during endurance events and races may enhance performance by sparing the body's limited glycogen stores. Other purported benefits of consuming MCTs, such as an increase in metabolism, less weight gain, and a lower level of body fat, have been demonstrated only in animals, using relative doses of MCTs that humans could not reasonably consume.

Possible Side Effects   Large doses (more than 30 grams) can cause intestinal discomfort, such as cramping and diarrhea. MCT is unsafe for athletes with diabetes or liver function problems. Essential fatty acid deficiencies can arise if MCTs are the sole source of fat in the diet.

Advice   MCT oil is expensive (US$60 to US$70 per quart), and it may be diluted with water or other ingredients. Try to find a product that contains only MCT oil. Start by stirring small doses into a carbohydrate-containing sports drink or experiment with a premixed MCT sports drink, such as Succeed! Clip2. Increase your intake gradually, because large doses can cause gastrointestinal problems, including cramping and diarrhea. Don't wait until race day to experiment with MCT oil. If you need extra calories while training, supplementing with MCT oil is a possibility. Just don't rely on it as the sole source of fat in your diet, because MCT oil lacks essential fatty acids.

Glutamine

As the most abundant amino acid in the body, glutamine plays a key role in maintaining a healthy gastrointestinal tract and immune system. Glutamine reserves (particularly in skeletal muscles) are depleted in times of stress, such as infections, surgery, trauma, and possibly even exercise. Prolonged strenuous exercise (running a marathon, for example) depresses blood levels of glutamine, with several hours of recovery needed for restoring proper levels.

Typically synthesized by the body, glutamine may become conditionally essential during illness and acute stress when the body can't make enough to keep up with its needs. Low glutamine levels have been measured in athletes suffering from overtraining syndrome. Glutamine supplementation may improve athletic performance by helping the body build and maintain muscle mass, by decreasing muscle damage and shortening recovery time, by strengthening the immune system, and by stimulating the accumulation of muscle glycogen.

Possible Side Effects   Glutamine may give athletes a false sense of security or lead them to abandon lifestyle factors that prevent poor health or overtraining syndrome. Free-form L-glutamine is unsafe for athletes with kidney or liver dysfunction.

Advice   No standard dose exists; however, research suggests potential benefits with 5 to 20 grams a day. Experiment with meal-replacement powders or nutrition bars containing glutamine mixed with other amino acids to aid absorption. To obtain an adequate dose, glutamine should be among the first five protein ingredients listed (many companies do not indicate the exact amount that the product contains).

Don't let the emerging role of glutamine as an indicator of exercise stress and overtraining lead you to abandon other healthy practices. Low blood levels of glutamine appear to be linked with the overtraining syndrome, but they do not necessarily cause it. Supplementing with glutamine isn't a substitute for time off from training, a healthy diet, adequate sleep, or learning how to manage stress appropriately.

Creatine Monohydrate

Creatine supplementation helps the body increase and rapidly replenish its stores of readily available energy (phosphocreatine and ATP)—the primary fuels needed for short, high-intensity efforts such as sprinting and lifting weights. For endurance athletes, creatine's ability to increase muscle strength and help buffer lactic acid buildup in the blood and muscles could improve the quality of interval workouts and other training efforts, which could ultimately translate into improved race performances.

Possible Side Effects   Creatine can cause weight gain (from tissues holding onto extra water), dehydration, and an increased risk of muscle cramps, tears, and pulls.

Advice   Humans need approximately 2 grams of creatine a day. Animal foods, such as meat, poultry, and fish, are rich sources of creatine. Our bodies also synthesize creatine from nonessential amino acids at the rate of approximately 1 gram a day. As far as endurance athletes are concerned, creatine supplementation has been shown to have no effect on maximal aerobic capacity ($\dot{V}O_2$max), nor has it been shown to improve endurance. Some researchers believe, however, that creatine supplementation might indirectly improve an athlete's ability to perform in endurance events. Creatine supplementation may lift an athlete's lactate threshold (the speed or intensity above which lactic acid accumulates in the blood, correlating with the percentage of aerobic capacity at which the athlete is able to perform), thereby allowing more intensive interval-type training. By facilitating strength and cardiovascular improvements in this manner, creatine supplementation could improve overall performances in endurance events.

Short-term creatine supplementation (up to 8 weeks) appears safe, but the American College of Sports Medicine recommends that all athletes first check with a physician. Be aware that although studies fail to support an increase in muscle cramps and pulls with creatine supplementation, anecdotal information from athletes abounds! Dehydration may be the culprit, so athletes who are taking creatine need to consume more fluids than usual during training and competition. The safety of prolonged creatine supplementation has not been completely established.

Two loading techniques that purportedly induce less water retention (and thus less weight gain) than the traditional 20-gram-per-day strategy include 6 grams per day over 5 to 6 days (.5- or 1.0-gram doses) with a maintenance dose of about 2 grams a day or 3 grams a day over 30 days. Supplementing with creatine will not build muscle or improve performance on its own. Coordinate creatine supplementation with your training schedule and start just before you begin a period of high-intensity training. Keep in mind that 20 to 30 percent of people fail to respond, even when creatine is taken correctly and an appropriate training program is followed.

Probiotics

Probiotics are live bacteria from certain foods or supplements that, when ingested, can enhance the growth of good bacteria in our intestines. The two most common species of probiotic bacteria are lactobacillus acidophilus and bifidobacterium bifidum, two species that already live in our intestines. Consuming extra probiotics should boost their numbers, and it may enhance the digestion and absorption of nutrients, reduce lactose intolerance, decrease allergies in susceptible individuals, and bolster the immune system.

Possible Side Effects   Consuming probiotics presents few, if any, risks for healthy adults. Upset stomach or bowel problems are a possibility, particularly in people with a history of gastrointestinal problems, such as irritable bowel syndrome or celiac disease.

Advice   As a preventive measure, eat more fermented milk products, such as yogurt (with live cultures), acidophilus milk, and kefir, on a daily basis. Probiotics are measured in colony-forming units (CFUs). For health effects, no official recommended dosages currently exist, nor are there established limits for safe consumption. According to the research to date, 1 billion CFUs are the minimum daily amount thought to benefit health. A *Consumer Reports* feature on probiotics found that yogurt products provided 15 billion to 155 billion CFUs per 6- or 8-ounce (175 g or 250 g) serving, and probiotic supplements supplied about 20 million to 70 billion CFUs per daily dose. Keep in mind that besides providing probiotic bacteria, yogurt products also dish up calcium, protein, and other nutrients.

Add probiotics (especially supplements) gradually to your daily diet, taking 2 to 3 weeks to build up to the recommended dose, especially if you suffer from constipation or other bowel disorders. Because probiotics pass through the intestine, a daily dose is needed. The shelf life of most supplements is a year, although probiotic levels probably drop significantly during this time. The American Academy of Pediatrics has no guidelines for probiotics use with children or teens. Women who are pregnant or lactating and people with severely suppressed immune systems should first check with their health care provider. Athletes may benefit from taking probiotic supplements when traveling to help ward off traveler's diarrhea, when under extra stress (after surgery, for example), or when taking antibiotics (which kill both bad and good intestinal bacteria).

Getting the Facts About Supplements

Dietary supplements fall into a special category that lies somewhere between food and drugs. Although they are required to carry a supplement's facts panel and an ingredient list similar to the Nutrition Facts label found on food packages, supplements don't have to meet the same tough standards regarding effectiveness and safety, truthful health claims, and safe manufacturing practices that apply to all drugs and food additives.

Before you reach for the latest magic potion, remember that just because the label says that the product contains certain ingredients doesn't guarantee that it does. Nor does it guarantee that substances that do not appear on the label couldn't have been deliberately added (or introduced by cross-contamination during manufacturing).

Do Your Homework

Taking supplements requires a consumer-beware approach, so where should you turn for guidance and sound advice? The supplement's facts panel is a good place to start. Look here to find a complete list of the ingredients found in the supplement (including the breakdown of magic formulas), the nutrients that these ingredients provide, and how these amounts compare with established daily values (DVs). You can also determine which part of the plant is used in an herbal or botanical supplement. A USP stamp of approval lets you know that the supplement will dissolve properly in your body, but it doesn't tell you how effectively it will be absorbed.

Don't rely solely on a supplement's facts panel or the health claims plastered all over the packaging. Unlike conventional foods, dietary supplements have no standard serving size. Dosage amounts and schedules have been left to the discretion of manufacturers (the people who want to sell the product), so remember this age-old advice: More is not always better. Some nutrients and substances don't have established recommended daily intakes. Stay alert for up-to-date information from reputable sources on safe doses.

Make Sure That It Is Legal, Safe, and Effective

When it comes to deciphering health claims, you'll need a healthy dose of skepticism and a bit of common sense to successfully navigate through the maze. You want to consider whether the supplement is legal, safe, and effective. Common sense tells you that securing this information requires looking past the promotional literature, advertisements, and anecdotal reports put out by manufacturers. Because of gaps in the Dietary Supplement Heath and Education Act, companies commonly exaggerate claims and rely on deceptive marketing techniques to sell products. Typical approaches used include presenting information that may not be accurate or that has been taken out of context; failing to provide scientific research when asked (it's ongoing or not available to the public); relying on testimonials from accomplished athletes and authority figures (for example, research scientists), who are most likely paid to endorse the product; and conducting and reporting their own research without publication in journals or evaluation by other scientists. Incidentally, obtaining a patent means that the product is unique, not necessarily safe or effective.

If you're a competitive athlete (including masters) subject to drug tests, you don't want to take a prohibited substance that can disqualify you from further competitions. You may also be interested in this information from an ethical standpoint, as were many of the outdoor purists I lived alongside in Boulder, Colorado. Stay abreast of updated guidelines and the most current list of banned substances by contacting your appropriate sports governing body, the National Collegiate Athletic Association, or the United States Anti-Doping Agency (see Selected Resources). If you're scientifically challenged, you may find the information opaque; however, the world's leading authority is the World Anti-Doping Agency (www.wada-ama.org).

You may not like what you find, though. You'll discover that some ingredients, such as DHEA (dehydroepiandrosterone) and ma huang (Chinese Ephedra), are specifically banned. Other than that, you're on your own when it comes to dietary supplements. Because no governing sports body can guarantee the purity or potency of all the supplements available, anything you take is at your own risk. Athletes in various sports have been tripped up by supplement manufacturers who contaminate nutritional supplements by adding banned substances, such as prohormones, to boost their effectiveness.

Furthermore, don't assume that you can resolve safety issues by buying high-priced versions or sticking with natural, drug-free herbal remedies. To begin with, you may not even be getting what you pay for. One study, for example, found that 60 percent of 64 "pure" ginseng products were worthless because they were so watered down with cheaper herbs.

Herbs fall under the same regulations in the United States as do other dietary supplements. This means that they may not be adequately tested to determine how safe or effective they are, especially if taken for longer periods than experts recommend.

For the most part, herbal dosages are manufacturer's recommendations or are based simply on historical use. The dosage listed usually applies to men, so children and women will likely need less. Remedies composed of a single herb are generally considered safer than herbal mixtures. Be sure to consult with your doctor about any herbal products that you use, especially

Banned Substances in Nutritional Supplements: Athletes Pay the Price

The Facts

1. The use of dietary supplements can and has led to positive anti-doping drug tests.
2. The use of dietary supplements can and has led to harmful health issues.

What Can a Consumer or Athlete Do?

Reduce the risks involved with taking dietary supplements as much as possible. (The only way to completely eliminate the risks is to avoid dietary supplement use all together.) Do your research, be aware, ask thoughtful questions, and become as fully informed as possible:

- U.S. Anti-Doping Agency (USADA): www.usada.org/supplement411
- NSF Certified for Sport program: www.nsfsport.com
- Informed Choice: www.informed-choice.org

if you are pregnant or trying to become pregnant, have a health problem, or take prescription medications.

Now comes the big question: How can you tell whether a supplement does what it claims to do? In other words, will you have more energy, lose weight, run faster, jump higher, and throw farther? Now is the time to pull out that healthy dose of skepticism that I mentioned earlier and remember the counsel "If it sounds too good to be true, it probably is." Be leery of general, broad claims, such as "slows aging" or "speeds up your metabolism," that promise to have a positive effect on what is a complex process in the body. Also be alert to "miracle," "secret," and "effortless" effects. Does it make sense, for example, that you could eat all you want and lose weight at the same time? When "scientific" mumbo jumbo appears, read it more closely. For example, aren't you a bit curious about the percentage of people who "may" be deficient and why you "may" be deficient rather than simply being deficient? Contact the manufacturer for more information about alleged benefits and request copies of, or references to, scientific articles reviewed in reputable medical journals.

Bottom Line

I'm not saying that supplements can't work. For some people, some of the time, to some degree, they can. After all, when it comes to the human body and enhancing athletic performance, the science often falls into a gray area.

Just keep in mind that we each represent an experiment of one, which may help explain why you don't notice any appreciable benefits from a supplement that a training buddy (or an elite athlete profiled in this book) may rave about or why you don't seem to get the same boost from an old favorite that you've taken for years.

You may also simply believe that a product works. Perhaps you started taking a supplement during a period of natural improvement that occurred because of other factors such as smarter training or better mental preparation. Maybe you simply experience a psychological lift (known as the placebo effect) when you take a certain supplement. This mental boost alone can be enough to power better performances. Of course, if prudent scientific evidence exists (such as the research supporting the use of sports drinks during exercise to stabilize blood sugar), or you're diagnosed with a nutrient-specific deficiency (iron-deficiency anemia, for example), then taking a supplement most likely will help.

Keep the definition of the word *supplement* in mind. A supplement should add to or fill out a sound diet and training program. Even if certain substances are shown to be of some benefit in improving athletic performance, keep the gains in perspective. Your inherited talent, mental attitude, training methods, eating habits, and equipment choices all play a far greater role in your success than could any dietary supplement. Maybe you even excel in spite of something that you take! You can't go wrong covering all these bases before you seek a safe, legal supplement.

Finally, make sure that you're willing to pay the price for taking supplements—literally and figuratively. It's tempting to take a supplement for a chronic health problem or for an injury that standard medical treatments fail to solve. Be prepared, however, to feel disappointed (less hopeful and motivated, too) whenever you invest in a supplement that doesn't live up to its claims. If you continue to train through an injury, relying solely on a supplement as the cure, consider the opportunities that you forfeit to try something else, such as another treatment plan, further medical help, or simply rest and time off. Even if you're just looking for an edge, don't let taking supplements distract you from doing what you might really need to do, such as revamping your training program or mastering basic cooking skills so that you can prepare healthier meals.

6

Solving Peak Performance Challenges

Within the last 10 years, an explosion of events designed to challenge the human condition by pushing athletes to more extreme environments, and for extended times and distances, has changed how these athletes compete and train. The training needed to compete in these new events bears little resemblance to the moderate levels of exercise that have been recommended for cardiovascular benefits. These new, more extreme challenges demand a new paradigm in providing care for these unique athletes.

Source: C. Asplund and C.J. Chang, 2011, "Care of the endurance athlete: Promotion, perception, performance and professionalism," *British Journal of Sports Medicine* 45(14): 1083-1084.

Just when you think you have everything under control, something pops up that snaps you back to reality—a tree root, a flat tire, a broken ski binding. Or you may be slowed by a common nemesis, such as depleted glycogen reserves, or bonking due to low blood sugar. On the other hand, the problem may be something that you're not as familiar with, such as anemia, newly occurring muscle cramps, or a food sensitivity. Female endurance athletes face additional challenges due to monthly hormonal fluctuations, as well as the physical and emotional changes associated with pregnancy and menopause. And, of course, veteran masters athletes must be prepared to face their own set of challenges and make adjustments. Smart nutrition strategies, in all these situations, can help you return to peak performance.

Muscle Cramps

If you've ever suffered with muscle cramps, you know that they seem to strike just when you need to pick up the pace. Unpredictable in nature, a cramp is a muscle contraction gone out of control, locking the muscle into a sustained and painful spasm. The exact cause of muscle cramps and how best to treat them remain unclear. Calf muscles seem to be most susceptible; however, a cramp can occur in any muscle.

Overexertion, or working a muscle to the point of exhaustion, is the most likely culprit; however, predisposing factors such as dehydration, an electrolyte imbalance, or a mineral deficiency may play a contributing role. Athletes, undoubtedly, tend to suffer muscle cramps more easily when dehydrated, so don't overlook an obvious solution. Start out adequately hydrated and closely monitor how much you're sweating during exercise, especially during prolonged efforts. Drink to match your losses (sweat and urine), ideally two to eight gulps or ounces, or 60 to 240 milliliters, every 15 to 20 minutes, and be sure to rehydrate afterwards. Use a sports drink containing at least 110 milligrams of sodium per 8-ounce serving if you're going longer than 60 continuous minutes.

A practical way to monitor fluid status during exercise is to look at your urine. No hard and fast guidelines exist for how often an athlete should urinate during prolonged exercise. If it's been more than a few hours, however, or if you can't urinate for several hours following exercise, you need to do a better job taking in fluid when you're on the move. Don't forget that you can lose 2 quarts (2 L) of sweat per hour during vigorous exercise in the heat. To avoid progressive dehydration, especially when training day to day in warm conditions, check your weight before and after you exercise. Assume that all the weight you lost is fluid that you need to replace that day. Rehydrate by drinking at least 2.5 cups of fluid for every pound (1.3 L for every kg) of body weight lost.

Besides drinking enough daily, choose foods that supply two important electrolytes, potassium and sodium. Potassium and sodium help maintain the body's water balance, and the electrical charges that they carry help trigger muscles to contract and relax. A potassium–sodium imbalance may lead to muscle cramps. Although you lose both potassium and sodium in sweat, you should have enough body stores of both to cover these losses. Most sports drinks intended for use during exercise, as well as foods typically eaten during ultralong events, provide both sodium and potassium.

Your best defense against muscle cramps is to eat potassium-rich foods daily and use the saltshaker liberally, especially if you sweat profusely, train in a hot environment, or are involved in ultraendurance events. Potassium-rich foods, such as pinto and kidney beans, potatoes, tomatoes, spinach, cantaloupe, orange juice, bananas, dried fruit, milk, and yogurt make good choices. Potassium supplements shouldn't be necessary, and they can be harmful if you consume large doses over a short period.

If you're in otherwise good health and don't have a family history of hypertension (high blood pressure), don't get tripped up by popular health guidelines calling for a restriction on salt (sodium). These guidelines target the general population, with the hope of reducing high blood pressure in sedentary and overweight people. As an endurance athlete, you may end up in the medical tent on race day if you subscribe to a salt-restricted training diet. Muscle cramps, especially if accompanied by fatigue and lethargy, can be due to a sodium deficit that develops during prolonged exercise. Many exercise physiologists and sports dietitians, in fact, believe strongly that sodium depletion is the major predisposing factor behind cramping during athletic performances, especially in warm weather.

Keep the saltshaker handy at the dinner table and answer salt cravings when they arise by consuming salty foods, such as pretzels, salsa and low-fat chips, beef jerky, pickles, soup, tomato juice, and canned foods. If you participate in ultraendurance events and suffer from recurring muscle cramps despite a daily liberal salt intake, consider experimenting with salt or electrolyte tablets. Be sure to take them with ample fluid during exercise; otherwise, you run the risk of causing gastrointestinal problems and dehydration.

A calcium deficiency, too, is often blamed for muscle cramps. Calcium, the most abundant mineral in the body, plays an essential role in normal muscle function. A calcium imbalance is unlikely to cause muscle cramps, however, because the body tightly regulates calcium blood levels. It does so by releasing calcium from the bones whenever enough dietary calcium isn't available; therefore, sufficient calcium for normal nerve conduction and muscle contraction always remains available.

Some athletes with calcium-poor diets, nevertheless, may see their cramps lessen or disappear when they eat more calcium-rich foods. To see whether more calcium makes a difference, consume at least two servings of calcium-rich foods daily. Dairy foods and other calcium-fortified foods, such as orange juice, soy milk, and tofu, make good choices. If your food choices consistently fail to provide enough calcium, round out your diet with a calcium supplement. If nothing else, the extra calcium will help protect your bones from becoming depleted.

If none of these nutrition strategies, in the end, helps in resolving muscle cramps, consult with a sports-minded physical therapist. Explore potential biomechanical causes of muscle cramps, such as leg-length discrepancy. A lack of flexibility or physical conditioning also can precipitate muscle cramps, so review your stretching and training techniques, too.

Runner's (Athletic) Colitis

Any endurance athlete may suffer from an intestinal problem, but runners appear to be especially vulnerable. Studies reveal that between 19 and 26 percent of marathon runners experience running-related diarrhea. Runner's colitis, or inflammation of the bowel during exercise, typically occurs during strenuous or prolonged exercise. It can cause cramping, diarrhea, and bleeding. A number of theories exist as to the possible cause of this problem, including ischemia (decreased blood flow, in this case, to the GI or gastrointestinal tract during exercise) and dehydration. In addition, the repetitive jarring action of running may injure the walls of the large intestine (colon), causing bleeding and diarrhea. Occasional episodes of runner's colitis, such as experiencing bad diarrhea during exercise but not at other times, should not cause chronic problems. If it does, see your physician immediately.

Making mindless food choices (what you eat), failing to plan ahead (how you think), and poorly timing snacks and meals around workouts (how you eat) are three very important factors to evaluate to prevent or resolve GI issues. Medications, supplements, and caffeine must be considered potential suspects, too. Your best defense against runner's colitis, however, is to drink plenty of fluids before and during exercise. Remember, during prolonged exercise, your body naturally diverts blood away from the colon to active muscles and to the skin to disperse heat. Being dehydrated aggravates the situation because a reduced blood volume means that even less blood is available to the large intestine. The lack of blood flow can potentially cause severe damage to the walls of the colon.

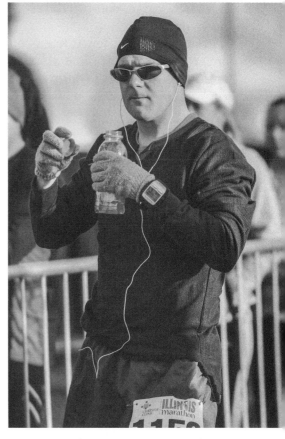

One elite female runner and two elite triathletes (one female and one male) have had parts of their colons surgically removed because of exercise-induced bowel problems. Concentrate on drinking fluids in the early stages of long races. As dehydration progresses, it becomes increasingly difficult for your body to absorb the fluids that you do drink.

Your day-to-day food choices do matter. Eating high-fiber foods, such as bran cereals and whole-grain products, too close to the time that you exercise (especially if you're nervous or anxious) also can cause diarrhea. Insoluble fiber causes the colon to retain water and soften bowel movements, which can result in diarrhea during the stress of competition.

The best defense against athlete's colitis is to drink plenty of fluid before and during exercise.

Caffeine is known to have a laxative effect, and artificial sweeteners, such as sorbitol and aspartame in candy and diet sodas, can cause diarrhea as well. Develop and stick to a prerace diet of foods that you have tested and know that you can tolerate. Check with your physician about the possibility that giardiasis (an infection of the small intestine caused by a parasite), medications, or herbal supplements are causing diarrhea during exercise. Your health care provider also can advise you on the use of antidiarrheal medications during prolonged exercise.

Iron-Deficiency Anemia

Iron-deficiency anemia, characterized by a low blood iron level, will slow even the fittest endurance athlete. Iron, although present in the body in relatively small amounts, plays a crucial role in the transport of oxygen. The body requires iron to form both hemoglobin and myoglobin. Hemoglobin, found in red blood cells, binds with oxygen in the lungs and then transports it (through the blood) throughout the body. Myoglobin, located in muscles, combines with oxygen and stores it until needed. If you suffer from anemia, your muscles receive less oxygen and, consequently, produce more lactic acid. As lactic acid builds up in your muscles, you fatigue prematurely when you exercise. Other possible signs and symptoms of iron-deficiency anemia include muscle burning and shortness of breath during exercise, nausea, frequent infections, sensitivity to the cold, respiratory illnesses, and a pale, washed-out appearance. Anemia also compromises our ability to think and carry out mental tasks.

Most of the iron in the body is incorporated into hemoglobin (60 percent) and myoglobin (10 percent), with a small amount (2 percent) involved in other intracellular components and enzymes. About 30 percent (less in women) is ferritin (storage iron), stored primarily within the bone marrow, liver, and spleen. If iron is lacking in the diet, the body draws from its reserve of stored iron (ferritin). When this reserve is depleted, however, the ability to form hemoglobin is compromised. Red blood cells are no longer able to carry enough oxygen to meet the body's needs. As a consequence, your capacity to train (especially intensely) or race drops off or, at best, plateaus. Once you register an outright low blood iron level, you are officially diagnosed with anemia. Don't be surprised, however, if your performances fall off well before this, due to increasingly depleted iron stores.

Iron Needs and Avenues of Loss

If you're a female athlete, your daily iron needs (18 milligrams) are higher than those of teenage boys (11 milligrams) and adult men (8 milligrams). This is due to the loss of iron through menstrual bleeding (the second largest cause of low iron levels in women). All athletes who suffer from recurring bouts of anemia should take a close look at their everyday eating. An iron-poor diet, particularly among active women, is the primary cause of most iron deficiencies. Even women who make smart food choices, however, often fall short of meeting their daily iron requirement. And female athletes who diet or restrict calories because they place a premium on having a lean physique will find it virtually impossible to consume enough iron. Both male and female vegetarian athletes also have a higher risk of developing anemia. The iron in plant foods is not as efficiently absorbed as the iron in red meat, poultry, or fish.

Endurance athletes lose iron through various other avenues as well. Iron is lost through GI bleeding that occurs with prolonged exercise, especially if diarrhea or cramping occurs during exercise. Less blood flows to the GI tract during exercise, especially during intense efforts, as more blood flows to active muscles. The lack of blood flow and nutrients in the lining of the GI tract causes cells to die and slough off. The result is occult, or hidden, blood in bowel movements. Some athletes suffer with bloody diarrhea occasionally, but in most cases, athletes are probably not even aware of GI bleeding and this mode of iron loss. Dehydration, an inevitable consequence of participating in endurance exercise, exacerbates GI bleeding by further reducing blood flow to the GI tract. Taking aspirin or nonsteroidal anti-inflammatory medications (Advil, ibuprofen, naproxen sodium, and so on) also may increase GI blood loss.

Iron lost through sweat and urine is usually negligible; however, these losses can add up with prolonged exercise. The physical jarring that the bladder endures during prolonged exercise, coupled with dehydration, for example, can result in visible blood in the urine. Daily exercise, especially if you're racking up the miles, also appears to impair iron absorption from the GI tract.

The body normally absorbs more iron in response to an iron deficiency. This compensatory response in athletes, however, appears to be blunted. One study, for example, found that iron-deficient runners absorbed only 16 percent of dietary iron as compared with the 30 percent absorbed by nonathletes. In real life, I frequently see endurance athletes struggle if they continue to train and push themselves despite being recently diagnosed with low-normal or depleted storage iron (low ferritin). Their iron stores take longer to rebound and nagging overuse injuries linger. These athletes actually perform suboptimally for longer compared to those who greatly limit or take a break from training altogether for several weeks.

Iron depletion also can result simply from the slow loss of iron associated with chronic injury to red blood cells. The repetitive trauma of hard foot strikes in high-impact sports such as running, for example, destroys red blood cells. Athletes involved in swimming and other nonrunning sports, however, also can have exercise-induced anemia. This has led to the theory that muscle contractions, acidosis (a decrease in blood pH), or the increase in body temperature associated with exercise may also damage red blood cells. Your liver recycles released hemoglobin from damaged red blood cells up to a point. Beyond that, the hemoglobin is excreted into the urine, thereby compromising your iron status.

Monitoring Your Iron Status

The loss of iron is divided into three stages according to the effect on the body's ability to make normal red blood cells. In stages 1 and 2, only ferritin (storage iron) decreases. *Stage 1* (iron depletion) is characterized by a serum ferritin level of less than 12 nanograms per milliliter, which indicates almost completely depleted iron stores. If iron depletion continues for several months, *stage 2* (iron-deficient erythropoiesis) can result, in which iron transport throughout the body and the production of red blood cells are affected. During both stage 1 and stage 2, a blood test will reveal a low serum ferritin level, but hemoglobin and hematocrit (percentage of red blood cells in the total blood volume) values will remain essentially normal. The mild anemia associated with stage 2, therefore, typically goes undetected. *Stage 3* (iron-deficient anemia) results when the lack of iron stores literally compromises the body's ability to produce normal red blood cells. In addition to ferritin being low, a blood test will now show below-normal levels of hemoglobin and hematocrit, which will result in a formal diagnosis of iron-deficient anemia.

The normal range for hemoglobin in female teenagers and adults is 12 to 16 grams per deciliter. For hematocrit, the normal range is 37 to 48 percent. For male teenagers and adults, normal values for hemoglobin range from 13 to 18 grams per deciliter. For hematocrit, the normal range is 45 to 52 percent. Athletes who live and train at higher altitudes typically have more red blood cells, resulting in slightly higher hemoglobin and hematocrit values. Being dehydrated when you have your blood drawn can also produce elevated levels.

When it comes to interpreting serum ferritin values, the general rule in the sports world is that levels below 12 micrograms per milliliter indicate completely depleted iron stores in the bone marrow, whereas values between 12 micrograms per milliliter and the lower limit of the normal range represent minimal iron stores. Diagnostic laboratories typically define normal, or adequate, iron stores as more than 20 micrograms per milliliter, whereas most exercise physiologists and exercise science researchers define serum ferritin levels of 35 micrograms per milliliter as the lower limit of normal for athletes.

You easily can monitor your iron status through specific blood tests that check hemoglobin, hematocrit, and serum ferritin levels. Hemoglobin and hematocrit are typically included in routine blood work during a yearly physical. Unless you have a sports-savvy physician, though, you'll most likely have to request to have your storage iron, or serum ferritin, checked.

To get the most out of monitoring your iron status, you'll want to determine your baseline values. Anemia is defined by a hemoglobin or hematocrit value that falls below the normal range. Normal and abnormal values overlap significantly, though, so compare your test results only to your personal baseline range. During my career as a competitive distance runner, for example, I always kept copies of my blood test results. Over time, I discovered that I perform poorly when my hemoglobin dips below 14 as my baseline runs closer to 14.5 grams per deciliter. A reading of 13 grams per deciliter, however, may not signal anemia for an athlete who has a lower baseline.

Most athletes, unfortunately, typically have blood work performed only when they feel poorly or when they aren't performing well. This approach means it will take a series of blood tests over time, correlated with physical symptoms as well as training and racing performances, to determine the ideal normal range. If you can swing it, have blood work performed when you're at the top of your game, too.

Treating Iron-Deficiency Anemia (Stage 3)

If you're diagnosed with iron-deficiency anemia (stage 3), treatment usually consists of 50 to 100 milligrams of elemental iron, two or three times a day. To reduce possible side effects, such as nausea, diarrhea, or constipation, gradually increase the amount that you take from once a day to three times a day as your tolerance increases. Ferrous sulfate, available in a liquid form, is absorbed better than most other varieties. Slow-release products help to reduce constipation.

Enhance how well your iron supplements are absorbed by taking them on an empty stomach, along with 500 milligrams of vitamin C or a cup of vitamin C–rich juice (like orange or cranberry). Take calcium and iron supplements a few hours apart, since calcium interferes with iron absorption. Allow at least 4 weeks of iron therapy before you have blood work repeated to confirm that your hemoglobin level is improving. By 8 weeks, the anemia is usually corrected, although every athlete responds differently. You may need to continue with iron supplements for as long as 6 months, however, to fully replenish iron stores, as evidenced by a normal ferritin level. Be sure to do this under the care of a physician.

Treating Iron Depletion

Athletes with low-normal or decreasing levels of serum ferritin, despite a hemoglobin reading in the normal range (stages 1 and 2), should consider iron therapy, too. Anemia impairs athletic performance by reducing the delivery of oxygen to tissues, but iron depletion can diminish your performance by a different mechanism. Iron-dependent metabolic processes at the cellular level, such as energy production in the mitochondria, may become impaired as your iron stores drop.

Studies of the effects of iron supplementation on performance in athletes with low iron stores have produced conflicting results. No improvements in $\dot{V}O_2$max have been shown, but other indicators of improved endurance, such as improvements in treadmill times and lower lactate levels during submaximal exercise, have been recorded. My personal experience and that of endurance athletes with whom I've trained suggest that low iron stores can hinder performance well before an official diagnosis of anemia. As with hemoglobin, an individual threshold, or optimal level of iron storage, most likely exists for every endurance athlete. While living in Boulder, Colorado, my serum ferritin levels fell to 21, most likely due to training at altitude. Although the physician considered this level normal, I began supplementing with iron. Another blood test 3 months later revealed that I had boosted my iron stores to almost twice that amount. More important, the chronic muscle soreness that I had been experiencing cleared up in just a few weeks.

Whether it helps immediately or not, boosting depleted (less than 12 micrograms per milliliter) and borderline-low ferritin levels by controlled iron supplementation makes good sense, as it can prevent outright anemia from developing. The recommended treatment consists of 50 to 100 milligrams of elemental iron once a day (taken with vitamin C) for 1 to 3 months, after which serum ferritin levels are rechecked. (Too much iron can be toxic for your liver.) Many times, the hemoglobin level will also increase, indicating that a mild anemia was already present although the initial hemoglobin level was technically in the normal range. Ideally, you want to maintain your iron stores as high as reasonably possible, as evidenced by serum ferritin readings of at least 50 micrograms per milliliter for women and 70 micrograms per milliliter for men.

Carefully plan blood tests around exercise. Your ferritin value can be artificially elevated for 48 to 72 hours following a prolonged bout of exercise such as a marathon or half Ironman (wait 1 to 2 weeks following an ultra) or if you're fighting an infection or experiencing inflammation. High-intensity training tends to decrease ferritin levels gradually, so keep this in mind as you interpret blood test results.

A chronic or reoccurring problem with iron depletion can be a red flag that your body is under too much stress. The effects of high mileage or intensity, underfueling (unintentionally or on purpose by dieting or fasting), and chaotic eating habits (skipping meals, for example), coupled with the effects of life stress, including insufficient sleep and recovery time, add up. Many exercise science experts, in fact, consider ferritin (and a new potential player, hepcidin) to be an indirect, but nevertheless, decent barometer of how the body is adapting to the training load put on it. Athletes who continue to try to train seriously and race while correcting low ferritin levels often end up being slowed by overtraining (or, as it is more accurately referred to today, underperforming) syndrome.

Hepcidin, a newly described hormone that's made in the liver, regulates cellular iron uptake. It also may represent another way that athletes lose iron. Hepcidin inhibits iron absorption and promotes sequestering it in macrophages in response to inflammation. Current studies are looking at whether inflammation caused by physical activity (military basic training, for example) elicits hepcidin release. If so, an increase in hepcidin could help explain the decrease in iron status observed in female military personnel during basic training, and perhaps apply to all athletes in training.

Preventing Anemia and Iron Deficiency

An emphasis on iron-rich foods will help prevent an iron deficiency from turning into anemia. The iron in animal foods, particularly from red meat, is far more absorbable than the iron in supplements or plant foods. (See Power Nutrient: Iron in chapter 1 for iron-rich food options.) Cooking in a cast-iron skillet also helps to boost iron intake, as will eating a vitamin C–rich food (fruits, vegetables, or juices) along with an iron-rich food. Female athletes who don't eat meat should consider taking at least a multivitamin with iron or a low-dose iron supplement (18 milligrams) daily.

Because iron deficiency is so common, especially among female athletes, I advise you to screen for it at least once a year. Be sure to request a serum ferritin blood test along with the routine tests that look at hemoglobin and hematocrit. Keep a record of your blood test results and record other pertinent information, too, such as the type and amount of training that you were doing, racing performances (if applicable), and comments on your general health.

Although you may be tempted to diagnose and treat yourself when you feel rundown and tired, no one should take appreciable amounts of iron without first seeing a physician. Some people are susceptible to iron overload, or hemochromatosis, which can lead to serious and irreversible damage to internal organs. Besides, taking iron supplements when you don't have an iron deficiency won't boost your performance, and consuming too much iron can impede the absorption of other minerals, such as zinc.

Understanding Sports Anemia

A low hemoglobin does not always indicate a problem. This is the case in dilutional pseudoanemia. Commonly referred to as sports anemia, dilutional pseudoanemia is the natural dilution of hemoglobin that occurs when endurance exercise produces an increase in plasma volume. Plasma, the watery portion of the blood, expands beyond its baseline in response to the exercise-induced release of various hormones. This increase in plasma volume artificially lowers hemoglobin and hematocrit readings.

Because the number of actual red blood cells remains normal (and increases proportionately during exercise as water is lost from the blood via sweat), the body's oxygen-carrying capacity is not compromised. Sports anemia doesn't usually last long. It frequently occurs in athletes who are

Tips for Avoiding the Common Cold

Your biggest fear may not be skiing through whiteout conditions or descending a steep mountain pass at 40 miles (64 km) an hour, but simply the thought of catching a cold. As an athlete, you probably know all too well that the common cold (or other upper respiratory infections) easily can prevent you from getting to the starting line, never mind the finish line, of your favorite activity. What can you do besides pay homage to vitamin C tablets? Plenty.

1. Eat a well-balanced sports diet. Keep your vitamin and mineral reserves at optimal levels so that your immune system will function at its best.

2. Don't shortchange yourself in the sleep department. Disrupted sleep has been linked to a suppressed immune system.

3. Avoid overtraining and chronic fatigue. When in doubt, leave it out, especially if you feel as if you're coming down with something. Give your body a chance to mount an attack without the extra stress generated by intense or prolonged physical efforts.

4. Wash your hands often. Viruses most easily enter your body when you touch germ-ridden hands to your eyes and nose.

5. Avoid large crowds and sick people whenever possible, especially before an important event or race. Consider getting a flu shot if you compete during the winter or if you travel a lot. You're particularly vulnerable to colds and other upper respiratory infections for 3 to 72 hours following an exhaustive bout of endurance exercise, so choose whom you hang out with wisely!

6. Consume a carbohydrate-containing beverage before, during (at least 30 grams of carbohydrate per hour of sustained exercise), and after all intensive training sessions and competitive efforts. This helps to lessen the negative effect stress hormones have on the immune system.

7. Don't try to drop weight quickly, especially not prior to a competitive event. Rapid weight loss stresses the immune system.

8. Keep other life stresses to a minimum. When this isn't possible, recognize that you're vulnerable to colds and infections, and moderate your training accordingly.

9. Be smart about supplements. Many athletes, despite credible evidence to the contrary, continue to believe in the herb echinacea to boost their resistance to colds, flu, and other upper respiratory infections. It's purported to stimulate certain white blood cells to

> continued

< continued

destroy invading organisms before they become infectious. Echinacea is most effective when taken at the first sign of symptoms (not beforehand) and then every 2 hours until symptoms are relieved. Take it for short periods—a few days to a few weeks at most. Continual use can actually suppress the immune system. (Don't take it at all if you're pregnant or nursing or if you have an autoimmune disease or allergies to ragweed.)

10. Sucking on zinc lozenges (the published research was done with zinc gluconate) at the first sign of sniffles may reduce the severity and duration of your cold. To avoid zinc overload, don't take lozenges for more than a week at a time. Avoid drinking citrus juices and soft drinks, which can interfere with zinc absorption, one half hour before and after taking the lozenges. To reduce feelings of nausea, don't take them on an empty stomach.

11. Taking vitamin C won't prevent you from catching a cold; however, it may help you feel better while you have it. Limit yourself to 1,000 milligrams a day, no more than 500 milligrams per dose. Larger doses might trigger diarrhea and, in some people, kidney stones. Athletes who participate in ultra events may be able to reduce oxidative stress to their immune system by supplementing with vitamin C (about 600 milligrams daily) for at least a week before the event.

12. If you do come down with a cold, comfort yourself with an 800-year-old remedy. A big bowl of hot chicken soup can improve coughing and help to clear the lungs.

Source: D.C. Neiman, 1998, "Immunity in athletes: Current issues," *Sports Science Exchange* 11(2). [Online]. Available: www.gssiweb.org/Article/sse-69-immunity-in-athletes-current-issues [April 24, 2013].

returning to training after being inactive for a while or when there is a jump in training intensity. Sports anemia doesn't respond to iron supplementation. It can be distinguished from iron-deficiency anemia because the lab workup will reveal that the red blood cells do not appear pale or small as they do in true anemia.

Food Allergies, Intolerances, and Sensitivities

Athletes often let self-diagnosed food allergies get in the way of eating a well-balanced, sports diet. About 25 percent of American adults believe that they have a food allergy, but only roughly 2 percent actually do. A food intolerance or sensitivity, on the other hand, can affect nearly everyone at some point. This next section provides strategies for dealing with both.

Food Allergies

What's the difference between a food allergy and a food intolerance or sensitivity? A reaction to food is deemed an allergy only if it involves or triggers the body's immune system. An allergen, usually a protein, in a food or ingredient causes the allergic person's immune system to overreact. Perceiving the allergen as harmful, the body produces massive amounts of immunoglobulin E (IgE), a type of antibody. IgE antibodies circulate in the blood and enter body tissues, stimulating other cells to release powerful substances, such as histamine. A reaction occurs within a few minutes (to up to a few hours later) and can include tingling or swelling in the mouth and throat, stomach cramps, vomiting, diarrhea, hives or a skin rash, or a runny nose, sneezing, coughing, and wheezing. In highly allergic people, anaphylactic shock, a severe and potentially fatal swelling of the throat, tongue, and airway that blocks breathing, can occur.

Eight foods cause almost 90 percent of all severe food allergy reactions. In adults, shellfish (shrimp, crayfish, lobster, and crab), peanuts, tree nuts (almonds, cashews, pecans, and walnuts), and fish top the list. Soybeans, eggs, wheat, and cow's milk round out the list. In general, if you're from a family in which allergies such as hay fever, asthma, or hives are common, you're more likely to be predisposed to developing a food allergy.

Having a food allergy is a rare and serious condition that warrants a proper diagnosis by a board-certified allergist. Try to find one who specializes in food allergies. Keep a detailed food journal of all food-related allergic reactions, including how much of the suspected food you ate before you experienced a reaction and how quickly the reaction occurred after you ate it. To narrow down the cause or help rule out a suspected food allergy, an allergist may perform various skin tests (PST, or a scratch or prick skin test) or blood tests (RAST, or radioallergosorbent test). Be aware that according to the expert panel convened by The National Institute of Allergy and Infectious Diseases, of the National Institutes of Health, one positive skin or blood test, by itself, isn't sufficient to make a diagnosis of a food allergy. (The PST, in particular, can be used to help identify foods that may provoke a reaction, but should not be used alone to diagnose a food allergy.) You must have a positive test to a specific allergen as well as a history of reactions that suggest an allergy to that same food.

Self-diagnosing a food allergy can quickly get you into trouble. Needlessly avoiding foods deprives you of food choices and important nutrients and it can make everyday eating a hassle. Incorrectly identifying an offending allergen is dangerous, too. In a true food allergy, even minute amounts of the allergen will cause a reaction. Once identified, the treatment consists of avoiding the food entirely. Allergy shots, as well as injections of small quantities of extracts from foods that you react to, are rarely effective in relieving food allergies.

Food Intolerances and Food Sensitivities

If you respond negatively to a food (experience digestive problems, for example), it's more likely a food intolerance or food sensitivity. You may suffer from many of the same or similar symptoms caused by a food allergy; however, your immune system is not involved (or if it is, not in the same way). A food intolerance or sensitivity tends to come and go in severity, and it is rarely life threatening. A prime example is lactose intolerance, which occurs when the body lacks enough lactase, an intestinal enzyme that breaks down the sugar (lactose) in milk. Stomach cramps, gas, and diarrhea signal this problem.

Another clear distinction from a food allergy is that a food intolerance or sensitivity will often allow you to eat varying amounts of an offending food without experiencing any symptoms. Lactose-intolerance sufferers frequently find that they can tolerate milk in other forms, such as yogurt, hard cheese, and ice cream. Using Lactaid tablets or drinking milk with added lactase can alleviate the problem, as well as drinking only small amounts of milk (4 ounces) with meals and never on an empty stomach. The good news is that in many cases, our bodies can learn to adjust to a troublesome food as we build up a tolerance to it. Studies show, for example, that people with lactose intolerance who commit to drinking 2 to 4 ounces (60 to 120 milliliters) of milk once a day (at mealtime) are able, over time, to handle larger amounts of lactose.

Gluten intolerance or celiac disease, an autoimmune intestinal disease, is an exception. Gluten is a protein found in wheat, rye, and barley (and possibly oats); therefore, it's in a wide array of foods, such as breads, crackers, and pasta. If you have celiac disease, ingesting even a small amount of gluten causes an autoimmune reaction that damages or destroys the villa in the small intestine, which hampers the absorption of nutrients. Left untreated, celiac disease leads to malnutrition, chronic iron deficient anemia, unhealthy weight loss, and osteoporosis. People with celiac also struggle with distressing GI symptoms, such as diarrhea, stomach upset, abdominal pain, and bloating.

The only effective treatment for celiac disease is a gluten-free diet—for life. It's often misdiagnosed because the onset of symptoms is usually gradual and characterized by a time lag of months or years after first eating gluten-containing foods. Celiac disease can be diagnosed through a specific blood test and an intestinal biopsy that shows damage to the villi.

Gluten sensitivity (GS), adverse reactions that result from ingesting gluten, is not as fully understood. It's not a wheat allergy, nor is it celiac disease. People with GS may have symptoms that resemble those associated with celiac disease, although non-intestinal symptoms prevail, such as bone or joint pain, muscle cramps, leg numbness, weight loss, and chronic fatigue. The small intestine of people with GS is typically normal. There's no reliable test, however, for non-celiac gluten sensitivity. It's diagnosed by ruling out or excluding other conditions, like a wheat allergy or celiac disease. If you think you react badly to gluten, see a doctor for celiac testing first, before starting a gluten-free diet. Otherwise, it's very possible to miss or delay a diagnosis of true celiac disease because the blood test will fail to detect the confirming antibodies.

Because gluten-free is the current hot trend, it seems as if a lot of people, athletes included, believe they will be healthier if they avoid gluten. Purported benefits of a gluten-free diet include automatic weight loss and better performances, even if you don't have an intolerance or sensitivity to gluten. It's estimated that about 1 percent of the population has celiac disease and another 6 percent or so have non-celiac gluten sensitivity, so it follows that 7 out of every 100 athletes—not 27 or 57—could definitely feel better gluten-free. As for preventing or treating other health conditions, such as irritable bowel syndrome or autism, no evidence exists that a gluten-free diet helps. If you simply believe that you feel better, perform better, or lose weight more easily when you don't eat gluten and gluten-containing foods, keep it in perspective. Going gluten-free typically means you eliminate a great number of processed and packaged foods, as well as fast food. Perhaps it is the avoidance of other qualities of the foods you eliminate, rather than the elimination of gluten, that makes you feel better.

Eating gluten-free isn't healthier if it's not done properly. Avoiding fortified breads, cereals, and grains for gluten-free products that tend not to be fortified, for example, can lead to deficiencies in iron, vitamin B_{12}, vitamin D, magnesium, and fiber. In addition, it's not as easy as simply filling up on gluten-free products that try to mimic their gluten-containing counterparts, because the gluten-free versions are typically higher in carbohydrate, fat, and sodium and lower in fiber. Work with a sports dietitian to design an eating plan that's built around wholesome whole grains (amaranth, quinoa, and pure buckwheat, for example) and that will meet your high energy needs. See table 6.1 for some gluten-free sports foods options.

If your list of intolerable foods keeps growing, other factors may be at play. Eating certain foods too close to exercise, for example, or when you're already feeling nervous or stressed may be the real problem. Athletes and coaches routinely blame dairy foods (especially milk), for example, for causing cotton mouth—dryness in the mouth accompanied by thick, white saliva. The most likely culprit behind cotton mouth, however, is a combination of emotional stress and dehydration—two factors that commonly occur during vigorous exercise and competition. Staying well hydrated before, during, and after exercise—rather than avoiding milk daily—is the best defense against cotton mouth.

Psychological triggers can be responsible for a food intolerance or sensitivity, too. For example, you may have experienced an unpleasant event as a child that's linked to eating a particular food. Or maybe you've convinced yourself that a certain food is associated with or responsible for a past poor performance. Whatever the case, when eating the food, you experience a rush of unpleasant sensations that can resemble an allergic reaction to food.

TABLE 6.1   Gluten-Free Sports Foods

Why consider going gluten-free? Athletes with celiac disease must avoid gluten or risk permanent damage to their small intestine. Others have a gluten sensitivity and experience distress when eating products that contain gluten, while others simply believe they feel and perform better on a gluten-free diet. Last, some athletes experiment and go gluten-free the 3 days prior to a long race in an attempt to reduce inflammation and GI distress. The following is a partial list of gluten-free sports foods.

Bars	Bonk Breaker, Clif Builder's, Clif C, Clif Kit's Organic, Kind, Lärabar, Odwalla, Perfect 10, PB & Whey, Picky, Simple, Soyjoy, Zone Perfect, SiS Go, Bumble, Enjoy Life snack bar, Elev8Me, Extend, Nonuttin' granola bar, Omega Smart bar, PureFit, thinkThin, Hammer Bars, Hammer Perpetuem, Perpetuem Solids
Chews and blocks	Carb Boom, Gu Chomps, Jelly Belly Sport Beans, Sharkies
Drinks	Ensure, Fluid Performance, Gatorade, Hammer Heed, Powerade, Generation UCAN, Ultragen
Energy gels	Carb Boom, Carboo4U, Crank e-Gels, Gu, Hammer Gel, Honey Stinger

If in doubt, check directly with the manufacturer to confirm that the item is gluten-free.

Finding a Solution

Eliminating a few foods from an otherwise balanced sports diet shouldn't cause a problem, especially if your everyday eating includes a wide variety of foods. Athletes often temporarily avoid certain foods, for example, as they approach an important competition. However, if you exclude entire food groups or struggle to eat more than just a few deemed-as-safe foods, it is more difficult to eat away from home and with others, and you miss out on key nutrients. If this is the case, seek help from a sports dietitian to help you make food substitutions and plan a well-balanced sports diet. If your symptoms are linked to food additives, such as MSG or sulfites (common in asthmatics), you should certainly avoid foods containing those substances. Check the ingredient lists on food labels and inquire how foods are prepared when dining away from home.

One way to investigate whether a specific food is the source behind your symptoms is to use an elimination diet. Keeping other factors the same, such as the amount and intensity of your training, eliminate one food at a time for several days. Monitor your symptoms for improvement. To confirm the connection, you need to eat the food again and see whether the symptoms return. Obviously, you can't do this without medical supervision if you've been experiencing severe reactions that you believe are food related. In addition, elimination diets aren't that useful if the symptoms that you experience occur infrequently.

Keep in mind that whenever you push your body to the limit, high levels of epinephrine (adrenaline) can interfere with the normal functioning of the GI tract. The rate at which food empties the stomach can be delayed, increasing the likelihood that you'll experience nausea and indigestion. Mental and emotional stress can also slow the time that it takes for food to leave the stomach. Eating smaller, more frequent meals composed of low-fat, familiar foods can help as you approach a competition or undergo periods of vigorous or stressful training. More often than not, modifying the timing of foods and fluids around exercise can make the difference.

No athlete wants to be slowed by bloating, flatulence, abdominal cramps, or diarrhea. Do your best to avoid abdominal discomfort before important events or races by staying well hydrated and avoiding gas-forming foods, such as carbonated beverages, beans, broccoli, cabbage, onions, and other problem foods that you've identified during training. Establishing a consistent eating pattern and regular bowel habits are your best bet in preventing abdominal and intestinal problems.

Female Athlete Triad

Female endurance enthusiasts, as well as recreational and elite competitors, are at risk for the female athlete triad. (Although not as clearly defined in the opposite sex, male endurance athletes are likely at risk too.) The triad is kicked off by an energy or caloric deficit that then leads to menstrual problems, such as hypothalamic amenorrhea (loss of three or more consecutive menstrual cycles or failure to start menses by age 15), and ultimately compromises bone health in the form of stress fractures and osteopenia (reduced bone mass). Individually, each of these conditions is worrisome; combined, they can do real damage to a female athlete's health.

Underfueling, or consuming fewer calories than your body needs to function properly, kicks off the triad. Some athletes engaged in strenuous training programs end up in an energy deficit by inadvertently expending more calories than they consume. More often, however, underfueling is the result of restricting calories in a deliberate effort to lose weight quickly in hopes of improving one's appearance or performance. Disordered eating (or chaotic eating patterns, as discussed in chapter 3), such as skipping meals, eating as little fat as possible, or periodically overeating and then purging (including exercising compulsively to burn off or cancel out calories), typically sets the stage. In response to eating too few calories, the brain signals the ovaries to produce less estrogen, and menstrual periods become irregular (or don't begin at all in young women).

Studies performed over the last three decades by research physiologist Barbara Drinkwater, PhD, and other female athlete advocates strongly support that menstrual irregularities (including amenorrhea) do not result from the stress of exercise or from having too little body fat. The definitive cause is low energy (caloric) availability. The good news is the medicine that's needed for reversing hypothalamic amenorrhea is food. A physically active woman initiates or restores her lost menstrual cycles by adequately replenishing daily the calories that she expends.

A prime concern with the triad is how it compromises bone health. Hormonal disturbances, such as a low estrogen level, accompany amenorrhea and interrupt the way that bones normally grow and develop. Without enough estrogen, especially during peak bone-building years (preteen to early 20s), bone is rapidly lost instead of being banked for the future. In other words, although an athlete may be in her mid-20s, she already could have the bones of a 60- or 70-year-old woman on the inside! This finding is particularly distressing, since Drinkwater and others have found that women and girls involved in sports normally present with a 10 to 15 percent increase in bone mass compared to their normal peers.

With lower-density bones comes an increased risk of stress fractures and soft-tissue injuries. And should you incur osteoporotic fractures (because of brittle bones that break easily), these changes in bone never reverse themselves. Amenorrhea can also interfere with a female athlete's future ability to become pregnant and, as ongoing research indicates, possibly put her at higher risk for heart disease.

Athletes, parents, and coaches should know that the American College of Sports Medicine considers amenorrhea to be the most recognizable symptom, or red flag, of the triad. Although certain medical conditions, such as hypothyroidism (an underactive thyroid), can cause amenorrhea, female athletes and those around them often view the absence of periods as a benign side effect of hard training. A 2004 survey undertaken by psychologists Roberta Sherman, PhD, and Ron Thompson, PhD, cochairs of the Athlete Special Interest Group of the Academy of Eating Disorders and consultants to the department of intercollegiate athletics at Indiana University for more than 20 years, confirms this sentiment. Of the almost 2,900 NCAA coaches of female athletes (representing 23 different sports) who responded, 37 percent viewed amenorrhea as normal. Fewer than half of the coaches considered amenorrhea to be abnormal and in need of medical treatment. In reality, a knowledgeable physician should evaluate any active woman with amenorrhea to determine the cause of the amenorrhea. The same advice applies to stress fractures, another easily recognizable sign of the triad.

Understand as well that not all three components—an energy (caloric) deficit, amenorrhea, and bone problems—need to occur simultaneously for the triad to be diagnosed. In reality, physically active girls and women tend to slide in and out of the triad, depending on how well they are doing at that time in achieving energy balance (calories consumed at least equal to calories expended). You don't have to be suffering from a full-blown eating disorder to induce amenorrhea; disordered eating habits can be enough. And the triad doesn't strike only elite athletes. Any active girl or woman who undereats, overexercises, or both is at risk for triad-associated complications. Experts recommend that girls and women presenting with one aspect of the triad should always be screened by a credible sports-minded health professional for the other two.

In 2005, the International Olympic Committee (IOC), which is responsible for the overall health and welfare of competitive athletes worldwide, took a more active stance regarding the female athlete triad. Speaking directly to the athletic community (sports medicine doctors, coaches, athletic trainers, and so on), the IOC released a first-time position stand that outlines practical and definitive steps to take in recognizing, treating, and most importantly, preventing the triad (for details, see Selected Resources).

Questions still remain about whether female athletes can catch up if they miss the window of opportunity to attain peak bone mass (puberty to adulthood, from ages 10 to 12 through 16 to 18). Oral contraceptives are frequently given to amenorrheic athletes to halt further bone loss. And they do work in that regard. This intervention, however, should be viewed, at best, as a stopgap measure; it's not enough to produce new bone growth. Rather, a female athlete with hypothalamic amenorrhea must work, supported by a treatment team (physician, sports dietitian, and possibly a therapist), to restore her natural menstrual cycle through good nutrition. Medications to promote building new bone (Fosamax, for example) are for postmenopausal women only. Women of childbearing age should not use them. Animal studies have shown that because of their long half-life, these drugs can cross the placenta and be absorbed by the fetus.

Male athletes, incidentally, are at risk for stress fractures and poor bone health as well. Consuming too few calories, especially in conjunction with endurance training, can lower testosterone levels. Insufficient testosterone (analogous to low estrogen levels in women), besides reducing fertility and sex drive, puts bones at risk.

Dietary changes alone, however, are rarely enough to reverse the triad. Lifestyle changes are necessary. If you've been diagnosed with hypothalamic amenorrhea, experts strongly recommend that in addition to consuming more calories, you reduce your training by 10 to 20 percent and restore or gain a modest amount of weight (2 to 3 percent of body weight) until you regain a normal menstrual cycle. Resistance training helps to strengthen bones, and you'll need to develop new skills and strategies for managing stress better. If you've been amenorrheic for a year or longer, a bone-density scan will let you know where you stand in regard to bone loss. If you're unwilling to make lifestyle changes or if making changes doesn't help your menstrual periods return (especially if you have a history of stress fractures or you've been amenorrheic for 6 months or longer), consider estrogen replacement therapy. Oral contraceptives are generally the recommended method.

When it comes to everyday eating, smooth out erratic eating habits and establish a schedule of consistent meals and snacks. If you constantly find yourself obsessed with food, or have an out-of-control sweet tooth, you most likely are eating too few calories. Also, if you've been avoiding meat, particularly red meat, you may want to reconsider. It's unclear why eating meat seems to protect a woman's menstrual periods, but it does. Include two or three small servings of red meat weekly (3 ounces each, or 85 grams, the size of a card deck). Remind yourself that fat is an integral part of a smart athlete's diet. Consume at least 20 percent of your daily calories as fat, which equates to 45 to 60 grams a day for most active women. You also need extra calcium and vitamin D at this point (1,200 to 1,500 milligrams of calcium and 400 to 800 IU of vitamin D daily), so choose foods rich in calcium and vitamin D, like milk. Add a supplement to make up the remainder. Calcium supplements alone are not enough to counteract the lack of estrogen associated with amenorrhea, and they don't prevent further bone loss. After menstrual periods resume, however, the extra calcium will help you build (up to age 30) and maintain bone mass.

Eating Disorders in Endurance Athletes

Being fit and athletic doesn't automatically protect you from eating disorders such as anorexia nervosa, bulimia nervosa, and binge-eating disorder. Numerous studies, in fact, suggest strongly that certain athletes, including some who participate in endurance sports, are at higher risk of developing eating disorders. Those most at risk include athletes involved in "appearance sports" such as gymnastics and skating, in sports in which low body weight is considered advantageous such as distance running and cycling, and in weight-category sports such as wrestling and rowing. A study of elite British teenage runners is a typical example. Seventeen of these 35 girls are believed to have suffered some form of eating disorder. Only four progressed through the ranks and made it to the senior national team.

Despite popular opinion in the sports world, eating disorders are not confined solely to female athletes. Men do suffer less from eating disorders than do women; however, at least 10 percent of all reported cases are among male athletes. Anorexia nervosa, moreover, is more likely to occur in male athletes than in other men. Male athletes also can become just as addicted to exercise, even in the face of illness or injury, as do some female athletes. Current statistics may continue to underestimate the problem, since few studies to date on male athletes have used the well-established criteria set forth by the American Psychiatric Association to diagnose varying degrees of eating disorders. On top of that, because eating disorders are perceived as a feminine disease, male sufferers typically seek help less often.

There's a growing awareness, however, that male athletes can be just as preoccupied with body size and shape as are many girls and women. One study examined eating, weight, and dieting practices in 162 competitive collegiate rowers: 82 heavyweights (56 women, 26 men) and 80 lightweights (17 women, 63 men). Lightweight rowers must meet weight restrictions as part of the sport. The findings (based on self-reported anonymous questionnaires) reveal that although female rowers exhibited more disordered eating behaviors overall, the male rowers also suffered with significant eating and weight concerns.

Roughly 12 percent of male rowers (and 20 percent of female rowers) in this sample reported having binge eating episodes at least twice a week. Binge eating is defined as the discrete consumption of large amounts of food coupled with a sense of loss of control and followed by emotional distress. Moreover, male rowers reported cutting weight (intentional rapid weight loss) more times per season than female rowers did (4.3 times versus .4 times), and they reported the frequent use of extreme methods to lose weight. Fifty-seven percent of the men reported fasting (compared with 25 percent of the women), and 2.5 percent reported vomiting (compared with 13 percent of the women). Male lightweights, in particular, are at risk for potential psychological and medical problems. They reported greater weekly and seasonal fluctuations in weight, cut weight more frequently, and were most likely to fast to lose weight compared with heavyweights or lightweight female rowers.

Before heading to the Olympic Games in Athens, Britain's leading middle-distance runner, Commonwealth 1,500-meter champion Michael East, sounded the warning in a July newspaper article. He claimed that many of the country's top male athletes were risking their health by starving themselves in an attempt to run faster. Why? East claims that they were doing so in a desperate attempt to recreate the glory days of the 1980s when Sebastian Coe, Steve Ovett, and Steve Cram led the world at middle-distance running. Bruce Hamilton, the British Olympic team's doctor, echoed East's concern. Hamilton agreed that disordered eating is common among male athletes and that inadequate dietary intake over time compromises all body systems, leaving runners prone to stress fractures, infections, and other problems.

As an athlete, male or female, committed to doing well in endurance sports, you're probably accustomed to doing things in the extreme—like rising religiously at five o'clock to train before putting in a full workday or spending a rainy Saturday running 30 miles (48 km) instead of going to the movies with friends. Not surprisingly, you also could be extreme in your attitudes and beliefs about body weight and eating behaviors, variables that certainly hold the promise of improving performance. Being competitive and compulsive (friends and family may have even referred to you as obsessive) contributes to your athletic success; however, it's also the very personality type that can lead to an eating disorder.

Causes of Eating Disorders

Eating disorders are complex in nature. They arise in a vulnerable person due to an inherited predisposition (genetics) that is ignited by a perfect storm or combination of precipitating factors. These may include family problems, long-standing emotional or psychological issues, major life transitions such as reaching puberty, for example, or going off to college, possible biochemical imbalances in brain chemistry, a history of dieting, and actual or perceived family, societal, or cultural pressures to be thin or have the perfect body. People with eating disorders don't set out to harm themselves. The eating disorder comes to serve as a coping mechanism, although it's an unhealthy one (similar to abusing alcohol, drugs, gambling, compulsive shopping, and so on). They turn to manipulating their food choices and their body (weight, shape, or size), in other words, as a way to cope with emotions that they don't know how to deal with in a healthier way. The eating disorder persists if they are allowed to or encouraged to practice the distorted behaviors and if the distorted beliefs they hold continue to be fed or strengthened by perpetuating factors (can be similar to or in addition to precipitating factors).

Simply being involved in a particular sport, by itself, rarely causes an eating disorder. We know this to be true because not every athlete who participates in a high-risk sport develops an eating disorder. Experts in this field have two theories to explain the high incidence of eating disorders associated with certain sports, such as gymnastics and long-distance running. First, people who have an eating disorder or are at risk of developing one seem to gravitate toward these sports. Second, being involved in these sports triggers or precipitates the development of an eating disorder in someone who is vulnerable or predisposed.

People who develop eating disorders typically share some underlying traits: They often feel unworthy or inadequate, have an intense need to be accepted, suffer from depression or anxiety, and lack sufficient skills to cope with unpleasant feelings and personal issues. Athletes, even the great ones, can suffer with these issues, too. Being involved in an endurance sport can further complicate the picture. You have a heightened awareness of your body (including perceived imperfections), and as a driven and disciplined competitor, you believe that you can always achieve more and do better (the win-at-all-costs attitude). On top of that, you may feel a loss of control over your daily activities as well as your goals. Besides pleasing yourself, parents and family members, friends, teachers, and bosses, you must also answer to coaches, teammates, sports associations and governing bodies, and perhaps even the media. Athletes who suffer with eating disorders typically speak of their weight as the only thing in life that they can control. Ironically, these athletes end up being controlled by the very thing that they desperately want to take charge of.

Anorexia Nervosa

Anorexia nervosa (AN) is characterized by distorted body image and excessing dieting that leads to severe weight loss with a pathological fear of gaining fat. Times of transition in early adolescence through early adulthood (12 to 24 years of age), such as puberty, going to college, a divorce in the family, or the death of a significant loved one, can precipitate anorexia in a vulnerable person. People with anorexia tend to be perfectionists with unrealistic goals, and much of their behavior can be viewed as compulsive or ritualistic.

There are two subtypes of AN: restrictive and purging. Someone who meets the criteria for AN and who binges and purges does not have bulimia nervosa; he or she has the purging type of AN.

The criteria for being diagnosed with anorexia include

- restriction of energy intake (calories) relative to requirements that leads to a significantly low body weight (less than minimally normal, or, for children and adolescents, less than minimally expected) in the context of age, sex, normal development, and physical health;
- intense and irrational fear of weight gain or becoming fat, or persistent behaviors that prevent weight gain, despite being at a significantly low weight; and
- extreme concern with body weight and shape including a disturbance in the way personal body weight or shape is experienced, undue influence of body weight or shape on self-evaluation, or persistent lack of recognition of the seriousness of the current low body weight.

The possible health complications of anorexia nervosa range from mild to severe enough to be life threatening, especially in physically active people:

- Slow pulse and low blood pressure
- Hair loss
- Severe loss of body fat and muscle wasting
- Cold intolerance
- Lanugo (fine hair on face and arms resulting from the body's attempt to provide insulation)
- Muscle weakness and fatigue or extreme hyperactivity
- Anemia
- Amenorrhea (loss of menstrual periods) and infertility problems
- Stress fractures, osteopenia (reduced bone mass), and early-onset osteoporosis
- Overuse injuries
- Inability to concentrate

- Depression and anxiety
- Insomnia
- Irregular heartbeat or other abnormalities
- Laxative dependence

Bulimia Nervosa

Bulimia nervosa is a secretive cycle of binge eating (although men often binge eat with others around) followed by inappropriate or unhealthy compensatory behaviors, such as self-induced vomiting; excessive exercise; or the use of laxatives, diuretics, or enemas. College-age students are particularly at risk; estimates are that one out of every five (20 percent) young women suffers from bulimia. Those with bulimia nervosa typically experience (and complain about) frequent or extreme fluctuations in weight. They cannot be identified solely by their weight, however, because an athlete suffering with bulimia could be fairly thin to normal weight or even slightly overweight. Excessive exercise, frequent trips to the bathroom after eating, laxative abuse, and strict dieting are potential signs to look for when someone is maintaining their weight despite frequently eating a larger-than-normal amount of food.

Criteria used to diagnosis bulimia nervosa include the following:

- Repeated episodes of bingeing (eating a large amounts of food in a short period) followed by purging (unhealthy compensatory behaviors), once a week for at least three months
- Feeling out of control during a binge
- Purging (using unhealthy compensatory behaviors) after a binge to avoid weight gain, including self-induced vomiting; fasting or strict dieting; vigorous or excessive exercise; or use of laxatives, diuretics, or diet pills
- Frequent dieting (restrained eating)
- Persistent overconcern with body weight and shape

The possible health complications of bulimia nervosa range from mild to severe enough to be life threatening:

- Swollen glands and sore throat
- Dental and gum problems
- Inflammation or tears of the esophagus
- Muscle cramps or weakness
- Edema or complaints of bloating
- Fatigue
- Electrolyte imbalances and dehydration
- Menstrual irregularities or amenorrhea

- Frequent stomach cramps, constipation, or diarrhea
- Laxative dependence
- Irregular heartbeat or other abnormalities
- Depression or social withdrawal
- Insomnia

Binge Eating Disorder

Binge eating disorder is characterized by recurrent episodes of eating an unusually large amount of food in a short period of time (2 hours, for example), accompanied by a sense of lack of control—feeling unable to stop eating or control what or how much he or she is eating. People with this disorder experience at least three of the following criteria:

- Eating much more rapidly than normal
- Eating until feeling uncomfortably full
- Eating large amounts of food when not feeling physically hungry
- Eating alone because of being embarrassed by how much one is eating
- Feeling disgusted, depressed, or very guilty after overeating

Binge eating is not the same as overeating. We all do that occasionally. The binge eater must be very distressed about his or her binge eating, binges must take place at least twice a week for at least six months, and there must be no inappropriate compensatory behaviors following a binge.

Health complications of binge eating disorder can include weight gain and related health problems such as high blood pressure or cholesterol, type 2 diabetes and heart disease, digestive problems, menstrual problems, joint and muscle pain, insomnia, and depression.

Anorexia Athletica

You may think that many of the athletes you coach, train with, or compete against are excessively concerned with their eating habits and weight. This obsession may be unhealthy, but it doesn't mean that they all have eating disorders. A growing body of evidence suggests, however, that more and more athletes (especially women) are suffering from a less severe or subclinical eating disorder called anorexia athletica. Although such athletes may not meet the strict medical criteria of being anorexic or bulimic, they nevertheless have serious eating problems and body-weight concerns. Dieting and maintaining a low body weight start out as the means to an end, typically to improve athletic performance; however, somewhere along the line, losing weight becomes itself the goal.

Researchers began by looking at this phenomenon in female athletes; however, considerable carryover applies to male athletes. One male recreational-level triathlete I counseled was weighing himself several times a day, although he appeared to be at a healthy weight. When questioned about it, he replied that he was assessing whether his training program was working. Eventually, he shared his true concern, which was an intense desire to lose 5 pounds (2 kg) from around his midsection. He was irritable and tired all the time from restricting himself to three small meals a day, although he worked a full day and trained daily. He repeatedly proclaimed, "If I didn't have to eat, I wouldn't." After spending time with him, it became apparent that losing weight had taken precedence over his athletic goals, since he now lacked the desire and energy to maintain his weekly training program.

Female athletes suffering from anorexia athletica have an intense fear of gaining weight or becoming fat even though they're underweight (5 to 15 percent below what is normal for their height) or have an extremely low body-fat level. These women generally don't suffer from the severe emotional distress seen in those who have anorexia and bulimia. Nevertheless, they view their bodies in a distorted way. They maintain their below-normal weight for at least a year by restricting the amount of calories that they eat (about 80 percent of what they expend or less), by severely limiting food choices and food groups, and by exercising excessively (beyond what is necessary for success or what other athletes of a similar fitness level do). Periods of binge eating followed by various purging methods, such as self-induced vomiting or laxative use, are typically also part of the picture.

Surprisingly, most of these athletes manage to maintain their weight (albeit low), although they eat far fewer calories than they expend. How this is accomplished is not completely understood, but it appears that the combined effects of chronic dieting and exercise may induce the body to conserve energy (calories) or become more efficient at using what limited energy is available. This phenomenon could spell further trouble in the future if these athletes find that they must resort to more extreme dieting measures to maintain their weight or lose weight. Even more important, research on elite female endurance athletes continues to point to prolonged dieting as the most important trigger for developing a full-blown eating disorder.

The implications of anorexia athletic are troubling. Although many athletes perform well initially—after all, that's the allure of losing weight—we know that they cannot do so forever. Even in the short term, however, anorexia athletica may be compromising an athlete's true potential. Whenever athletes are chronically low in energy and other nutrients, they are more likely to suffer from dehydration and electrolyte imbalances, chronic fatigue, anemia, upper respiratory infections, poor healing, and longer recovery times.

Common Warning Signs of an Eating Disorder

No athlete wakes up on a Monday with anorexia or comes down with bulimia following a hard workout or race, as might happen with the common cold. Warning signs exist far earlier that indicate that eating and weight-related concerns have taken over the athlete's life. These warning signs include a marked increase or decrease in weight not related to a medical condition, intense preoccupation with weight and body image (that is, frequent comments about weight, size, or shape), compulsive or excessive exercising beyond purposeful training, narrowing of food choices and development of abnormal eating habits (refusing to eat with others, maintaining a list of forbidden foods, engaging in bizarre food rituals such as moving food around the plate with utensils without actually taking a bite, and so forth), self-induced vomiting (bathroom visits after meals), periods of fasting or dieting, amenorrhea, and abuse of laxatives, diet pills, or diuretics. A vegetarian eating style may also be a red flag for eating disorders, particularly among young, athletic women (see chapter 7).

Weight-preoccupied athletes tend to be highly self-critical. They may appear anxious, irritable, or depressed, and they often withdraw from people and activities that they normally enjoy. Fatigue or denial of obvious fatigue, dizziness, chills, abdominal discomfort when eating, insomnia, and shin splints are all typical day-to-day complaints along with more frequent stress fractures. Bulimia, with its secretive cycle of binge eating and purging, can be harder to identify because athletes with bulimia typically don't lose excessive weight or experience amenorrhea as do athletes who suffer with anorexia. Some signs that do indicate bulimia include "chipmunk cheeks" (from swollen glands), bloodshot eyes (from the force of vomiting), knuckle scars, and worn-off tooth enamel (discovered during dental visits).

If you or someone you know suffers from anorexia or bulimia nervosa, understand that it is a serious medical condition with potentially irreversible consequences. One study, for example, found that 53 percent of patients with anorexia nervosa also have osteoporosis—a condition characterized by brittle bones that fracture easily. It can be even worse. An estimated 1,000 women die each year of anorexia nervosa. In fact, together anorexia and bulimia cause more deaths than any other psychiatric disorder. Many of the previously mentioned behaviors or signs by themselves aren't proof that an athlete is suffering from an eating disorder. Nevertheless, because the best chance of a complete recovery lies with early intervention, ignoring a potential problem isn't wise. For more information on national organizations that provide help, see Selected Resources.

Seeking Help

What should you do if a training partner, teammate, or someone you coach is struggling with weight or body image? Don't wait for the person's performance to fall off or for a serious medical problem to develop to prove you're right. Common blood tests typically won't show a problem either. Immediately seek out someone you trust who is qualified to provide help. A sports medicine physician, a sports dietitian (a registered dietitian who specializes in sports nutrition), or a sports psychologist or therapist who specializes in eating disorders are all good bets. The more serious the eating disorder is, the more likely it is that a team approach (physician, sports dietitian, and therapist) will be needed for promoting a complete recovery.

Be sure that you approach friends, teammates, or athletes under your guidance privately and tactfully. Don't mention their weight, talk about calories, or tell them to "just eat normally." Rather, express your concern about their health. Tell them what you see as they train and perform that frightens or disturbs you—for example, skipping meals, having lapses in concentration at work or school, experiencing frequent colds and nagging injuries, not being able to complete workouts or finish strongly, withdrawing from teammates and social activities, and not having fun while pursing fitness or athletic goals. Judging or criticizing behaviors or giving simple solutions isn't helpful, and it ignores or minimizes the emotional struggle that the person is caught up in. Your goal or responsibility is not to change their behaviors or to fix the problem, it's to get them into treatment.

Don't be surprised if the person turns down the help that you offer or avoids the issue altogether. Denial is a primary defense mechanism used by people with eating disorders to protect themselves. Athletes caught in the throes of an eating disorder cannot simply give up their distorted beliefs or change their behaviors overnight. The person first must learn to communicate in a healthier manner (using their voice, not their body) and develop new coping skills to deal with unpleasant emotions and situations. Routinely express your concerns and offer to accompany the friend, teammate, or athlete under your guidance to seek medical help or attend a support group. Athletes often find that meeting with a sports dietitian for a simple nutrition checkup is a nonthreatening first step. Should the athlete refuse to seek professional help during a negotiated time span, share your intention to approach someone else, such as a coach, parent, or spouse (whoever is most appropriate). Coaches, obviously, can insist that an athlete get a complete eating disorder evaluation from a knowledgeable team of sports-minded health professionals before being allowed to (or allowed to continue to) train and compete. Never forget the fact that although people do recover from eating disorders, they rarely do so without professional help.

Preventing Eating Disorders in Athletes

The best treatment for eating disorders is prevention. Promote and model the message that food is fuel and that serious athletes respect their bodies by eating the necessary calories and nutrients. Emphasize strength and stamina, not a certain idealized body weight or look. The next best step is to intervene early before an athlete's distorted beliefs about food, weight, and body shape and size become firmly entrenched. If you're involved with athletics in any way, you need to send a clear message that an athlete's physical and mental health always takes precedence over sports performance. Don't minimize or ignore early warning signs, such as disordered eating and compulsive exercise. Eating disorders, after all, don't happen overnight. An athlete doesn't simply catch anorexia or wake up one morning with a case of bulimia—the red flags have been waving for a while. Treat athletes who struggle with their weight as you would an injured athlete. Provide the same medical help and guidelines for safe participation.

If you are a parent or coach, take a close look at your own attitudes regarding weight, body size and shape, and athletic ability. Body-image distortion and disordered eating go hand in hand and are pervasive in the sports world. Do you constantly diet to try to obtain an unrealistic weight or size? Are you perpetuating the oldest myth in the book that the thinner an athlete is, the faster he or she will be? Do you label foods as *good* or *bad* or routinely use these terms to describe yourself or others after eating them? It's not appropriate for you as a parent or coach to weigh athletes. If concerns are that great, make certain the athlete has appropriate resources and access to sports-minded health professionals who can help. Listen to the experts' recommendations regarding setting a healthy weight range, including a minimum weight that must be maintained. Discussions about weight are personal, so always approach the athlete in private.

Female fitness buffs and athletes (and coaches who work with them), in particular, need to accept genetic differences, including how much weight or body fat a person is predisposed to carry. If you're an athlete who struggles with disordered eating, focus on feeling good about yourself. This starts with accepting your natural body type. Although you may not be able to completely ignore cultural and sports-specific pressures to look different, you can work on how your body image influences your current behaviors and, more important, the rest of your life.

Special Nutrition Concerns for Female Athletes

Female athletes can face unique challenges related to their menstrual cycle, pregnancy, breastfeeding, and menopause. It's not surprising, since the body and mind are experiencing enormous hormonal shifts at these times. The following sections provide nutrition strategies that help female athletes better manage premenstrual syndrome, as well as advice on how to feel your best and remain fit and active while pregnant, breast-feeding, and approaching menopause.

Premenstrual Syndrome

If you feel that your ability or desire to train or perform suffers at certain times of the month because of your menstrual cycle, you're not alone. One likely cause is premenstrual syndrome (PMS or PMDD–premenstrual dysphoric disorder), a condition that affects 90 percent of women to some degree, especially those in their 30s and 40s. Although exercise can help curb the symptoms of PMS, an athlete in touch with her body may be more aware of or sensitive to monthly hormonal fluctuations.

Women of all athletic abilities, from fitness enthusiast to elite, can be affected by PMS. A complex mixture of emotional, behavioral, and physical symptoms that appears on a regular, recurring basis that correlates with the timing of your menstrual cycle (1 to 2 weeks before the onset of menstruation) indicates PMS. The symptoms vary widely among women, but tend to fall into four categories: anxiety (mood swings, irritability, sense of being out of control), cravings (increased appetite, craving for sweets or salty foods, fatigue, headache, dizziness), edema (weight gain, breast swelling or tenderness, abdominal bloating), and depression (forgetfulness, crying, insomnia). With PMS, the symptoms resolve quickly (within 4 days) after the onset of menstrual bleeding. During the teenage years and early to mid-20s, symptoms may be minimal and barely noticeable. As you get older, the symptoms may gradually become worse from year to year or may rapidly increase in intensity following the birth of a child.

The exact cause of PMS remains unclear. An imbalance in one of the two female hormones, estrogen and progesterone, or an imbalance of the ratio between these hormones, as well as alterations in brain chemicals, appears to play a role in susceptible women. Not all women suffer to the same degree with premenstrual symptoms. Athletic women may feel particularly hampered by physical symptoms, such as fluid retention, weight gain, and breast tenderness. Many also complain of feeling clumsy, less coordinated, and more susceptible to muscle or skeletal injuries. Mood swings, uncharacteristic fatigue, or the energy lows associated with PMS can also make it feel hard just to get out the door.

Diet and Supplements

Although nutrition issues alone most likely don't cause and can't cure PMS, modifying your diet may help alleviate symptoms. No single treatment has proven effective for all women, so you may need to try various strategies to find relief. In some cases, it may take a few menstrual cycles to see any effects.

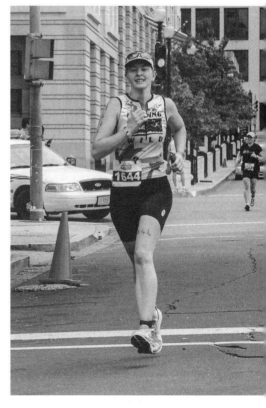

Solid nutritional strategies can help female endurance athletes mitigate and cope with the impact of physiological changes on performance.

Here are some recommended strategies:

- Eat small, frequent meals based on wholesome complex carbohydrate during the two weeks before your period is due. Going long periods of time without food causes your blood sugar to plummet, which accentuates many PMS symptoms. Eat six small meals a day, about 3 hours apart, to help keep your blood sugar level on a more even keel. Include plenty of foods with complex carbohydrate, such as pasta, baked potatoes, whole-grain cereal, crackers and bread, rice dishes, and vegetables. Choose whole-grain versions rather than sugary foods.

  When blood sugar levels get too low, adrenaline is released, which may interfere with the normal metabolism of progesterone. In addition, the extra adrenaline can make you feel more anxious, tense, or aggressive. Eating complex carbohydrate also increases the production of serotonin, a brain chemical that leaves you feeling satiated, as well as less depressed and less irritable.

- Limit your consumption of simple sweets. Resist the urge to self-regulate your mood or energy level with sugar. Simple sugars found in baked goods, soda, and candy can cause rapid swings in blood sugar levels. You may feel better and temporarily have more energy only to find yourself in need of another sugar fix a short while later. Enjoy these foods in moderation at a meal, not on an empty stomach.

- Stay well hydrated. Dehydration can make PMS symptoms worse, especially feelings of fatigue. Limit or avoid alcoholic beverages.

- Avoid caffeinated beverages and other sources of caffeine. Try to eliminate, or at least substantially cut back on, the caffeine in your diet throughout the entire month. We don't know for sure why it may contribute to PMS, but as a stimulant, caffeine also induces the release of adrenaline. Many women find that eliminating caffeine is particularly helpful in alleviating breast tenderness or pain.

- Monitor your sodium intake. Traditional advice always has been to cut back on sodium (10 days before your period) so that you retain less water, which may help some women alleviate the bloating, tender breasts, and headaches associated with PMS. Hormonal fluctuations, however, most likely induce the body to retain water (whether or not you eat salty foods) and even cause some women to lose sodium before their periods. Increase your sodium intake slightly to see whether doing so makes a difference, particularly if you typically crave salty foods.

- Boost your calcium intake. During certain phases of the menstrual cycle, fluctuations in calcium-sensitive hormones that regulate calcium levels may set off a host of PMS symptoms by interfering with the brain chemical serotonin. If you don't get 1,200 milligrams of calcium a day by eating calcium-rich foods (see Power Nutrient: Calcium in chapter 1), boost your intake to the recommended level with a daily calcium supplement (in divided doses of 500 to 600 milligrams at a time). Daily calcium supplementation has shown promise in reducing symptoms of mild to moderate PMS, including generalized aches and pains, food cravings, water retention, depression, and mood swings. You may need two or three menstrual cycles to see positive effects.

- Boost your magnesium intake. Magnesium also plays a role in the synthesis of brain chemicals, so make sure that you regularly eat plenty of magnesium-rich foods. Good sources include legumes, whole grains, dark green leafy vegetables, nuts and seeds, tofu, and seafood. Supplemental doses (200 milligrams) may help some women with mild symptoms of PMS, such as bloating.

Here is some advice on other popular treatments for PMS:

- Use caution with vitamin B_6 supplements. Vitamin B_6 is involved in the synthesis of brain chemicals, such as dopamine and serotonin, and in the way that the body metabolizes hormones. Some women report relief of PMS symptoms with supplementation, although most studies do not find it superior to a placebo or sugar pill. Doses as low as 200 milligrams a day, taken for an extended time, may cause irreversible nerve damage, including tingling or numbness of the hands or feet and difficulty walking.

  To derive the possible benefits, eat foods rich in vitamin B_6, including whole grains, soybeans, soy milk, potatoes, salmon, poultry, spinach, broccoli, bananas, and cantaloupe. If you choose to take a supplement, take an entire vitamin B complex containing no more than 50 milligrams of vitamin B_6. Take doses over 100 milligrams a day only under the supervision of a physician.

- Many women find relief from female problems by turning to herbal remedies. Black cohosh and chaste berry tree are purported to reduce PMS by balancing hormone levels, Saint-John's-wort supposedly does the same by acting as a natural antidepressant, and valerian root may reduce PMS by serving as a mild tranquilizer and sleep aid. To reduce possible side effects, try one herbal remedy at a time. Check with your physician first, especially if you take any medications, including oral contraceptives, estrogen, or antidepressants.

Managing Your PMS Symptoms

When it comes to PMS, your best bet is to establish healthy eating patterns, modify your training and racing schedules as needed, and seek healthy ways to manage daily stress. Avoid remedies that promise to cure PMS if you abstain from eating long lists of offender foods, such as refined white sugar, white flour, and so on. Such an extreme diet has not proved effective. It is difficult to follow, and can create more anxiety than it's worth.

Keeping a daily chart of your three to five most severe symptoms will help you recognize the effects of PMS on your appetite and athletic performance. Record the absence or presence of your symptoms, their severity, and the day of your menstrual cycle (day 1 starts with menstrual bleeding). Ovulation (approximately days 12 to 14 of a normal menstrual cycle), for example, boosts a woman's daily energy needs by 100 to 200 calories. You'll be less anxious, less irritable, and less prone to food cravings if you're aware that an increase in appetite is natural and normal at this time.

If self-help techniques such as healthy nutrition habits, dietary supplements, and a stress management program prove to be ineffective, explore other treatment options with your physician. Oral contraceptives or antidepressants may also be indicated to help alleviate the emotional and physical symptoms associated with PMS.

Nutrition and Pregnancy

Even if your pregnancy was planned, your goals may not include sitting around for 9 months waiting for the baby to arrive. Many female athletes desire to, and are able to, retain a high degree of fitness during pregnancy. A timely return to competition following the birth of a child is also a powerful motivator for many female endurance athletes. Listening to your body and maintaining healthy eating habits before, during, and following your pregnancy are the keys to ensuring a healthy baby and a healthy, fit mom.

Prepregnancy Diet Concerns

Pay attention to your diet before you plan to conceive to reduce your risk of having a baby born with a birth defect that affects the brain or spinal cord (neural tube defects), such as spina bifida or anencephaly. The first eight weeks after conception are the most crucial time in your baby's development. By the eighth week, the developing fetus has a complete nervous system, a beating heart, a fully formed digestive system, and the beginnings of facial features. Neural tube defects occur during the first month of pregnancy when the neural tube is forming. As many as half of all pregnancies are unplanned, so many women, including female athletes, don't realize that they are pregnant at this time. Weight gain can be minimal during these first few weeks, and a woman may attribute a late or missed menstrual period to hard training efforts or the stress associated with competitions.

Consuming 400 micrograms a day of the B vitamin folate or folic acid will help your developing baby form and develop new and normal body tissues. (Folate is used when the vitamin is found naturally in foods; folic acid is used when it is found in supplements.) Natural sources of folate include legumes, such as lentils and dried beans, leafy green vegetables (especially spinach and broccoli), whole grains, orange juice, and some fortified breakfast cereals. Grain products, such as breads, pasta, rice, cornmeal, and enriched flours, are now being fortified with small amounts of folic acid, too. Nevertheless, most women do not consume adequate amounts of folate in their diet.

If you're contemplating pregnancy, see your doctor before you try to conceive and begin taking a prenatal vitamin–mineral supplement as directed to obtain the folic acid that you need. Because many pregnancies are unplanned, the March of Dimes, a research organization that studies birth defects, recommends that all women of childbearing age, whether planning to become pregnant or not, take a multivitamin with 400 micrograms of folic acid daily and eat folate-rich foods. (Avoid taking a daily multivitamin containing more than 5,000 IU of vitamin A. Excessive levels of vitamin A can be toxic to a developing baby.)

Abstaining from alcohol makes sense too. No safe level of alcohol consumption has been determined for pregnant women. Consuming limited amounts of alcohol after conception but before becoming aware that you're pregnant shouldn't cause distress. Regularly consuming alcoholic beverages, however, does affect the developing fetus. Having one to two drinks per day can result in a smaller baby. Drinking greater amounts can lead to birth defects associated with fetal alcohol syndrome. The earlier you eliminate alcohol, the better off your baby will be.

Dealing With Morning Sickness

Weight gain, food cravings, fatigue, and morning sickness are issues that all pregnant women have to deal with. Most female athletes are prepared to slow down as they gain weight throughout their pregnancy. You may even be looking forward to satisfying a craving or two. You may not be prepared, however, for the slowdown caused by morning sickness and fatigue during the first few months of your pregnancy.

Morning sickness, characterized by nausea with or without vomiting and fatigue, affects 50 to 90 percent of pregnant women to some degree. Despite being studied for at least four thousand years, the exact cause of morning sickness remains a mystery. Fluctuating hormonal levels, dehydration, and a trigger of some sort most likely combine to produce the nausea. It's usually worse in the morning when rising, although it can occur anytime throughout the day. Morning sickness usually resolves itself by the end of the first trimester (week 13), but don't worry if you still experience it into the fourth or fifth month.

Because every pregnancy is different, what triggers morning sickness will also vary from woman to woman. You'll have to experiment to find what works for you in reducing or alleviating the symptoms of morning sickness. Some age-old remedies that have stood the test of time include keeping soda crackers near your bed to nibble on before you get up and not brushing your teeth right after eating. You may find that eating a snack before you go to bed or when you awaken during the night may ward off nausea in the morning. A heightened sense of smell is typical during pregnancy, and smells or odors may play a large role in triggering bouts of morning sickness. Try to sleep with the window open. Avoid cooking odors, perfume, aftershave, and cigarette smoke. If the smell of some foods makes you sick, avoid them.

Be prepared to eat small meals every 2 to 3 hours to keep your blood sugar from getting too low, which may induce nausea. Don't worry about craving or only being able to tolerate junk food during bad periods of morning sickness. The goal is to find foods that you can eat and keep down. Your favorite workout food, the one you can stomach during a hard effort or in the middle of a long race, might just do the trick. Concentrate on eating nutritious foods after the nausea and vomiting pass. Eating typically causes you to drink more, which will help you avoid becoming dehydrated. Drink beverages slowly and between meals to combat nausea. Of course, you'll want to pay particular attention to drinking enough fluids before, during, and after exercise.

Weight Gain and Energy Needs

You may be surprised that eating for two requires only an extra 300 calories a day, primarily during the second and third trimesters. That's not much— in fact, three glasses of low-fat milk will do the trick. As you reduce your training, you may not even need to eat any extra food to meet your energy needs. Let your rate of weight gain be your guide. You'll want to gain at least 25 to 35 pounds (11 to 16 kilograms) during your pregnancy to reduce the chance of complications, such as having a baby that weighs too little or is born prematurely. Pay particular attention to eating 2 to 3 hours before you exercise, as well as immediately afterward, to minimize exercise-induced falls in blood sugar. Keep supplemental carbohydrate (for example, sports drinks, energy gels, and energy bars) on hand to ingest during exercise as needed, even during short sessions when you typically wouldn't need anything.

Gaining less than 5 pounds in the entire first 3 months can be perfectly normal. Typical gains are about a pound per week after that. Athletic women may easily gain more than the recommended range, particularly if you're lean and enter your pregnancy with a low body-fat level. If that's the case, don't worry about what the scale says. If you're eating healthy foods and continuing with your exercise routine (with modifications as necessary), your baby will profit from the extra weight that you gain.

Nutrient Needs and Food Cravings

During pregnancy, you need more of certain nutrients. Besides folic acid, active women need to pay particular attention to getting enough calcium, iron, and protein. Your calcium needs jump to 1,200 milligrams a day, or the equivalent of four servings of dairy foods (see Power Nutrient: Calcium in chapter 1). As your baby's bones calcify, calcium moves out of your bones and across the placenta. Without adequate calcium stores, you run the risk of weakening your bones. This increases your risk of developing a stress fracture when you return to training, and for developing osteoporosis earlier in life.

Pregnancy doubles your iron requirement to 30 milligrams a day, because you need to make hemoglobin for extra red blood cells for yourself and the developing fetus. Along with the inevitable loss of iron that occurs with blood loss at birth, your iron stores will also be used to create your baby's iron stores. Because many female athletes, particularly those involved in endurance sports, have low iron stores, have your iron status checked early in your pregnancy and at regular intervals thereafter. Although pregnant women commonly experience fatigue, especially during the first trimester, iron-deficient anemia only makes matters worse.

You also require an extra 10 grams of protein daily—the amount supplied by one glass of low-fat milk and a piece of whole-grain bread. Most female athletes easily can meet their increased protein needs through food alone; however, supplementing with calcium and iron makes sense. Incidentally, individual food cravings do not typically reflect any particular nutrient deficiency. Go ahead and appease your cravings within reason. Food aversions and cravings probably arise during pregnancy because of changes in your sensitivity to tastes and smells.

Foods to Avoid While Pregnant

Food safety during pregnancy is simple. Just be careful about ingesting anything that you wouldn't serve your baby. Besides alcohol, watch out for caffeine, artificial sweeteners, contaminants from pollution or bacteria, and herbal supplements. Restrict your daily intake of caffeine (considered a necessary substance by many athletes!) to 300 milligrams or less, about the amount in two cups of brewed coffee. Some studies suggest that drinking more than that may increase your risk of giving birth to an underweight baby. Although artificial sweeteners appear to be safe for pregnant women to consume, relying on natural sweeteners, like sugar, honey, or molasses, is a safer route to follow.

Skip soft cheeses such as feta, blue cheese, Brie, Camembert, and Mexican-style cheeses during your pregnancy. These items, as well as hot dogs, luncheon meats, and cold cuts, can be contaminated with a bacteria called listeria, which causes a flulike illness. Transmitted across the placenta, listeriosis food poisoning can lead to premature delivery, miscarriage, stillbirth, or serious health problems for your newborn child. Because of the risk of bacterial contamination, you should also stay away from raw or undercooked meat, poultry, and shellfish; sushi; unpasteurized milk or juice; and raw eggs found in homemade ice cream, eggnog, and raw cookie dough. Because of their potential mercury content, restrict your intake of tuna and swordfish to twice a week.

As for herbal supplements, few if any of these products have been tested for safety during pregnancy or lactation. If you're considering taking herbal supplements during your pregnancy (or while breast-feeding), consult with your physician first.

Breast-Feeding

Breast-feeding, not pregnancy, is the time more aptly referred to as eating for two. Your body requires an additional 600 or more calories a day to produce enough milk. Studies have shown that most breast-feeding women who exercise seem to increase their daily food intake spontaneously by 400 to 500 calories to cover their increased energy needs. The rest of the energy comes from fat stores accumulated during pregnancy for that purpose.

Dieting or excessively restricting your calories to speed up the process of returning to your prepregnancy weight doesn't make sense. You'll end up irritable and low on energy just when you need it the most during the first few months when you're fighting off the effects of sleep deprivation and adjusting to a new schedule. Don't try to lose more than 2 pounds (1 kg) per week. You took nine months or more to gain the weight, so you will likely need at least nine months to lose it, although regular exercise can speed up the timetable.

To keep up with your baby's demand for milk, you need to consume enough calories, adequate carbohydrate, and plenty of fluid. Plan to have a mini meal each time that you nurse, such as a piece of fruit or half a sandwich, plus at least 8 ounces (240 ml) of fluid, such as water, milk, or juice. A poor diet is more likely to decrease the quantity, not the quality, of the milk produced. If you're having trouble producing enough milk, reevaluate your food choices and boost your calorie intake. (A baby who gains 4 to 8 ounces, or 112 to 230 grams, a week the first month, and 1 to 2 pounds, or .5 to 1 kilogram per month the first six months, is getting enough milk and gaining weight appropriately.) Your calcium needs remain high (1,200 milligrams per day) while breast-feeding, and you should continue to monitor your iron stores (serum ferritin) and supplement with iron as needed. Women often find it helpful to continue taking a prenatal vitamin–mineral supplement while breast-feeding.

Dehydration can be a problem until you recognize how much your fluid needs have increased. Drink enough so that you feel you have to urinate every time you feed your baby. The clearer your urine, the better hydrated you are. Don't plan to exercise strenuously if your urine isn't clear. Dark, concentrated urine indicates that you're already dehydrated.

Substances such as alcohol and caffeine enter breast milk, and large amounts consumed in a short period can affect your nursing infant. Intense exercise efforts also affect breast milk composition by decreasing immunoglobulin A, a substance important for a healthy immune system, and by increasing the amount of lactic acid that appears in breast milk. The increase in lactic acid causes a sour taste that your baby may find unpleasant. Within

90 minutes after exercise, however, breast milk returns to normal, so these changes don't appear to be significant. If your infant appears to react to your breast milk following exercise, try breast-feeding your baby before you head out to train.

Menopause

While menopause is certainly a normal and natural phase of life, it can wreak havoc in the lives of some athletic women. Menopause usually occurs about the age of 50 (age range is 35 to 59), but the menopause transition (perimenopause) may last 5 to 10 years. And it's taking place at the same time that age-related changes are kicking in. Fatigue, waning motivation, and a fear of runaway weight gain often drive women at this time to try fad diets or unrealistic workouts in an attempt to thwart body changes. As estrogen levels fluctuate and progressively fall, however, changes will occur.

In terms of midlife weight gain, only about 5 pounds can be attributed to the effects of menopause. Due to a more malelike hormonal pattern (less estrogen, so the effects of existing testosterone are greater), it tends to be deposited around the abdomen as belly fat. Beyond that, however, research points to less exercise (less volume and often far less intensity) and a surplus of calories as the real culprit, rather than reduced hormones. Young athletes with amenorrhea (thus, the same reduced hormones), after all, don't get fat.

A less active lifestyle at this stage in life is a double whammy for women. Besides reducing the calories you require, it also leads to a decline in muscle mass (women have less to begin with than men). Less muscle means a slower metabolism and fewer calories being burned.

On top of that, changing midlife sleep patterns and sleep-disrupting night sweats can quickly leave you exhausted and unmotivated to train. Sleep deprivation also is known to increase appetite (leptin, the hormone that curbs appetite, is reduced and ghrelin, the hormone that increases our appetite, becomes more active), and it is associated with weight gain. At the same time, women who've been dieting for years often say "no more," which means "yes, please!" to many more foods. Add in successful careers featuring travel and pleasurable meals as well as opting for fine dining (and wines) and plush vacations more often, and it's easy to end up with more calories and less exercise.

Obsessing about body changes and losing weight (neither under your direct control) does little good. Focus instead on what is under your control. Firmly establish a regular eating schedule—three meals and two snacks—to cut down on late-night eating. Build in fun foods to avoid deprivation-driven binges. And treat your body right by getting what you need from real foods. Recent research published in the *Journal of the American Medical Association* shows no benefits of soy supplements in terms of reducing bone loss or menopausal symptoms. Calcium and vitamin D supplements by themselves are not an insurance policy against osteoporosis, either. As revealed by the

Women's Health Initiative (a clinical trial which followed over 36,000 normal, healthy middle-aged and elderly women for 7 years after randomly assigning them to the preventive strategy of taking 1,000 milligrams of calcium and 400 international units of vitamin D daily or to a placebo), any effect of taking calcium and vitamin D supplements to prevent osteoporosis is extremely modest at best. Your best bet is to obtain calcium (1,200 to 1,500 milligrams daily) by eating dairy foods and calcium-fortified soy foods, like tofu. Lastly, if you've had a distorted view of food or your body all your life, it's never too late to seek help from a qualified dietitian or therapist. Midlife happiness, otherwise, will truly elude you.

Regular exercise also can play a positive role for women in contributing to the quality of life during menopausal or middle-aged years. Be sure to pursue both aerobic exercise (to strengthen the heart and lungs) and strength training. Strength training is a must to maintain or build muscle mass and to maintain bone density by decreasing postmenopausal bone loss. Along with your training diary, keep a detailed record of all physical (fatigue, insomnia, joint pain, muscle pains, headaches, hot flashes, or excessive sweating) and emotional (depression, anxiety, poor memory, or irritability) symptoms you experience (absent to severe) in an effort to understand how your changing hormonal status influences your exercise performance.

Competitive sportswomen may be particularly frustrated during peri-menopause as natural estrogen levels progressively drop. Limited scientific research exists, however, on how menopause-induced hormone depletion definitively affects athletic performance. Many competitive female athletes, nevertheless, report deterioration in performance, an inability to maintain the same quantity and quality of training sessions, an inability to perform skills due to fatigue and strength loss, and significant heat intolerance. A greater chance of getting injured is a possibility, too.

The Medical and Science for Women in Sport group of Sports Medicine Australia supports hormone replacement therapy (HRT) as likely the best option for women who are interested in maintaining their best possible athletic performance. The choice, obviously, is one for each woman to make in consultation with her doctor, since there are risks associated with HRT for some women. (Keep at least a 3-month diary of symptoms, effects on training, and so on before your consultation.) HRT usually includes estrogen with progesterone added, and estrogen alone for women who have had their uterus removed. It also could include testosterone for surgical menopause and conditions not responding to estrogen alone. Drug testing is now part of masters competitions, however, and testosterone is a banned substance.

Whether you elect HRT or not, be confident in what you know to be true for your body. Learn to recognize the symptoms of hormonal depletion and how they affect your performance, and have the confidence to make adjustments to your workouts. Modifications can include training less, working out less intensely, building in more frequent and longer recovery periods, cross-training, and racing shorter distances or removing the stress of competition altogether.

Remember, endurance training is stressful to the body, and so is menopause. If stress is short lived, our bodies can adapt efficiently. A continually stressed body, however, breaks down. In stressful situations, the body releases a powerful hormone called cortisol. An overload of cortisol can depress the immune system and induce weight gain as the hormone directs the body to store fat. Do what you can during menopause to manage—or better yet, decrease—other areas of stress in your life. And certainly don't allow your training or racing choices to become a source of stress.

Unique Challenges Faced by Veteran Masters-Level Athletes

Reaching the age of 40 has special significance for endurance athletes, since it denotes being eligible for a new (and often highly competitive) age group category. From this point on, however, other significant changes are occurring, too. Most notably, maximal aerobic capacity ($\dot{V}O_2max$) steadily declines, dropping by as much as 10 percent per decade. $\dot{V}O_2max$ is a direct measure of the heart's overall power as an oxygen pump and of the ability of muscle cells to utilize oxygen sent to them through the cardiovascular system. The higher your $\dot{V}O_2max$ is, in other words, the higher the rate at which your body can produce energy to sustain endurance activity.

It's been challenging to determine how much of this loss is due to normal aging. More recent research, such as a study that followed 42 masters athletes for 8 years, suggests that the decrease in $\dot{V}O_2max$ is less related to aging and more related to the adoption of a more sedentary lifestyle. Being less aerobically fit due to a reduced volume of exercise or a less intense training program, in other words, appears to be the primary culprit. Life gets more complicated and different priorities arise for the masters athlete who is juggling career, family, and social obligations. Shifts in body composition occur with aging, too, and a decrease in muscle strength mirrors the decrease in muscle mass. The good news is that endurance-trained masters athletes who continue with regular vigorous exercise can prevent the glucose intolerance and insulin resistance problems associated with aging.

In terms of metabolism, evidence suggests that energy or caloric needs decrease with age due to a drop in basal metabolic rate (one-third responsible) and reduced physical activity. This frequently cited data, however, did not include people who vigorously exercise. In the few studies that have tried to quantify the energy needs of masters athletes, results have shown no differences compared to younger athletes. Regular aerobic exercise (such as running) thus appears to attenuate the expected age-related decrease in metabolism. This means you can't rationalize or blame those extra pounds on turning 50 (or 60 or 70), because the main factor predicting calorie needs is your training volume (which influences how much muscle you retain), not aging per se. Training does tend to decrease in older athletes, so be honest with yourself. If you're doing less (expending fewer calories) these days compared to in the past, you will need to eat less to maintain the same weight.

Other than adjusting caloric intake when training volume decreases, no scientific reason exists currently for separate nutrition recommendations for masters athletes. Carbohydrate, protein, and fat recommendations are the same as for younger endurance athletes, as is the need to consume adequate carbohydrate, fluid, and sodium during prolonged exercise. Older athletes also will benefit from consuming carbohydrate and protein in the early recovery phase (first 15 to 30 minutes) following endurance exercise to maximize glycogen resynthesis.

Older adults (age 50 years and up) do have an increased need for some micronutrients. The Dietary Reference Intakes (DRIs) for vitamins D, B_6, and B_{12} and the mineral calcium are higher for older adults. (The only reduced DRI is iron for older women.) Adding a daily multivitamin or mineral supplement for seniors can help ensure an adequate intake of key nutrients like vitamins B_{12}, B_6, and D, folate, zinc, and magnesium. (You still may need an additional calcium supplement.) Masters athletes older than 60 especially may benefit from taking synthetic forms of vitamin D and vitamin B_{12} because normal aging tends to lessen the body's ability to absorb and use natural forms. (For a listing of current DRIs, see appendix B.)

If you take medication for a chronic medical condition (cholesterol-lowering medications, thiazide diuretics, and nonsteroidal anti-inflammatory drugs are just a few examples), ask your health care provider about potential nutrient–drug interactions that can cause the loss of minerals and other key micronutrients. Compensate by consuming food-rich sources and, if necessary, by taking a supplement. Be aware, also, that many medications used to treat medical conditions common in older adults are on the banned substance list. If you're a masters athlete who competes, check with your governing body or organization regarding drug testing procedures and therapeutic use exceptions. Otherwise, you may be in violation of doping regulations.

Fluids and heat tolerance may be the most critical issues that a masters athlete needs to monitor. Older athletes have less body water compared to younger counterparts. As we get older, our ability to detect thirst diminishes. The kidneys' ability to concentrate urine also decreases with age, meaning that more water is needed (lost) for removing waste products. As our skin ages, sweat glands change, with each gland producing less sweat. These are all normal age-related changes. Coupled with an athlete's need for additional fluid, however, it's easy to see how masters athletes can get into trouble quickly. Since plenty of variables already threaten to distract an athlete's focus while training and racing, a programmed schedule of drinking can reduce the risk of dehydration. Be sure to use a sports drink to replace both the fluid and the sodium you lose in sweat.

Many masters athletes report significant problems exercising in the heat. Heat intolerance could be related to the decline in sweating capacity. The research suggests, however, that it's less a function of aging than of overall fitness. Older athletes who are well conditioned and acclimatized to the heat, in other words, are less likely to suffer adverse effects of warm-weather endeavors. Allow yourself to acclimatize fully (it takes about a week). During this time, reduce your usual training by one-half initially, and then build back up slowly. Follow a programmed drinking schedule during exercise and be alert for any signs of heat illness. (See chapter 14 for more on performing in extreme heat.) Last, use common sense. If you're worried that it's too hot to exercise (especially if you're trying to decide whether or not to compete), it probably is.

7

Endurance Eating
for Vegetarians

Well-planned vegetarian diets seem to effectively support parameters that influence athletic performance, although studies on this population are limited. Because plant proteins are less well digested than animal proteins, an increase in intake of approximately 10 percent protein is advised. Very low fat diets or avoidance of all animal protein may lead to a deficiency of essential fatty acids.

Source: N.R. Rodriguez, N.M. DiMarco, and S. Langley, 2010, "Nutrition and athletic performance," *Medscape Today News.* [Online]. Available: www.medscape.com/viewarticle/717046 [April 24, 2013].

Endurance sports and vegetarianism have much in common. Guidelines exist for each discipline; however, there's more than one path to follow to successfully accomplish the task. Although you certainly can jump recklessly into either venture, a little planning goes a long way to maintaining peak athletic performance.

If you choose a vegetarian sports diet while training for and competing in endurance and ultraendurance events, you can obtain the necessary nutrients that your body demands. But you must be as committed to meeting your nutrition needs as you are to fulfilling your athletic goals.

Following a vegetarian, even vegan, eating style doesn't have to be complex or life consuming, but it does require some effort. By reading this chapter, you will become more aware of the potential challenges and pitfalls endurance athletes face when following a vegetarian eating style. You'll also learn how to best fulfill your everyday nutrient needs using plant-based foods. Nonvegetarian athletes can benefit, too, by learning how to incorporate more health- and performance-promoting plant foods into their meals and snacks.

Defining Vegetarianism

Today's vegetarian is not the stereotypical tofu-eating hippie of years past. Today *vegetarian* is an umbrella term that refers to people who have many different reasons for choosing to eat variety of diets, including vegan, fruitarian, pescetarian, lacto-ovo vegetarian, macrobiotic, raw, and even flexitarian (or semi-vegetarian), which occasionally includes meat.

Athletes also cite different reasons for eliminating animal products from their diet. A vegetarian eating style may be undertaken to improve health, boost performance, adhere to spiritual or cultural guidelines, protect the environment, or to abide by a love for animals.

The following terms describe the general categories of vegetarian diets:

- *Vegans* (or strict vegetarians) eat only plant foods, such as grains, beans, fruits, vegetables, nuts, and seeds, and consume no animal products (meat, fish, poultry, seafood, eggs and egg products, and dairy foods, such as milk and cheese).

- *Lacto-vegetarians* eat dairy and plant foods, but eliminate all meat, poultry, fish, seafood, and eggs.

- *Ovo-vegetarians* eat eggs and plant foods, but avoid meat, poultry, fish, seafood, and dairy foods.

- *Lacto-ovo vegetarians* include eggs, dairy, and plant foods in their diet, but exclude all meat, poultry, fish, and seafood.

- *Pescetarians* are open to eating fish and seafood but exclude all other meat.

- *Flexitarians,* or semi-vegetarians, seek to decrease the amount of meat they eat, primarily for health reasons; however, they will occasionally eat red meat.

Risks and Rewards of a Vegetarian Diet

With careful planning, a vegetarian eating style can improve your health and, potentially, your athletic performances. Simply eliminating animal foods without finding appropriate substitutes, however, results in an unbalanced diet that does more harm than good. As a vegetarian athlete, be prepared to put more thought and planning into your everyday food choices. The goal is to incorporate alternative sources of key nutrients like calcium, iron, zinc, and protein. Otherwise, your health and performance will suffer.

Rewards

Opting for a vegetarian eating style is, for the most part, a healthy path to follow. Health experts continually urge us to eat more plant foods and fewer animal products, which lack fiber and tend to be high in fat and cholesterol.

Consider the contents of My Plate. The recommendation for someone who requires 2,000 calories a day includes 6 ounces (90 g of carbohydrate) of grains supplied by bread, cereal, rice, and pasta, and the like; 2 1/2 cups of vegetables; 2 cups of fruit; 3 cups (750 ml) of dairy products; and 5 1/2 ounces (supplying 40 g of protein) of protein foods such as meat, poultry, fish, beans, and eggs. Adding it up, that's a prescription for eating far more servings of plant foods than animal foods. Planning meals around grains, beans, soy foods, vegetables, and fruit definitely supports optimal health. Several recent studies show that compared with the general public, vegetarians have lower rates of hypertension and certain cancers, as well as much lower risk of developing heart disease and diabetes. Eating a plant-based diet can also make it easier to maintain a healthy weight.

Plant-based diets supply plenty of carbohydrate that can be used to replenish glycogen stores—a prerequisite if you work out daily, train more than once a day, or want to keep moving for hours on end. Endurance athletes need to consume about 60 percent of their daily calories from carbohydrate-rich foods. Foods from the grain group, fruits and vegetables, as well as beans, soy foods, milk, and yogurt fit the bill. If you're filling up on these foods, you're most likely already adopting a vegetarian or near-vegetarian diet. You should be able to obtain the rest of the nutrients that you need, including enough high-quality protein, if you eat a variety of foods daily and make some savvy substitutions for the foods that you eliminate.

Risks

Despite all the benefits associated with a vegetarian eating style, I find it difficult to comment specifically about whether endurance athletes perform better on meatless diets. The vegetarian theme includes too many variations. Many athletes eat healthy, well-balanced vegetarian diets, but others struggle to get what they need from diets that are too restrictive. The bottom line is that you can't automatically assume improvements in health or performance simply because you eliminate red meat or other animal products. A vegetarian lifestyle, in fact, has been linked to menstrual abnormalities, and in some athletic women, vegetarianism may even be a red flag that signals an eating disorder.

I've counseled numerous vegetarians who make poor food choices and end up with diets low in protein, iron, zinc, and calcium. How does this happen? Try this eating plan on for size: no red meat; few if any eggs, dairy, or soy foods; and sporadic amounts of fish, poultry, and beans. Survival depends on eating lots of bagels, salad, pasta, frozen yogurt, energy bars, and desserts or snack items. You're likely to end up in this rut if you make little effort to shop and prepare snacks and meals, if you aren't keen on trying new foods, or if you live in a carnivorous (meat-eating) household and routinely eat only the starchy parts of family meals.

Consuming the nutrients and calories that you need to partake in endurance endeavors becomes more difficult as you eliminate foods and food groups. Vegan diets pose the greatest challenge. Eliminating two food groups increases the risk for deficiencies, especially of some key nutrients such as vitamins B_2 and B_{12}, iron, zinc, and calcium. Endurance athletes often struggle to meet their high-calorie needs on vegan diets as well.

Special Nutrition Concerns for Vegetarians

Vegetarians typically define themselves by the foods that they don't eat. You will commonly hear a vegetarian say, "I don't eat meat," but how often do you hear one say, "But I do eat bok choy, tofu, and garbanzo beans?" To reap the benefits of vegetarianism, you must seek alternative sources of nutrients for the foods that you choose to eliminate. The easiest way is to focus on including a wide variety of foods in your daily diet, such as whole grains, dark green leafy vegetables, beans, and soy foods.

If you're curious about how your vegetarian eating style measures up, ask yourself a couple of questions: Do you, or are you willing to, explore new foods to meet your nutrient needs? Do you, or are you willing to, plan balanced meals and snacks to meet the high energy needs of being an endurance athlete? If you can answer yes to both questions, you're on your way to eating a healthy, well-balanced vegetarian diet.

Calories, Carbohydrate, and Fat

Vegetarian athletes typically have little problem eating enough carbohydrate. Breads, cereals, pasta, rice, fruits, vegetables, beans, lentils, some soy foods, and milk and yogurt all supply carbohydrate. By their nature, vegetarian diets rank higher in complex carbohydrates and fiber and lower in saturated fat and cholesterol than diets containing meat. Eating enough whole grains, however, can be a challenge for some vegetarians. Developing a taste for barley, brown and wild rice, bulgur, couscous, kasha (buckwheat), millet, and quinoa is particularly important for vegetarian athletes. Besides supplying complex carbohydrates, these foods provide protein, iron, zinc, and other trace minerals. An easy first step is to switch to eating whole-grain cereals and whole wheat bread, crackers, and pasta.

Your daily fat requirement (at least 20 percent of total calories) doesn't change if you follow a vegetarian diet. In fact, many vegetarians assume that eliminating animal products ensures a low-fat diet. Not necessarily. You can easily rack up fat calories if you rely too heavily on nuts and seeds, cheese and other whole-milk dairy foods, and high-fat snack and convenience foods. If this is an area that you need to work on, read food labels and choose low-fat alternatives whenever possible. If you rely heavily on nuts and cheese for protein, consider leaner options, such as beans (e.g., black, kidney), lentils, and soy foods. Don't forget that you can always cut back on how much or how often you eat a particular food.

Plant foods are bulkier and usually lower in calories than animal foods, so some athletes end up feeling full before they consume enough calories. Vegan diets, in particular, are high in fiber and low in fat. If you're having trouble consuming enough calories, don't skip meals or snacks (plan to eat six or more times a day), and concentrate on including plenty of high-calorie, nutrient-dense foods such as nuts and seeds, nut butters, fruit juices, dried fruit, and dairy foods. Cooking with modest amounts of fat or oil also will help boost your calorie intake. Desserts and snack foods supply loads of calories. Just be sure that you first eat foods that are more nutritious.

Protein

Getting enough protein is a common concern of vegetarian athletes. Because endurance athletes have higher protein needs, sprinkling a few chickpeas on a salad or crumbling a little tofu into a vegetable stir-fry won't get the job done. Most female endurance athletes need 65 to 90 grams of protein a day; active males typically require 95 to 120 grams daily.

Keeping up with your protein needs requires a two-pronged approach: Eat a variety of plant foods daily and consume enough calories to maintain your weight. Consuming too few calories means that protein gets used for energy rather than for building, repairing, and maintaining body tissues, including muscle. If you continue to eat adequate amounts of poultry, fish, eggs, and dairy products, getting enough high-quality protein won't be a problem. Animal foods provide all the essential amino acids (which must be supplied by one's diet because the body cannot make them) that we consistently need to have on hand. The body constantly recombines amino acids to create the new proteins that it needs. Plant sources of protein, such as grains, dried beans and peas, nuts, seeds, and vegetables, are considered lower quality because they contain low levels of one or more essential amino acids. Soybeans are the exception. They contain certain key amino acids in higher amounts than found in other beans. Ounce for ounce, soybean protein is equivalent in quality to animal protein.

In the old days, vegetarians were advised to combine specific plant foods, such as rice and beans, within a meal. Eaten together, these foods would complement each other by providing all the essential amino acids needed for building new complete proteins. Today we know that combining plant foods at the same meal isn't necessary. The body can assemble its own complete proteins from a small pool of free amino acids that it maintains for this purpose. If you are a vegetarian, however, this system is effective only if you eat a variety of plant foods, as well as enough calories, every day. Of course, bean burritos, lentil soup with corn bread, and peanut butter sandwiches made with whole wheat bread taste good, so you still have a valid reason for eating these combination foods.

To boost your protein intake and avoid the carbohydrate-overload trap, consciously include a protein-rich food at all your meals and snacks (see table 7.1). Lacto-ovo vegetarians, for example, can add milk products (regular or soy) or eggs to any meal or snack. Eat hot or cold cereal with milk, dunk a bran muffin into yogurt, snack on a slice of cheese pizza, or prepare French toast for breakfast. Another good strategy is to make sure that you don't eat your grains plain. Smear nut butters, low-fat cottage cheese, or hummus on a bagel. Vary your pasta toppings by using canned spicy beans one night and a vegetable and tofu stir-fry another. Keep in mind that anything made for pasta can just as easily be spooned over brown rice or instant couscous or rolled in a tortilla.

Vegetarians who eliminate animal foods without substituting traditional vegetarian staples have the most trouble meeting their protein needs. A good rule to follow is to eat dried beans and peas (and lentils) and soy foods daily. Quick-fix beans (precooked canned varieties) and meat substitutes made from soybeans provide easy and simple ways to get the protein that you need. Choose hearty soups and stews made with lentils, split peas, and beans. Try baked beans on your next baked potato or serve a quick meal in a can such as vegetarian chili. When it comes to soy foods, experiment with

TABLE 7.1 Protein Content of Commonly Eaten Foods

Food	Typical serving	Protein (grams)
Meat (red meat, poultry, fish)	3 oz (85 g) cooked	21–25 g
Cottage cheese	1/2 cup (115 g)	13 g
Milk or yogurt	1 cup (250 ml)	8 g
Cheese	1 oz (~28 g)	7 g
Egg	1 medium	6 g
Lentils	1 cup, cooked	18 g
Beans (black, kidney, and so on)	1 cup, cooked	12 g
Edamame (boiled soybeans)	1 cup, cooked	22 g
Soy nuts	1 oz (28 g)	11 g
Soy milk	1 cup (250 ml)	10 g
Tofu	3 oz (85 g) (1/5 block)	10 g
Peanut butter	2 tbsp	8 g
Nuts or seeds	1 oz (28 g)	5 g
Bread	1 slice	3 g
Pasta or grain	1 cup, cooked	6 g
Potato	1 small	2 g
Starchy vegetables (peas, corn, winter squash)	1/2 cup, cooked	2 g

different forms. Serve meat substitutes (check the freezer section in natural food stores and the health food section of grocery stores) and use textured vegetable protein in dishes that traditionally call for ground meat, such as chili and tacos.

Keep in mind that animal foods provide a more concentrated dose of protein than plant foods do. A typical small hamburger or chicken breast (3 ounces, or the size of a card deck) supplies 25 grams of protein. You'll have to eat a generous cup of cooked beans plus a cup of a cooked whole grain or 2 cups of pasta topped with 3 ounces (85 g) of tofu to match that. You can determine the amount of protein in frequently eaten foods by checking the Nutrition Facts label on food packages. Be certain to compare the serving size against the portion that you actually consume.

In terms of soy and the risk of breast cancer, animal studies have shown mixed effects on breast cancer with soy supplements. In humans, however, studies have not shown harm from eating soy foods. Consuming a moderate amount of soy foods (tofu, tempeh, edamame, and veggie burgers), in other words, appears safe for the general public. The 2012 American Cancer Society Guidelines on Nutrition and Physical Activity for Cancer Survivors, written by a panel of experts and based on research to date, also found no harmful effects to breast cancer survivors from eating soy. Both the guidelines for prevention and the guidelines for survivors, however, recommend against taking soy supplements until more research is done. Soy supplements contain much higher levels of isoflavones, which are chemically similar to estrogens, than what you would normally find in the foods you eat. Plus, they haven't been rigorously tested.

Eating More Whole Soy Foods

You've seen plenty of soy foods in the grocery store, but how do you eat the stuff? Or at least sneak some into your (and your family's) diet? The following list offers simple suggestions to get you started.

1. Drink soy milk (fortified with calcium and vitamin D), pour it over cereal, and use it in place of low-fat milk in recipes for soups, muffins, pancakes, waffles, and pudding.

2. Create smoothies by blending fresh fruit (bananas and strawberries work well) with vanilla-flavored soy milk.

3. Add diced firm tofu or chunks of tempeh to your favorite spaghetti sauce, chili, vegetable soup, stew, stir-fried dish, and casserole.

4. Combine soft tofu with cottage cheese or ricotta cheese in lasagna and stuffed shells or use it as a cheese substitute in pasta dishes.

> continued

< continued

5. Blend soft tofu into low-fat sour cream for a baked-potato topping or use it instead of sour cream or yogurt.

6. Crumble tofu into scrambled eggs during the last minute of cooking.

7. Snack on roasted soy nuts (found in most supermarkets).

8. Prepare tempeh on the grill. Steam it first, marinate in barbecue sauce, and then grill until brown. Add cubes of firm or extra-firm tofu to shish kebab.

9. Snack on steamed, lightly salted edamame (eat the soybeans right from the pod); stock up on frozen shelled edamame and add to soups, salads, and side dishes.

10. Try tofu dogs (soy hot dogs), soy burgers, and other meat alternatives; replace ground meat with textured vegetable protein in tacos, spaghetti sauce, chili, meatballs, and meat loaf.

To estimate your daily protein requirement in grams, multiply your weight in pounds by .55 to .75 (in kilograms by 1.2 to 1.7). Athletes who primarily eat vegetarian foods should select the higher end of the range, especially those participating in ultraendurance events.

Refer back to table 7.1 for the protein content of commonly eaten foods. Use this list as a reference to keep track of your daily protein intake.

Iron and Zinc

Athletes who eat a meatless diet run a greater risk of getting too little iron and zinc. Even marginal deficiencies can hamper performance. With an iron-poor diet, you won't form enough hemoglobin and myoglobin, the oxygen-carrying molecules in the blood and muscles, which will leave you feeling weak and fatigued. Female athletes, in particular, are at greater risk for low iron levels because of smaller reserves and greater losses through menstruation. Athletes need adequate zinc to fight off infections and help wounds and injuries heal.

Absorbability is a key issue when it comes to getting enough iron and zinc. About 20 to 30 percent of the iron in meat (heme iron) is absorbable, compared with only 2 to 8 percent in plants (nonheme iron). The zinc from animal sources is also generally more absorbable because fiber and compounds called phytates found in whole-grain foods can interfere with zinc absorption.

All types of meat, not just red meat (although it's the best source), contain the more easily absorbed heme iron. You'll benefit by including poultry (especially the dark meat), fish, and seafood in your diet. Don't rely on dairy foods or eggs to come through in this department because both are poor sources of iron. Some better plant sources of iron include fortified breakfast cereals; wheat germ; cooked beans, peas, and lentils; leafy dark green vegetables like spinach, kale, and collard greens; tofu and textured vegetable protein; nuts and seeds; dried fruit; and prune juice.

Vitamin C enhances iron absorption, so serve foods rich in vitamin C along with the iron-rich plant foods listed earlier. Foods high in vitamin C include strawberries, kiwi, cantaloupe (rock melon), citrus fruits, red and green peppers, broccoli, and tomatoes, to name a few. Drink a glass of orange juice along with a bowl of iron-fortified cereal, for example, or cook beans in a tomato sauce. Cooking in a cast-iron pot or skillet will also raise the iron content substantially because the mineral leaches into the food. Meat contains MFP factor, a compound that also promotes the absorption of nonheme iron, so if you do eat meat, have iron-rich vegetables and meat together.

Animal foods (especially oysters) contain abundant amounts of zinc, whereas plant foods provide only moderate amounts. You need to make an effort to include several servings of zinc-rich foods in your diet every day. If you consume enough protein, you're most likely getting enough zinc. Significant plant sources of zinc include lentils, beans, whole grains, whole wheat bread, wheat germ, nuts, soy and dairy foods, and some fortified breakfast cereals.

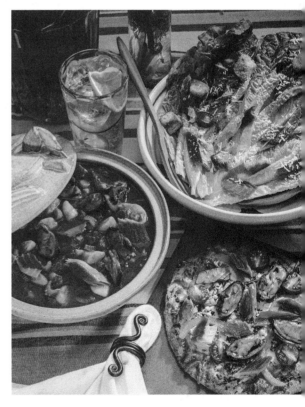

Don't be too quick to reach for supplements that provide beyond 100 percent of the reference daily intake (RDI) for iron and zinc. Clearly, if iron-deficiency anemia is a problem, additional iron will help. You should start, though, by monitoring your iron levels through routine blood tests that look at your hemoglobin, hematocrit, and serum ferritin (storage iron) levels. Too much supplemental iron can interfere with the absorption of zinc and copper, and cause constipation. Oversupplementing with zinc may cause a relative deficiency in other minerals, such as copper, because they all compete for absorption. Eating plant foods rich in iron and zinc, however, won't cause any problems. Play it safe—make the effort daily to include good meatless sources of iron and zinc.

Enjoy a wide variety of vegetarian meals, featuring soy foods and dried beans and peas (legumes) to meet your iron, zinc, and calcium needs.

© PhotoDisc

Calcium and Vitamin D

Besides building strong bones and teeth, calcium helps muscles to contract and relax, nerves to send messages, and blood to clot properly. Vitamin D aids in the absorption of calcium and phosphorus, nutrients essential for healthy bone tissue. Daily calcium needs vary depending on gender, age, and, for women, menstrual status. Shoot for at least 1,000 milligrams a day. If you eat dairy foods, you can get plenty of calcium from fat-free and low-fat milk, yogurt, and cheese. Plant foods that contain calcium include dark leafy greens (such as kale, mustard, collard, and turnip greens), bok choy, broccoli, beans, dried figs, soy nuts, sunflower seeds, and other calcium-fortified foods, such as orange juice, cereal, breakfast bars, tofu (processed with calcium

Vegetarian Calcium Sources*
1 cup (250 ml) of milk
1 cup of fortified soy milk or rice milk
1 cup of yogurt
1.5 oz (45 g) cheese
1 cup of tofu (made with calcium sulfate)
1 1/2 cups of cooked dark leafy greens—kale, collard, turnip greens
2 cups of cooked bok choy
3 cups of cooked broccoli
1 1/2 cups of canned baked beans
1/2 cup of soy nuts
11 dried figs
3 tbsp of sesame seeds
4 oz (115 g) of canned salmon or sardines (with bones)
1 cup of fortified orange juice
Fortified breakfast cereals (varies)
*at least 300 milligrams of calcium per serving.

sulfate), and fortified soy or rice beverages. If you occasionally eat animal foods, canned sardines and salmon (be sure to eat the bones) are also good calcium sources.

Check the Nutrition Facts label on your orange juice, soy and rice beverages, and tofu. If you're relying on these foods for calcium, be sure to select calcium-fortified varieties and tofu prepared with calcium sulfate. Green leafy vegetables can provide adequate calcium, but only if you eat enough of them to make it count. You need to eat 3 cups of broccoli or 1.5 cups of kale, for example, to equal the calcium in one glass of milk or a cup of yogurt. (Don't forget, at 300 milligrams a cup, you need the equivalent of at least three glasses of milk a day to reach the daily goal of 1,000 milligrams of calcium.) If you think that calcium supplements are the answer, be aware that a diet low in calcium is also likely low in protein and vitamin D. Calcium supplements won't help with that. To increase absorption, take calcium supplements with meals, in doses of 500 milligrams or less at one time, and not along with an iron supplement.

Few foods are naturally high in vitamin D. Our bodies usually make enough when our skin is exposed to sunlight (at least 15 minutes several times a week). Fortunately, athletes routinely spend a great deal of time outdoors wearing little clothing! Keep in mind that our skin becomes much less efficient at making vitamin D as we age, however, and sun exposure is inadequate in northern climates during much of the year. Good food sources of vitamin D include fattier fish (like salmon), egg yolks, and fortified foods such as milk, butter, margarine, breakfast cereals, and soy beverages. Vegans, especially, should consider taking a daily vitamin D supplement (teens and adults up to age 70, 600 IU; over age 70, 800 IU per day.) For more information on vitamin D, see chapter 5.

B Vitamins

If you eat a well-balanced vegetarian diet, full of whole grains, enriched grains, legumes, nuts, seeds, fruits and vegetables, and enough calories, you should have little trouble meeting your need for thiamin, riboflavin, niacin, vitamin B_6, and folic acid. Vitamin B_{12} is needed for maintaining healthy red blood cells and nerve fibers. Vitamin B_{12} is a unique vitamin, produced by bacteria in the soil and in animals. Unless they are in the habit of ingesting soil along with their greens (as animals do), most people meet their needs by eating animal foods, so you're covered if you consume eggs, dairy products, fish, or poultry. Deficiencies are rare, even in vegetarians, because the daily requirement is small (2 micrograms a day), and the human body carefully hoards and guards its supply.

The only plant foods that are reliable B_{12} sources are fortified foods such as soy milk, soy burgers, and certain breakfast cereals (such as Total or Product 19). Nutritional yeast (e.g., Red Star brand T-6635), not regular baking yeast, is also a reliable source. Don't count on tempeh, spirulina, sprouted legumes, miso, sea vegetables, or umeboshi plums; these foods don't contain the active form of vitamin B_{12}. Vegans who don't routinely eat fortified products should take a supplement because subtle neurological damage can occur before you know that you have a deficiency.

A Day in the Vegetarian Life

Here is a nutrition-packed, one-day vegetarian menu. Preparation time for each meal is under 10 minutes.

BREAKFAST

1 cup of quick oatmeal, topped with 1 cup of fat-free vanilla yogurt and 2 tbsp of raisins

2 slices of hearty grain bread with 1 tbsp of peanut butter

8 oz (250 ml) of orange juice

LUNCH

1 soy burger on a whole-grain bun, with sliced tomato and onion

1/2 cup of pasta and bean salad

Handful of baby carrots dipped in yogurt salad dressing

> continued

< continued

SNACK

1 cup (250 ml) of calcium-fortified soy milk

1 soft pretzel

DINNER

1 cup of black bean chili, over top of 1 cup of cooked Mexican-style rice and corn mix

Dark green salad with 1 tbsp (15 ml) of low-fat dressing

1 cup of frozen yogurt with 1/2 cup of fresh or frozen strawberries

TOTAL: 2,660 calories

60% carbohydrate, 15% protein, 25% fat

400 g carbohydrate, 100 g protein, 74 g fat

Special Health Concerns for Vegetarians

A meatless diet does not guarantee good health and better performances. Unless you stick to some basic guidelines and stay up with your daily calorie and nutrient needs, you're likely to encounter some difficulties. Two particular problems that have been shown to slow vegetarian athletes are amenorrhea in females or a too-low testosterone level in males, as well as disordered eating habits.

Amenorrhea, Suppressed Testosterone, and Vegetarianism

Female athletes who adopt vegetarian diets may be at higher risk for amenorrhea, a serious medical condition characterized by low estrogen levels and the loss of menstrual periods. Male vegetarian athletes may be at risk for an abnormally low testosterone level. Women who follow a plant-based eating style typically have lower levels of hormones that affect menstruation, such as estrogen and prolactin, than do nonvegetarian women. Male athletes with diminished hormonal function are subject to the same fatigue, weight loss, frequent infections, increase in injuries, and diminished performances as their female counterparts. Early research on altered sex-hormone levels appeared to point to some component characteristic of a vegetarian diet as the cause; possibilities include high fiber intake, low fat or protein content, or the presence of weak plant hormones. More recently, however, studies point to an energy deficit or failure to consume enough total calories as the likely culprit.

Because amenorrhea, as well as suppressed testosterone levels in males, also are linked with extreme or extensive exercise, an altered hormonal status may be especially prevalent among vegetarian athletes. High rates of

Quick and Healthy Vegetarian Snacks and Meals

Items to prepare

Whole-grain pancakes

Whole-grain muffins or cookies

Graham crackers, rice cakes, whole-grain crackers, tortillas

Instant macaroni and cheese, couscous with lentils, polenta, or mashed potatoes

Instant brown rice or other whole grains

Bagels or whole-grain bread with nut butter

Oatmeal or cold cereal with milk

Dried fruit—raisins, apricots, dates, figs, papayas, apples

Frozen juice bar

Bean taco, burrito, or enchilada

Lentil or split-pea soup

Fruit shakes or smoothies

Low-fat cottage cheese, low-fat cheese (dairy or soy)

Yogurt (dairy or soy)

Canned beans, vegetarian chili

Ethnic frozen meals—Mexican, Chinese, Thai, or others

Tofu hot dogs

Soy burgers

Quick mixes of tabbouleh, hummus, refried beans, or black beans

Roasted soy nuts or other nuts

Vegetable pizza

Items to take when traveling

(Request hot water at mealtimes or prepare dehydrated items in room by adding hot water.)

Hemp or brown rice protein powder

Protein-rich energy bars

Freeze-dried or dehydrated tofu, dehydrated hummus, and instant lentil, split-pea, or other dried-bean soup mixes

Concentrated liquid calories in the form of protein-based beverages

(e.g., Power Dream soy energy drink, Boost, Ensure, Carnation Instant Breakfast drink/mix)

amenorrhea have been reported in vegetarian female athletes, particularly in runners. In one study, vegetarians made up 25 percent of the female runners with amenorrhea, but only 11 percent of the runners who had regular menstrual periods. In a study of eight male endurance athletes, following a lacto-ovo-vegetarian diet for 6 weeks led to a slight decrease in total testosterone levels.

If you develop amenorrhea (or fail to start your menstrual cycle by age 15) or your testosterone level is suppressed, don't ignore it. You're three times more likely to develop a stress fracture, and low levels of estrogen in females and testosterone in males at any age lead to premature bone loss. Examine your current eating habits. Often, gaining (you're actually restoring if you've lost weight) as little as 2 percent of body weight (2 pounds for a 120-pound woman and 3 pounds for a 160-pound man, or 1 kilogram for a 54.5-kilogram woman and 1.4 kilograms for a 73-kilogram man) and maintaining this healthier weight as you train is all that is needed for restarting menstrual periods or boosting a low testosterone level.

As an endurance athlete, you can easily burn off large amounts of calories exercising, so as indicated earlier, amenorrhea or a too-low testosterone level most likely results because of an energy imbalance. You simply aren't consuming enough calories daily to sustain your high energy expenditures. If your current vegetarian eating style doesn't keep up with your calorie needs, you'll need to eat more energy-dense foods and adequate fat (at least 20 percent or one-fifth of total calories) and protein, as well as cut back on fiber-rich foods that fill you up too quickly. Be prepared to initially cut back on how intensely you exercise, too, and to reduce your weekly training volume by 10 to 20 percent (possibly even more if you're a woman trying to conceive).

Along with eating a wide variety of plant proteins daily, be certain that you consume adequate high-quality protein, such as that provided by soybeans, milk, and egg whites. Other vegetarian foods lack one or more of the essential amino acids the body needs for efficient tissue growth and repair. The research suggests that athletes with amenorrhea, for example, tend to have diets low in protein compared with athletes who menstruate regularly. Some studies show that adding meat (red meat in particular) has a protective effect on menstrual periods, although it's unclear why. A similar scenario appears true for male athletes. A study that compared strength and muscle gains in men doing resistance training who were eating either a vegetarian diet or an omnivore diet, for example, found that meat eaters lost 6 percent fat mass and gained 4 percent muscle mass compared to the vegetarians.

Obviously, whether you include or exclude meat in your daily diet is a matter of personal choice. Depending on your individual needs and your long-term goals, however, you may want to reevaluate the effect that including small portions of meat several times a week could have on your health and performance.

Disordered Eating and Vegetarianism

Some vegetarian athletes, male and female, inadvertently consume too few calories to sustain their high energy output. Others, however, consciously restrict the foods that they eat under the guise of vegetarianism. In other words, they choose (or choose to continue) a vegetarian eating style as a way to control their weight and cope with pressure to be thin. These athletes may feel better about themselves or superior to others when they eat differently, or they may feel more perfect if they don't eat certain foods.

Some hallmark behaviors to look for are vegetarians who narrow their protein choices to a few items they feel are acceptable; avoid fat by shunning nuts and seeds, nut butters, dairy products, and other higher-fat items; and skip meals or elect not to eat in social settings rather than prepare or search out vegetarian fare. If you, or someone you train with or coach, pursue vegetarianism primarily as a politically correct means to lose weight or to achieve a lean appearance, heed the warning signs. Such harmful and ineffective eating behaviors set you up for anemia, stress fractures, and possibly a full-blown eating disorder.

Parents and coaches of teenage athletes need to be especially vigilant when it comes to young people and vegetarianism. Evaluate the reasons that teens give for renouncing foods and the effectiveness with which they replace those foods with healthy substitutes. Girls, in particular, may adopt vegetarianism as a socially acceptable way to mask their disordered eating habits.

Researchers at the University of Minnesota surveyed high school students across Minnesota and found that teenage vegetarian girls are twice as likely to diet, four times as likely to induce vomiting, and eight times as likely to use laxatives as are their meat-eating peers. These findings support a reverse study of 116 patients who suffered with anorexia nervosa (self-induced starvation): 54 percent avoided red meat, although only 4 percent had done so before the onset of their eating disorder.

One of my clients, a 13-year-old who adopted a vegetarian diet at age 5, played soccer, swam, ran, and participated in gymnastics during a typical week. When a swim coach at a summer camp delivered the erroneous message that athletes should avoid eating fat, my client began to count calories and fat grams, skip meals (saying that she was not hungry or that the vegetables tasted terrible), and exercise twice a day. After she lost 10 pounds (4.5 kg) and her menstrual periods stopped, her parents took action.

When I met her, I found that besides not eating meat, she didn't like fish, rarely drank milk, ate eggs only if they were prepared for her, and wrinkled her nose at the mention of beans or tofu. Obviously, with this approach, she wasn't meeting her everyday protein, iron, and calcium needs. She also wasn't consuming enough food (calories) to match the calories that she expended daily through exercise. Fortunately, a strong desire to continue her sports activities motivated this teen to restore the lost weight. She ate more of the foods that she liked, and after a few months, she began to eat some foods that she had previously considered forbidden.

A vegetarian diet can be either a healthy way to eat or a haphazard eating style that comes up short in many key nutrients. To reap the benefits of vegetarianism, you must be willing to do two things: stock your kitchen with some vegetarian staples (and know how to prepare them!) and invest some time and energy exploring new foods that will help you meet your nutrition needs.

LEARNING FROM THE BEST:
VEGETARIAN OR VEGAN EATING FOR ENDURANCE EATING

Scott Jurek, a vegan, a three-time Ultrarunner of the Year, and the author of *Eat and Run: My Unlikely Journey to Ultramarathon Greatness,* contends that following a vegetarian, even vegan, eating style doesn't have to be complex or life consuming. What it takes is planning and willingness to solve problems—to figure out what you need to do and to be creative about doing it.

Jurek won the Western States 100-Mile Endurance Run seven straight times and the Badwater Ultramarathon twice. He currently holds the U.S. all-surface record in the 24-hour run with 165.7 miles (267 km)—6.5 marathons in a day. Read on for his tips on how to excel at meeting your nutrition needs as a vegetarian or vegan endurance athlete.

1. Think about quantity as well as quality. The biggest downfall of vegetarian and vegan endurance athletes, especially ultra athletes, is often just not getting in enough calories. If you're a vegetarian who eliminates and doesn't replace, that is, you don't look for alternative sources, you will suffer the consequences of consuming too few calories. Although eating as clean as possible is important, this does not mean starving yourself.

2. Plan your protein. As recommended, Jurek relies on heavy hitters—tofu, tempeh, and legumes, eating a serving of each at least once a day. Smoothies also contribute valuable protein in the form of soy yogurt and added hemp or brown rice protein powder. He cautions athletes not to rely on heavily processed soy protein powders.

3. Don't fear fat. Endurance athletes don't need to shy away from fat. Jurek meets his high energy needs by getting 20 to 25 percent of his daily calories from healthy fats—avocados, olive oil, almond butter, and almonds are his favorites.

4. Don't make excuses, even on the road. At home, keep quick-fix staples on hand. When feasible, take a small cooler with you when traveling (as Jurek routinely does). Be creative when dining in restaurants, such as asking for a commonly stocked alternative protein source such as extra nuts and seeds on the side or canned garbanzo or kidney beans. Look for these items on salad bars too. Asian restaurants are the best bet for dense-protein foods such as tofu. Jurek also travels with protein-rich energy bars, such as Nectar bars and Lärabars, as well as freeze-dried or dehydrated tofu, dehydrated hummus, and instant lentil, split-pea, or other dried legume soups. These items travel well, and you can eat them after your restaurant meal or easily prepare them at the table by requesting hot water.

5. Embrace food. Jurek loves to eat and prepare food. He relishes the psychological boost that comes from knowing that he has taken the time and energy to fuel his body adequately. He challenges endurance athletes to think of food as a life source, allowing them to do what they love to do.

6. Fuel up during supported races. Vegetarians and vegans will find plenty of options for race foods among what is typically offered at aid stations. Almost all drinks and foods are vegan, and therefore provide exactly what an endurance athlete needs—a steady supply of carbohydrate. For concentrated liquid calories, Jurek drinks rice milk and soy protein drinks (e.g., Power Dream soy energy drink). During ultraendurance races, calorie-rich energy bars help too.

8

Meal Planning for Endurance Athletes

In 2011, 1.3 million pounds of pasta were sold in American grocery stores. If lined up, 1.3 million pounds of 16-ounce spaghetti packages would circle the Earth's equator almost nine times.

Source: Agricultural Council of America, www.agday.org/education/fun_facts.php [April 24, 2013].

Unless you've been completely technology-free and training in isolation, you most likely have plenty of nutrition knowledge. Most of the sports-minded people I meet, in fact, have more than enough information. Many still lament, however, that they don't know what to eat. Making smart everyday food choices requires that you translate the science (what we know to be true) into eating habits that you practice, and ultimately master. Whether you need to reduce or expand your food selections to better meet daily nutrient and energy needs, learning (or relearning) to eat regular meals and snacks is the most effective first step. A steady, consistent influx of calories boosts the body's metabolism and immune system and gives you more energy during the day when you need it most. Besides, ignoring hunger signs and skipping meals makes eating well more difficult because it leads you to make poor choices and overeat at the next meal.

If you eat at least three times a day, you'll need to make a decision about what to eat more than a thousand times a year. I find that active people, even elite athletes, are too caught up in *what* to eat, and would benefit tremendously from putting more of their energy into *how* to eat. What you choose to eat will vary from day to day and situation to situation. You may plan to eat chicken at dinner only to arrive at your friend's home to find sirloin steak being served. A slice of pizza may be the best choice at two o'clock, well before an after-work run, but not at four o'clock. Eating a bagel some mornings might be enough; other mornings, it won't be. And while downing a few energy gels and an energy bar or two may be the most supportive thing you can do on a Saturday ride, it might not be a wise choice to sit at your desk on a weekday afternoon.

In other words, eating a smart sports diet is both a science and an art. Although recommendations about what to eat do exist, they are situational. Just as you decide what shoes and clothing to wear on a long bike ride or what pace to maintain in the first half of a race, you must choose foods based not only on your current needs, but also on long-term goals. No one else, including the latest diet guru, can tell you what to eat, nor can you determine beforehand exactly what and how much you will need to eat on any given day. For people used to tracking the seconds with stopwatches, measuring distances to the 10th of a mile, and following workout plans determined by others, eating smart may be challenging, confusing, and even anxiety provoking. It doesn't have to be.

Five Guidelines on Eating for High Performance

To provide some structure (and much needed calmness regarding food), I've developed some guidelines for athletes on how to eat. These guidelines work whether you are eating in (at home) or out, at work, at school, or while on the road. They are designed to help you consistently eat in a way that leaves you physically ready and mentally prepared to embrace and enjoy your workouts, your relationship with food, and life in general.

1: Plan to Eat Every Three to Four Hours While Awake

In other words, don't let yourself get too hungry. Eat every 3 to 4 hours (while awake) to maintain a steady blood sugar level. This keeps the brain well fueled. You won't perform to your full potential, otherwise, physically or mentally. Allowing yourself to get too hungry means that when you do eat, you're apt to toss good intentions out the window and simply eat whatever food is in sight, which may not be the healthiest fare.

Eating regularly scheduled meals and snacks is an essential habit of people who are able to maintain their weight in a healthy manner. Eating enough during the day helps you to avoid back-loading calories at night. You eat, that is, during the day when you need the energy the most (and are most likely to burn off the calories) instead of running on fumes during the day and then shoveling in the majority of your calories between dinner and bedtime. Besides, if you don't start eating early in the day, it's nearly impossible to get in all the nutrients that you need. Are you realistically going to have, for example, 3 cups of vegetables, 2 cups of fruit, and 3 cups (750 ml) of milk (or the equivalent) at dinner alone?

2: Eat Well at Mealtimes

The timing of meals is up to you since it depends on when you work out, your work or school schedule, and any other commitments you may have. Eating three well-balanced meals, however, is a given. When thinking about or planning a meal, including as you wait in line at your favorite eatery, apply this guideline: Eat a minimum of three food groups at mealtime. At lunch and dinner, make it three food groups plus a protein food. (Incidentally, you don't have to stop at three food groups—challenge yourself to include appropriate-sized servings from four or even all five food groups.)

And be honest with yourself about amounts—it needs to equate to at least a serving as defined by Choose My Plate. (For a review of what counts as a serving, see chapter 1.) In other words, 2 tablespoons of milk in coffee doesn't count, nor does the lettuce leaf or two that's found on the typical sandwich. Some athletes take this concept a step further and create their own daily meal plan. To do this, take your recommended My Plate servings (as estimated in chapter 1) and divide them up among meals (three) and snacks (at least two). Use

> ### Breakfast on the Run
>
> **10 quick no-cook healthy breakfast ideas for when life wants to get in the way**
>
> Breakfast parfait: low-fat dairy/soy milk + fruit + high-fiber cereal
>
> Breakfast trail mix (nuts, dried fruit and high-fiber cereal) + string cheese
>
> Peanut butter on brown rice cakes/whole-grain toaster waffles + apple (whole/slices) + 1 cup milk
>
> Breakfast smoothie (fresh/frozen berries, yogurt/silken tofu, 100% juice) + whole-grain mini bagel
>
> Breakfast fruit wrap: whole wheat tortilla + low-fat ricotta cheese + little fruit spread and sliced fruit + chopped nuts
>
> Breakfast roll-up: whole wheat tortilla (warmed up) + peanut butter + sliced banana + drizzle of honey
>
> Whole wheat pita bread + hummus + fresh fruit/small box of raisins
>
> Whole wheat pita + chopped hard-boiled egg + grated cheese + sliced ham
>
> Cottage cheese + fruit + chopped nuts
>
> Muesli: overnight soaked grains + nuts + dried fruit + yogurt

this written plan to guide your everyday food selections. It also can help you stay focused on the big picture or long-term goal (e.g., mastering high-performance eating habits) versus getting bogged down in day-to-day details.

When it comes to eating breakfast, it's a habit—either you learned to do it, or you didn't. If it isn't a well-established habit for you, invest in making it one. Breakfast eaters routinely report being able to perform better at school or work, and it's an essential habit of people who lose weight and keep it off at least a year. Making time to eat lunch can reduce stress, enhance productivity, and recharge you for the afternoon, especially if you train at the end of the day. And finally, it isn't necessary that you prepare a gourmet meal for dinner; however, sitting down to eat it is. You deserve a break at the end of a long day, and sitting down for dinner can be an enjoyable way to reconnect with family and friends. Besides, you also want to adequately refuel for tomorrow. Remember, many poor training days are the result of poor eating days.

Here are some simple action steps to take to establish the habit of eating regular meals:

- **Choose to eat breakfast.** If you've gotten out of the habit or conditioned your body not to be hungry, rethink the importance of this meal. If you're not hungry in the morning, examine your current eating habits. You're most likely eating too much or too late at night. Stop eating an hour earlier at night. Keep cutting down the time until you wake up hungry enough to eat breakfast. Anything goes for this meal, from traditional breakfast fare to leftovers from last night's dinner. The ultimate quick on-the-go breakfast is a cup of 100 percent fruit juice, a carton of low-fat milk, and a baggie of fiber-rich dried cereal.

- **Make lunch a priority.** Again, anything goes. Brown bagging has the advantage of availability, especially if you can't get away from your desk or have other commitments. Pack your lunch the night before and keep stashes of nonperishable items (instant oatmeal, peanut butter, crackers, dried soup mixes, dried fruit, energy bars, and so forth) in your briefcase, locker, or desk drawer for the days that you forget to bring a lunch. Drink liquid lunches, such as meal-replacement supplements or instant breakfast drinks, when you're really pressed for time or need more calories. If you eat out or at a cafeteria, do your best to make wise choices. Concentrate on eating fiber-rich complex carbohydrate and lean protein foods, not fat-laden lunches. Compensate at other meals or snacks for what you don't eat or can't get at lunch.

- **Sit down for dinner.** Eating out is no longer a special occasion (i.e., once or twice a month) for most people, especially time-crunched athletes. But the guidelines still apply. Keep My Plate in mind and aim to fill out the food groups as you would at home. Be smart about choosing the restaurant or eatery, and you'll have plenty of options. If you use some creativity, even convenience-store cuisine can offer acceptable fare. Although some endurance athletes can afford (or actually require) higher-fat items, the list in appendix C (Eating on the Run: Dining Out) emphasizes higher-carbohydrate, lower-fat selections for those who eat out regularly.

To help meet the challenge of what to eat for dinner when eating in, save time and mental energy by planning ahead. This approach will help you be more creative when it comes to deciding what to eat. Eating the same few foods or too much of any single food can be boring and can lead to trouble. Furthermore, if you get too hungry or don't have the right ingredients on hand, you'll end up doing what we all do—grabbing whatever is the easiest.

Quick Meal Planning When Eating at Home

1. Work out a system beforehand, especially if you're feeding a family. Plan five simple meals for the upcoming week, for example, concentrating on what the main entree will be. (Between leftovers and eating out, you should be covered for the week.) As dinnertime approaches, simply select one. Other athletes do well with a set routine, for instance, chicken every Monday, pasta on Tuesday, fish or seafood on Wednesday, and so on. To add variety, prepare the entree a different way or vary the side dishes that you serve it with (for example, couscous or instant stuffing instead of rice).

2. Keep staples on hand to throw together quick, nutritious meals: milk and whole-grain cereal, scrambled eggs and toast or toaster waffles, baked potato (use the microwave) topped with baked beans or cottage cheese, pasta and meat sauce, bean-based soup and sandwich, canned chili and crackers, and so on. Round out the meal with some fresh, frozen, or canned fruit or juice, or fill half your plate with vegetables (raw or cooked).

3. Keep a running list of kitchen staples that need to be restocked. Add to it any ingredients or foods that are needed that week for preparing special meals. Take the list with you when you shop. (Try out a cell phone app so you don't have to worry about misplacing the list.) A well-stocked kitchen is the key to assembling healthy, good tasting, time-saving meals. Shop at a familiar store so that you can locate items quickly. (For staples to keep on hand, see Eating on the Run: Stock Your Kitchen in appendix C.)

4. Buy part of dinner and prepare the rest. Buy a rotisserie chicken or meat loaf, for example, and add your own healthy sides, such as instant mashed potatoes and microwaved or steamed vegetables. Alternatively, take advantage of prepared foods, such as boneless, skinless chicken breasts, cubed or sliced cooked turkey, skinned fish filets, peeled shrimp, canned beans, instant-cooking grains, salad-bar produce or salad from a bag, and grated cheese.

5. Have fun at mealtimes. Experiment by buying one new food from the grocery store each week or try a new recipe once a month. Don't get bogged down by thinking that you have to create an entire new meal; just make or purchase one new item and serve it with some familiar standbys. Be willing to experiment. Keep the winners and toss the rest.

6. Cook for more than one meal. Cook meals in bulk on the weekends and then date and freeze them in family-size or individual-size

> continued

< continued

containers. Alternatively, prepare at least enough extra at dinnertime so that you have leftovers to eat at another meal the following day.

7. Stock your kitchen with all or some of these time-saving devices: a sharp knife, cookware that can go from freezer to microwave, small electric or hand-operated food chopper, blender, vegetable steamer (no pots to watch), rice cooker, toaster oven (toasts, bakes, or broils small amounts of food), microwave, and a Crock-Pot or slow cooker (requires more preparation time in the morning, but dinner is ready when you arrive at home).

3: Eat a Protein-Rich Food and Some Healthy Fat at Every Meal

Carbohydrate supplied by our daily food choices provides energy; however, not even endurance athletes can live on carbohydrate alone. Including protein at mealtime (at least 20 grams at both lunch and dinner, which you can obtain from 3 ounces of lean meat, poultry, or fish, or the equivalent in soy foods, eggs, or cooked beans) sustains us, but it's fat that really satisfies. Fill up on carbohydrate, and you can easily find yourself either eating too much or getting hungry again in just an hour or two. For most busy and active people, this approach isn't desired or practical.

To meet daily nutrient needs and keep your blood sugar level steady for a longer, more reasonable period of time, include a protein-rich food at mealtime. This is especially vital at lunch and dinner. (See the Go Lean With Protein section in chapter 1 for a review of protein-rich foods.) One way to remember to include protein at mealtimes is this mantra: Don't eat your grains plain. Smear a bagel with peanut butter, toss baked beans over noodles, or throw seafood or chicken into your favorite sauce and pour it over pasta, rice, or couscous.

Fat, however, is what really satisfies us—both physically and mentally. Judicious use of healthy fats (see the Choose Healthy Fats (Oils) Over Unhealthy Fats section in chapter 1 for a review)

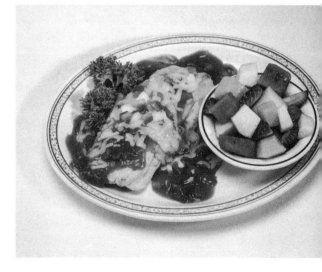

Meals that provide lean protein, complex carbohydrate, and fat are the cornerstone of high-performance eating.
© PhotoDisc

is much more productive in the long run than trying to avoid all fat or not paying any attention at all to the type or quantity of fat you eat. Because it is digested much more slowly, meals (and snacks) that contain fat slow the rise and fall in blood sugar that occurs after we eat. This means that we feel full longer and can last 4 to 5 hours before needing (at least physiologically) to eat again. Fat also makes the foods that we eat taste good, satisfying our mind and our taste buds. Extras or fun foods like sweets, chips, and French fries also provide fat and play an important role in a smart sports diet. For more on that, keep reading.

4: Design Snacks That Feature Foods From Two Different Food Groups

Do your body a favor and think of snacks as mini meals or opportunities to get the nutrients and fuel that you need. (Selecting foods that are more nutritious is particularly important if you tend to graze throughout the day instead of eating defined meals.) For active people who juggle workouts around their other commitments, well-designed snacks or mini meals are often the only way to accomplish the job. As much as possible, snack on

---

Performance-Enhancing Snacks

Peanut butter and jelly or banana sandwich (half or whole)

Trail gorp (nuts, raisins, dried fruit, and so on)

Instant oatmeal with dried apricots

Cereal or low-fat granola with fruit and yogurt

Banana, pumpkin, or date bread and a carton of milk

Cookies (oatmeal raisin, fig bars, vanilla wafers, gingersnaps, animal crackers, or graham crackers) and milk

Low-fat cheese and crackers or rice cakes

Tuna fish and crackers

Pita bread with low-fat cheese

An English muffin or bagel topped with peanut or other nut butter

Low-fat muffin with milk, yogurt, or juice

Rice cakes or crackers and hummus

Slice of pizza (thick crust and vegetable toppings)

Baked potato topped with salsa, cottage cheese, or low-fat cheese

Cup or bowl of soup and crackers

Three-bean, pasta, or potato salad (with low-fat dressing) and a roll

Raw vegetables dipped in low-fat salad dressing or salsa

Nonfat refried beans or salsa and baked chips or crackers

Piece of fresh fruit and pretzels or low-fat popcorn

Fresh fruit dipped in yogurt or chocolate-flavored syrup

Frozen fruit juice bar or low-fat frozen yogurt

Angel food cake with fresh berries or dipped in yogurt

Half a papaya or cantaloupe filled with yogurt or cottage cheese

Breakfast drink or shake made with low-fat milk, ice cream, or yogurt

Fruit smoothie (fruit, yogurt, and milk or juice)

Meal-replacement drink

foods that come from the five food groups. Select at least one food from a food group, or even better, put together foods from two different food groups, such as whole wheat crackers and cheese or yogurt and fruit. See Performance-Enhancing Snacks for more ideas.

Save fun foods like cookies, cake, chips, and ice cream to have at meal-times. It's easy to overeat fun foods on an empty stomach (especially if you've gotten too hungry), and they can crowd out healthier fare. Physically active people often obsess about a fun food's fat or calorie count the entire time that they're eating it. Focusing more on the food than on how you feel, however, dilutes the pleasure of eating these foods. And it sets you up to miss the "I'm full" signal and eat too much. Build sweets and treats in at mealtimes (you know that you're going to eat them anyway). Slow down and allow yourself to savor and enjoy foods you simply want, rather than need. You'll be much more likely to consume an appropriate amount. Also, keep in mind the 80–20 rule. If you're making smart choices most of the time (8 times out of 10 or 80 percent of the time), then go easy on yourself the remainder of the time (20 percent).

Do Energy Bars Fit Into a Smart Sports Diet?

Run this by your taste buds: carrot cake for breakfast, an almond brownie as an afternoon snack, and a chocolate praline following your evening workout. This diet is possible—thanks to the seemingly endless supply of energy bars available. You may even have come to believe that energy bars (also called sports or endurance bars) are, well, real food.

Containing more than simple and complex carbohydrate, today's energy bars typically include varying amounts of protein, fat, vitamins, and minerals, as well as antioxidants, herbs, and other potentially performance-enhancing substances (although little evidence exists that these substances have any effect on athletic performance). You may also be consuming items that you don't want, such as caffeine, palm-kernel oil (a saturated fat common in coated bars), or high-fructose corn syrup (a refined sweetener).

My Plate was designed with real foods in mind. From that perspective, energy bars don't fit neatly into any food group. Despite being fortified with vitamins and minerals, carbohydrate-rich bars are often high in added sugar, and they contain little or no fiber. Balanced bars may provide protein, but without the accompanying iron and zinc found in protein-rich foods. Some bars, in reality, aren't much different from a candy bar or a bunch of fat-free cookies combined with a vitamin pill.

Having an occasional energy bar, even up to one a day, isn't likely to do you any harm in terms of nutrition (if you can afford the calories). Most will count as at least two servings from the grain group; if they contain protein, 7 grams is the equivalent of 1 ounce of meat. Beyond that, however, think about energy bars as extras. They function best as a sports food or a fuel supplement to an otherwise balanced diet based on real foods.

Bear in mind that a food is more than just the sum of its parts. The nutrients in a food work together and produce an effect greater than that which a single nutrient could produce. It's still not clear exactly which quantity or combination of nutrients our body requires. Some potential health boosters, like the phytochemicals (plant chemicals that appear to help the body ward off aging and disease) found in fruits and vegetables, haven't yet been fully identified, so they can't possibly be in your favorite bar. For these reasons, routinely replacing meals or snacks with processed foods doesn't make sense from a health or performance perspective.

Fill in or round out your diet with energy bars, but don't make them the main part of it. At their best, energy bars supply a convenient dose of energy. They work well as an easily digestible preworkout or prerace meal, as fuel during exercise (as tolerated), and as a way to help replenish muscle glycogen stores following exercise. You might also rely on energy bars (meal-replacement products, too) as a backup, perhaps on busy days or while traveling when you would otherwise miss or skip a meal or snack. To be sure of what you're getting and what you're missing out on, check the nutrition label and ingredients list of whatever bar you choose. Many bars lack substantial amounts of some key nutrients that athletes are often low in, such as vitamins A and C, calcium, iron, and fiber.

5: Drink a Healthy Beverage With Every Meal or Snack

As an athlete, the time to think about being well hydrated is not right before you head out the door. Make life easy. Attend to your fluid needs throughout the day simply by drinking a healthy beverage with every meal or snack. You might drink water or, depending on the situation, you might choose 100 percent fruit or vegetable juice, low-fat milk, herbal tea, or a sports drink. (See chapter 1 for a review of healthy beverages.)

No Time to Cook? Seek Nutritious Fast Food

Smart eating is not about being a gourmet chef or about getting caught up in trying to eat perfectly. Smart eating is about balancing nutrition, convenience, and pleasure. Learn to assemble quick, healthy, good-tasting meals from foods you stock in your pantry, fridge, and freezer, as well as those purchased from a favorite deli or take-out eatery. Keep it simple: Eat a minimum of three food groups at mealtime. At lunch and dinner, make it three food groups plus a protein food.

> continued

< continued

Grains

Instant brown rice

Instant oatmeal

Whole-grain bread and crackers

Whole-grain cereal

Quick-cooking grains, salads made with whole grains (deli)

Whole-grain toaster waffles

Tortillas (corn and flour)

Lentils

Baking potatoes (microwave)

Pasta

Fruits and Vegetables

Prewashed greens from a bag

Precut veggies, stir-fry fixings (salad bar)

Frozen vegetables

Spaghetti sauce, salsa

Fruit salad (deli/salad bar)

100 percent fruit and vegetable juices

Dried fruit

Protein Foods

Eggs

Canned beans

5-bean salad (deli)

Canned chili

Canned tuna, chicken, fish

Rotisserie chicken or precooked chicken strips

Frozen entrees (e.g., Kashi)

Edamame (deli/salad bar)

Peanut butter

Cottage cheese

Dairy Foods

Low-fat milk

Low-fat shredded cheese

Greek-style yogurt

Fats and Oils

Low-fat salad dressing

Light mayonnaise

Avocado

Olives

Nuts, seeds

Sample Meal Plans for Endurance Athletes

Look at the following sample meal plans to view how endurance athletes can enjoy a variety of tasty foods and fulfill their nutrition requirements on a typical training day. When you exercise—first thing in the morning, at lunchtime, or after work—will determine exactly which foods are best to eat. Eating three well-balanced meals, supplemented by at least two healthy snacks, however, remains constant. What varies is the amount of food that you eat at a sitting and the actual time that you choose to eat your meals and snacks. In the following example, for instance, you may eat breakfast, and at lunchtime, eat the baked potato wedges and only half the sandwich. If you've already worked out (or time allows for adequate digestion), saving the other half for a midafternoon snack makes sense, especially if you tend to eat dinner late or if special circumstances call for a late dinner.

Notice also that active people and athletes at all calorie ranges (especially those racking up long distances) need to spend some of their calories on foods and drinks appropriate for use during and after exercise. The goal isn't to skimp on beneficial sports drinks and energy gels (or other sports food needed for fuel) during or after training bouts so that you can spend the calories on extra sweets, alcohol, and foods high in fat like French fries and cream cheese. Remember, athletes who eat in a way that leaves them physically ready and mentally prepared are the ones consistently able to train at a high level.

Sample Calorie Meal Plans for Athletes

2,200-Calorie Meal Plan

BREAKFAST

1 cup (250 ml) of orange juice

1 cup low-fat milk

or 6 oz (170 g) of low-fat flavored yogurt

Black coffee or tea

Note: Orange juice, milk, or yogurt can be saved for a midmorning snack.

Breakfast burrito

1 flour tortilla (8 in., or 20 cm, diameter)

1 scrambled egg (in 1 tsp of low-fat soft or tub margarine)

1/3 cup of black beans

2 tbsp of salsa

> continued

< continued, **2,200-Calorie Meal Plan**

LUNCH

Water or unsweetened beverage

3/4 cup of baked potato wedges

with 1 tbsp of ketchup

Roast beef sandwich

1 whole-grain (2.5 oz, or 70 g) sandwich bun

3 oz (85 g) of lean roast beef

2 slices of tomato

1/4 cup of shredded romaine lettuce

1.5 oz (42 g) of part-skim mozzarella cheese

1 tsp of yellow mustard

DINNER

1 cup low-fat milk

1/2 cup of flavored white rice

with .5 oz (14 g) of slivered almonds

1 cup of steamed broccoli

1 cup of low-fat ice cream

Stuffed, broiled salmon filet

3 oz (85 g) of salmon, cooked

1 oz (28 g) of bread stuffing mix

1 tbsp of chopped onions

1 tbsp of diced celery

2 tsp (10 ml) of canola oil

EXTRAS AND FUN FOODS

1 cup of cantaloupe

Energy bar (200 calories)

or 4 cups (1 liter) of rehydration sports drink

or 3 fig bars and 4 oz (112 ml) of 100% fruit juice

TOTAL: 2,235 calories
58% carbohydrate, 20% protein, 22% fat
325 g carbohydrate, 109 g protein, 55 g fat

2,600-Calorie Meal Plan

BREAKFAST

1 cup of orange juice

1 cup of low-fat milk

or 6 oz (170 g) of low-fat flavored yogurt

Black coffee or tea

Note: Orange juice, milk, or yogurt can be saved for a midmorning snack.

Breakfast burrito

- 1 flour tortilla (8 in., or 20 cm, diameter)
- 1 scrambled egg (in 1 tsp of low-fat soft or tub margarine)
- 1/3 cup of black beans
- 2 tbsp of salsa

LUNCH

Water or unsweetened beverage

3/4 cup of baked potato wedges

with 1 tbsp of ketchup

Roast beef sandwich

- 1 whole-grain (2.5 oz, or 70 g) sandwich bun
- 3 oz (85 g) of lean roast beef
- 2 slices of tomato
- 1/4 cup of shredded romaine lettuce
- 1.5 oz (42 g) of part-skim mozzarella cheese
- 1 tsp of yellow mustard

DINNER

1 cup of low-fat milk

1/2 cup of flavored white rice

with .5 oz (14 g) of slivered almonds

1 cup of steamed broccoli

1 cup of low-fat ice cream

Stuffed, broiled salmon filet

- 4 oz (112 g) of salmon, cooked
- 1 oz (28 g) of bread stuffing mix
- 1 tbsp of chopped onions
- 1 tbsp of diced celery
- 2 tsp (10 ml) of canola oil

EXTRAS AND FUN FOODS

1 cup of cantaloupe

Energy bar (200 calories)

or 4 cups (1 liter) of rehydration sports drink

or 3 fig bars and 4 oz (112 ml) of 100% fruit juice

1 tbsp of peanut butter

1 oz (28 g) of whole wheat crackers

or 2 full graham crackers

1 cup (250 ml) of 100% fruit juice

or 5 oz (140 ml) of wine

TOTAL: 2,640 calories
58% carbohydrate, 19% protein, 24% fat
381 g carbohydrate, 124 g protein, 69 g fat

> continued

3,000-Calorie Meal Plan

BREAKFAST

1 cup of orange juice

Black coffee or tea

Breakfast burrito

1 flour tortilla (8 in., or 20 cm, diameter)

1 scrambled egg and 2 egg whites (in 1 tbsp of soft or tub margarine)

1/2 cup of black beans

2 tbsp of salsa

MIDMORNING SNACK

1 cup of low-fat milk

or 6 oz (170 g) of low-fat flavored yogurt

1 cup of cold whole-grain cereal

or 1 packet of instant oatmeal

LUNCH

Water or unsweetened beverage

3/4 cup of baked potato wedges

with 1 tbsp of ketchup

Handful of baby carrots

Roast beef sandwich

1 whole-grain (2.5 oz, or 70 g) sandwich bun

4 oz (112 g) of lean roast beef

2 slices of tomato

1/4 cup of shredded romaine lettuce

1.5 oz (42 g) of part-skim mozzarella cheese

1 tsp of yellow mustard

AFTERNOON SNACK

1 cup of cantaloupe

1 tbsp of peanut butter

1 oz (28 g) of whole wheat crackers

DINNER

1 cup of low-fat milk

3/4 cup of flavored white rice

with .5 oz (14 g) of slivered almonds

1 1/2 cups of steamed broccoli

Stuffed, broiled salmon filet

5 oz (140 g) of salmon, cooked

1 oz (28 g) of bread stuffing mix

1 tbsp of chopped onions

1 tbsp of diced celery

2 tsp (10 ml) of canola oil

EXTRAS AND FUN FOODS

1 energy bar (250 calories)

or 16 oz (500 ml) milk shake (made with skim milk)

2 cups (500 ml) of rehydration sports drink

1 energy gel

or 8 oz (250 ml) of 100% fruit juice

or 2 cups (500 ml) of rehydration sports drink

or 1 medium banana

TOTAL: 2,995 calories
56% carbohydrate, 21% protein, 23% fat
418 g carbohydrate, 157 g protein, 77 g fat

3,500-Calorie Meal Plan

BREAKFAST

2 cups (500 ml) of orange juice

Black coffee or tea

Breakfast burrito

1 flour tortilla (8 in., or 20 cm, diameter)

1 scrambled egg and 2 egg whites (in 1 tbsp of soft or tub margarine)

1/2 cup of black beans

2 tbsp of salsa

MIDMORNING SNACK

1 cup of low-fat milk

or 6 oz (170 g) of low-fat flavored yogurt

1 cup of cold whole-grain cereal

or 1 packet of instant oatmeal

LUNCH

Water or unsweetened beverage

3/4 cup of baked potato wedges

with 1 tbsp of ketchup

Handful of baby carrots

> continued

< continued, **3,500-Calorie Meal Plan**

Roast beef sandwich

1 whole-grain (2.5 oz, or 70 g) sandwich bun

4 oz (112 g) of lean roast beef

2 slices of tomato

1/4 cup of shredded romaine lettuce

1.5 oz (42 g) of part-skim mozzarella cheese

1 tsp of yellow mustard

AFTERNOON SNACK

1 cup of cantaloupe

1 tbsp of peanut butter

1 oz (28 g) of whole wheat crackers

DINNER

1 cup of low-fat milk

1 cup of flavored white rice

with .5 oz (14 g) of slivered almonds

2 cups of steamed broccoli

with 2 tbsp (30 ml) of regular salad dressing

Stuffed, broiled salmon filet

5 oz (140 g) of salmon, cooked

1 oz (28 g) of bread stuffing mix

1 tbsp of chopped onions

1 tbsp of diced celery

2 tsp (10 ml) of canola oil

EXTRAS AND FUN FOODS

1 energy bar (250 calories)

or 16 oz (500 ml) milk shake (made with skim milk)

2 cups (500 ml) of rehydration sports drink

1 energy gel

or 8 oz (250 ml) of 100% fruit juice

or 2 cups (500 ml) of rehydration sports drink

or 1 medium banana

1 beer (12 oz, or 355 ml)

or 6 oz (175 ml) of wine (~150 calories)

TOTAL: 3,500 calories
55% carbohydrate, 19% protein, 24% fat
482 g carbohydrate, 163 g protein, 92 g fat

How Do Kenyan Runners Eat?

Kenyan runners are widely considered to be some of the best endurance athletes in the world. About half of all of the male athletes in the world who have ever run 10 kilometers in fewer than 27 minutes, for example, hail from Kenya. The eating habits of these Kenyan runners, which must play a key role in their success, however, had not been extensively studied until recently. Since nutrition is a science, Yannis Pitsiladis of the International Centre for East African Running Science in Glasgow, Scotland, along with 1972 Olympic 800-meter bronze medalist Mike Boit, Vincent Onywera, and Festus Kiplamai from the exercise and sports science department at Kenyatta University in Nairobi and the department of foods, nutrition, and dietetics at Egerton University in Njoro, Kenya, took up the task of scientifically figuring out what the Kenyans eat. Over a seven-day period, they monitored everything that 10 elite Kenyan male runners (several Olympic medalists as well as champions from two recent world championships) ate while attending a training camp near Kaptagat, Kenya.

What they found was that the Kenyans are doing things right when they sit down at the dinner table. Their staple edibles were carbohydrate-rich foods such as boiled rice, bread, poached potatoes, boiled porridge, cabbage, kidney beans, and ugali (a well-cooked cornmeal paste that is the national dish of Kenya). Ugali provided 23 percent of daily calories, followed by copious amounts of plain white sugar, mostly in tea (20 percent), rice (14 percent), and full-fat milk (13 percent). With 76 percent of their 3,000 daily calories supplied as carbohydrate (about 4.7 grams per pound of body weight, or 10.4 grams of carbohydrate per kilogram of body mass), they amazingly consumed 600 grams of carbohydrate every single day—thus, consistently restocking their glycogen stores. The rest of their diet met the recommended guidelines for athletes, too, supplying adequate protein, mostly from 3.5-ounce (100 g) portions of beef, eaten four times a week, (75 total grams daily or 1.3 grams of protein per kilogram of body weight) and a modest amount of fat (61 percent from full-fat milk added to tea). The Kenyans took no dietary supplements of any kind, relying instead on regular foods (three meals and two snacks daily) to fuel their efforts.

Another golden rule of sports nutrition that these amazing runners adhered to related to timing. The Kenyans always ate within 1 hour after workouts. (They trained twice daily, running 75 high-quality miles, or 120 kilometers, for the week in preparation for the Kenyan cross country season.) This means they consistently took advantage of the postworkout period when glycogen resynthesis rates can be maximized (provided the athletes regularly consume adequate carbohydrate).

> continued

< continued

Overall, the Kenyan meal plan strongly resembles the eating habits of another group of outstanding distance runners known for their ultrarunning expertise—the Tarahumara Indians of the Sierra Madre Mountains in Mexico. Research reveals that the Tarahumaras also consume about 75 to 80 percent of their total daily calories from carbohydrate, 12 percent from fat, and 8 to 13 percent from protein. Like the Kenyans, the Tarahumara Indians eat plenty of beans, as well as copious quantities of cornmeal.

The bottom line: Design an eating plan that works for you; however, make sure it's based on sound, credible sports nutrition principles. In other words, don't ignore the science.

Source: O. Anderson, n.d., "Eating practices of the best endurance athletes in the world." [Online]. Available: www.active.com/running/Articles/Eating_practices_of_the_best_endurance_athletes_in_the_world [April 24, 2013].

PART II

Nutrition Plans for Specific Events and Conditions

9

Shorter-Range Endurance Events

Professional cyclist Frank Schleck wore a drink pack on his chest when riding a 7-kilometer time trial to finish 12th and win the overall title in the 2011 Critérium International. A hydration pack worn on the front versus the back purportedly can give an advantage of two seconds per kilometer in a time trial.

> From 1 April 2012: If a rider uses a camelback or similar hydration equipment, it must be worn on the back only, not on the chest. The contents must be limited to 0.5 liters.

Source: International Cycling Union Sport and Technical Update, March 2012.

Perhaps you're just getting started as an endurance athlete, or you've figured out that you excel on the relatively shorter end of endurance-related activities. Having a defined goal, whether it is to tackle local hiking trails or to put it on the line in a 10K road race or a sprint triathlon, can be motivating and can keep life interesting. Despite popular opinion, having a well-thought-out nutrition plan is very much part of the equation for achieving success in these shorter endurance ventures. And, if you have any plans to participate or compete in longer events, you will need to practice and hone your nutrition strategies during these higher-intensity, shorter-range efforts.

This chapter will help you explore or work at excelling in higher-intensity, shorter-range endurance endeavors, such as the following:

Running: 5K, 8K, 10K, and 10-mile (16 km) road races, or these distances as a single leg of a team relay race, or shorter trail races (those that take up to 2 hours to complete)

Duathlon or triathlon: sprint distance, Olympic distance

Cycling: short amateur and pro–am road races and time trials (lasting 3 hours or less), standard cyclo-cross and mountain-bike races (lasting 2 hours or less), the cycling leg of a triathlon or mountain-bike team relay race, or organized rides taking 2 to a leisurely 4 hours to complete

Multisport or adventure racing: short 2- to 3-hour multisport adventures, undertaking a single leg of an adventure team relay race

Hiking or trekking: forays of up to 4 hours, especially if at a moderate to fast pace, such as fastpacking

Winter sports: recreational cross-country ski and snowshoe outings and races lasting 1 to 3 continuous hours, shorter Nordic ski races (lasting 90 minutes or less)

Keep in mind that designating these activities as shorter-range endurance events based on time of exertion or distance is somewhat arbitrary because both criteria are heavily influenced by fitness level and experience—what might be a shorter-range effort for a highly trained competitive endurance athlete could be a long-distance effort for a fitness enthusiast.

What separates shorter-duration events from going out simply for a run (or ride, swim, or ski), as well as from long-range and ultraendurance competitions, is the shorter time frame and the higher intensity (faster pace) that you plan (hope) to undertake and maintain. If you're a serious competitor, you'll be putting in hours of training for a race or activity that will take a fraction of that time to complete. Training specifically for the activity is essential. Race-day strategy, including going out at the proper pace, is also extremely important. Keep in mind that carbohydrate provides most of the energy used by working muscles and that a faster pace (especially going out at a fast pace, settling in, and then picking up or kicking in to finish strong) dictates that both anaerobic and aerobic energy systems play a role. (See chapter 2 for a review of energy systems.) If you're serious about competing, don't underestimate the benefits of sound nutrition planning and execution in higher-intensity, shorter-range endurance efforts.

Just as important, you may want to enjoy yourself as much as possible and make it to the finish or end of your outing. Let's face it—some active people, including recreational athletes, never quite complete all the recommended hours or miles of training. They then undertake athletic challenges that exercise scientists would categorize as being beyond what they have physiologically prepared for. In this case, paying attention to nutrition needs before and during the event or race is crucial to your ability to enjoy yourself and finish (and avoid becoming sick or getting injured). Being physically underprepared coupled with making poor nutrition decisions is not a winning combo.

Pre-Event Nutrition Game Plan

If you've followed a smart sports diet going into the race or event, carbohydrate loading is not necessary. You should have more than adequate glycogen stored in your muscles (up to 400 grams of glycogen, or 1,600 calories) and liver (100 grams, or 400 calories) to fuel the anaerobic and aerobic demands placed on working muscles during the actual competition. In other words, before shorter-range endurance races, especially those lasting 90 minutes or less, you don't need to superload your muscles with glycogen as do marathoners, Ironman triathletes, or cyclists who are attempting a century ride (100 miles, or 160 kilometers).

Some athletes preparing to compete, however, do run a greater risk of gradually depleting their glycogen stores if they never allow their muscles to regain their full potential supply. Most at risk are athletes involved in heavy training who don't rest adequately before races, those who follow low-carbohydrate diets, or those who are overly concerned about maintaining a desired weight. In these circumstances, an athlete may enter a shorter-range endurance competition with glycogen stores that are insufficient to sustain an all-out competitive effort. Remember, you burn proportionately more carbohydrate as your pace quickens and oxygen becomes less available to working muscles. (And carbohydrate is the only fuel the body can burn during flat-out efforts.) Likewise, you also burn more carbohydrate during fast starts, surges, ascents of hills, and sprints to the finish line. (Review chapter 4 on how to maintain adequate muscle glycogen stores from day to day.)

One or Two Days in Advance and Dinner the Night Before

This close to an endurance endeavor or race, the nutrition focus is three-fold: Hydrate adequately, top off glycogen stores, and avoid getting ill from something you eat. This can be accomplished easily by eating snacks and meals composed of familiar foods that you like and by drinking a healthy beverage along with each meal and snack. (See chapter 8 for a review of these guidelines.)

As for dinner the night before, you can relax! No magical or preferred prerace dinner exists. The only rule is to stick with familiar foods that you enjoy. This is not the time to be adventurous. You don't want to be up all night making trips to the bathroom. Although you will most likely naturally tend toward carbohydrate-rich foods like pasta, rice, tortillas, and potatoes, keep in mind that athletes have competed successfully after eating all kinds of foods. (For carbohydrate-rich meal ideas, see table 4.3 in chapter 4.) One thing is certain—stuffing in carbohydrate at this time is unnecessary. Eat at a reasonable time for you, consume appropriate-sized portions, and know that you can eat again, if need be, before bedtime (for example, milk and cereal or an energy bar).

Some athletes become obsessed with having the perfect prerace meal or the same foods every time. To keep your stress level in check, become comfortable with a variety of acceptable foods and meals, especially if you travel to compete, because you will not be guaranteed to get the same foods every time. Remind yourself that this last supper is only one of many factors that go into your preparation for the next day's event or race.

Last, but not least, prepare and pack any nutrition essentials that you plan to consume during the event or race, such as sports drinks, energy gels and bars, and foods that have previously passed the test in training (as well as a recovery drink or bar and food for afterward). Double-check that any equipment you plan to use, such as hip packs or bum bags, water bladders, and gel flasks, is in good working order. Fill up your drink bottles (or hydration system) the night before so that you can just grab them in the morning (during warm weather, you can freeze bottles beforehand).

Morning of the Event

Eat breakfast. No matter how early you plan to hit the trail or how early a race goes off, eat something. You might choose something as simple as toast with jam or honey, a glass of juice, or a banana. If need be, get up early, eat, and go back to bed. Eating breakfast tops off glycogen stores in the liver (your brain fuel), which have been depleted by half or more overnight, and settles the stomach, meaning that you won't be distracted by or become anxious about hunger pains or falling blood sugar as you're waiting to begin. Liquid breakfasts, such as a meal-replacement beverage (see chapter 5), are good for sensitive or nervous stomachs, as well as for those with long drive times to get to the starting line. To avoid surprises, stick with foods that you typically eat.

You will need to time when you eat breakfast so that you don't end up stranded in the bathroom beforehand or feel uncomfortably full while racing. Athletes vary widely in what they can tolerate, but resist the urge to skip breakfast altogether, especially if you will be on the go at a moderate to fast pace for more than an hour. In general, the more time you have beforehand, the more solid food you should be able to tolerate and the more you can (and most likely will need to) eat. No concrete recommendations exist, but most people do well with .5 grams of carbohydrate (2 calories) per pound of body weight (1.0 gram carbohydrate or 4 calories per kilogram) if they eat 1 hour before the event (for example, a canned liquid meal or energy bar that provides 100 to 300 calories) and up to 2.0 grams of carbohydrate per pound 4 hours before (for example, a hearty breakfast that holds you over). Keep in mind that liquid foods clear from the stomach faster than solid foods.

Drink plenty of familiar (well-tolerated) fluids such as water, sports drinks, fruit juice, and milk up to 2 hours before the start. Doing so will give you time to urinate any excess. If you choose not to eat breakfast, drinking carbohydrate-containing beverages such as sports drinks or juice becomes even more important. If you're used to having tea or coffee in the morning, don't skip it today. Drink another cup of water or a sports drink 5 to 15 minutes before the start. (For energy gel users, this is the time to consume a packet with a few gulps of water.)

Treat any sports foods that you will use during the race or event as you would any other piece of equipment that you rely on. First, don't leave home without them. Second, don't wait to the last minute when you're nervous or excited to figure out what you need to do. Double-check that your bottles are on your bike or in your knapsack, that fluid is flowing easily through the bladder hose, or that your hip pack or bum bag is loaded with an energy gel or two. You can also carry single energy gel packs in a pocket, pinned to the inside of your shorts, or tucked into your cycling shorts or sports bra.

During the Event

During these relatively shorter events and races, your main job is to monitor your fluid needs and prevent dehydration, which can lead to a more dangerous situation, such as heat exhaustion. Elite runners, sprint triathletes, and time-trial cyclists often will not drink during shorter endeavors. Most competitors, however, as well as completers, either will need to drink or would benefit greatly from drinking during shorter events and races. The benefits of drinking during the event are particularly significant for those who sweat heavily, underprepared athletes, and those who are competing at altitude or in warmer or more humid conditions than they're accustomed to.

Remember, this isn't about what you can do, such as ride 30 miles (48 km) or race a 10K, without needing any water. This is about working with your body to be as physically and mentally prepared as possible to enjoy and conquer the upcoming challenge. If you'll be on the move for a couple of hours or longer, maintaining a normal blood sugar level will affect your ultimate success. Shorter-range events and races also provide opportunities to practice techniques and strategies for eating and drinking while on the move that won't be optional if you move

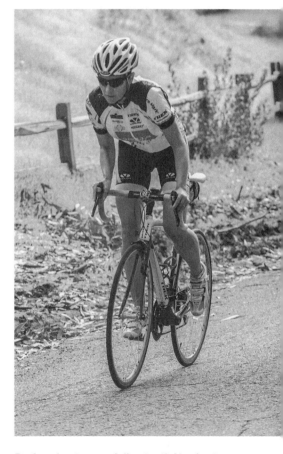

Performing to your full potential in shorter, higher-intensity efforts requires that you fully support your body. Base your fluid and fuel intake on your personal needs.

up in distance. (For more sports-specific tips and strategies, see chapters 10 through 13.)

Drinking water should be adequate in most situations, especially if you'll be on the move for an hour or less. Don't be afraid, however, to consume a sports drink. No law exists that states sports drinks may be consumed only if you're going longer than 60 minutes. In fact, the carbohydrate boost from sports drinks (and gels) may be just what makes the difference (especially if you didn't eat breakfast) in your ability to kick, or finish strongly, at the end of a shorter-endurance race or event. Remember, merely rinsing your mouth with a carbohydrate-containing beverage during shorter-duration exercise has been shown to delay fatigue and boost performance (see chapter 4 for more details). Overall, individual fluid needs vary widely—from a gulp or two to several ounces every 15 to 20 minutes from the time you start.

For events and races lasting longer than 60 continuous minutes, sports drinks are strongly recommended because they efficiently provide what's needed most—fluid and carbohydrate. Supplemental carbohydrate—from sports drinks, gels, chews, and blocks, and energy bars and real foods, if appropriate—helps you maintain a normal blood sugar level and ward off hypoglycemia (low blood sugar), or bonking, as the event or race unfolds. The effort that you are putting out will seem easier and your goal more doable when your brain is receiving a steady supply of fuel. Table 9.1 provides the approximate carbohydrate content of some commonly used sports foods.

Individual needs vary widely, depending on your fitness level, pre-event glycogen stores, and pace, as well as the activity, the weather, and course conditions. The general rule is to consume at least 30 grams of carbohydrate (100 carbohydrate calories) per hour of activity after the first hour.

For most adults, one gulp of fluid roughly equates to drinking about 1 ounce (30 ml). Novice competitors need to realize that slowing down, walking, or even stopping altogether to drink enough fluid is far better than dropping out of the race (or getting injured or feeling miserable the entire time) because of being dehydrated or glycogen depleted. The more comfortable you are drinking on the move, the more likely you are to meet your fluid needs. The only way to become proficient is to practice, practice, practice!

TABLE 9.1   Sample Carbohydrate Counts of Common Sports Foods

1 cup (8 oz or ~8 gulps) of standard sports drink	12–15 g
1 energy gel packet	25 g
1 package (1.58 oz, or 45 g) of Sharkies (energy sports chews)	36 g
Glucose tablets	4–5 g each
6 Clif Shot Blok energy chews	48 g
1 packet (1 oz, or 28 g) of Jelly Belly Sport Beans	25 g

- **Runners**—Simply grabbing a cup or two off an aid station table isn't good enough; you must get the fluid down. Practice the following favored technique: Grab a cup, pinch or crush it lightly to form a funnel, and take one or two gulps at a time. In self-supported running adventures and trail races, use bladders, hip belts, or other bottle carriers specifically designed for runners.

- **Cyclists**—Use your common sense when drinking on a bike. Concentrate on the road, look ahead for hazards, and slow down if necessary. When riding one-handed as you reach for a water bottle (or energy gel or food), keep your bike from veering by gripping the center of the handlebar next to the stem with your stronger arm. Always empty your down-tube bottle first and then switch it with your full seat-tube bottle. Keep in mind that rapidly evaporating sweat can give a false sense that fluid losses are minimal. In addition, the windchill factor that occurs during cycling may prevent you from feeling warm or overheated, which also masks or delays the need to drink.

  Depending on your goals as a road cyclist, you may need to master drinking in a variety of situations—reaching with either hand; taking bottles from a jersey pocket, another rider, or a support vehicle; and while braking, riding in a pack, climbing, riding in a pace line, or at a feed zone.

  Some situations, such as mountain bike and cyclo-cross races, favor hands-free drinking. Use a bladder hydration system designed specifically for cyclists. From a safety standpoint, a bladder system is superior because your hand will be off the handlebars for only a split second while you grab the drinking tube. In organized rides, bladders allow you to carry a large volume of your preferred drink to meet your needs between supported rest stops. On rides in which you have access to water along the way, save weight by packing baggies of premeasured powdered sports drink.

- **Triathletes and multisport adventurers**—Keeping a sleek aerodynamic bike on the road is challenging, especially in windy conditions. Triathletes spend the most time in a race cycling, which makes becoming proficient at drinking while on the bike a priority. Figuring out how to carry it is an individual, almost personal choice from standard water bottles to aerodynamic bottle systems. Be sure to practice with your hydration system at your intended race pace.

  Multisport athletes who use water bottles need to keep them easily within reach—not buried at the bottom of a pack. A hands-free bladder system that is hardy (puncture resistant) and nonrestrictive may be an option.

- **Hikers and other winter sports athletes**—Although you may not feel thirsty when exercising in cold weather or may want to avoid making pit stops, hydration remains a priority. If using bottles, always keep them easily accessible—not buried at the bottom of your pack. A water-bottle carrier with insulated water bottles (fill with prewarmed drinks in cold weather, if feasible) or a bladder system that is insulated, lightweight, and nonrestrictive may work well for you. Keep in mind that tubes and valves in fluid-delivery systems designed for winter use can still freeze up in cold temperatures, so old-fashioned insulated water bottles are often the best way to go if you expect extreme conditions.

Ski marathoners need to practice the following favored drinking technique. On a slight downhill (a flat section can work too, if you can keep moving without using your arms), whip your bottle carrier around to the front, pull the bottle out, and tuck the pole on that side under your arm. The idea is to remain aerodynamic by drinking in a tucked position. Take advantage of your position in a racing pack. If you're in front, gliding and drinking helps prevent people from passing. If you're drafting off others in a pack, you can drink while being shielded from the wind and maintain your pace.

Postevent Recovery Plan

Your job isn't quite finished when you cross the finish line. Be mindful of the carbohydrate window and jump-start the recovery process by rehydrating with a carbohydrate-rich beverage (or food) within 30 minutes of finishing. Aim for at least .5 grams of carbohydrate per pound (1.0 grams per kilogram) of body weight. Numerous options in liquid form are available if you don't feel like eating immediately after vigorous exercise: sports drinks (14 to 19 grams per cup, or per 250 milliliters), fruit juice (25 to 40 grams per cup), high-carbohydrate or meal-replacement beverages (check the label, some provide as many as 50 grams per serving), milk or fruit smoothies made with low-fat milk (12 grams per cup), or non-diet soda (40 or more grams in a standard-size can).

Jump-start muscle repair and recovery by consuming, if possible, a small amount of protein (10 to 15 grams, found in some recovery drinks and energy bars, as well as in yogurt and milk) within this same period. At the very least, include quality protein at your next meal—eggs, meat, poultry, fish, beans, dairy, or soy—within 2 hours of your finish. (See the section titled Protein Intake in chapter 2 for review.)

Drinking alcohol following all-out efforts can easily impede your recovery by hampering your efforts to rehydrate (as a diuretic, alcohol causes your body to lose fluid) and by interfering with the body's ability to replenish glycogen stores. Your best bet is to make rehydrating with nonalcoholic beverages a top priority. Furthermore, after an intense physical effort, your body may not be able to tolerate or process alcohol as well as it normally does, so indulge in moderation.

While the details are fresh in your mind, jot down some notes about the sports drinks and foods that you consumed during your race or adventure—what worked, what didn't, and what you want to try next time.

LEARNING FROM THE BEST: COMPETING IN SHORTER-DISTANCE TRIATHLONS

Boulder-based triathlete Cameron Dye, 28, was named the 2012 Non-Olympic/ITU Triathlete of the Year by USA Triathlon after winning six races during the season, a triathlon feat almost unheard of at the professional level. He credits a foundation built from years of progressive work that started with swimming at age 8 and running cross-country in high school. It was as a young age-group swimmer, in fact, that Dye quickly learned the value of listening to his body and giving it the fuel it needs.

Read on as Dye, who specializes in non-drafting Olympic distance races—the standard triathlon distance of 1.5 kilometers (0.93 mile) swim, 40 kilometers (25 mile) bike, and 10 kilometers (6.2 mile) run—shares his winning nutritional tips for getting to the finish line as quickly as possible in shorter, higher-intensity endurance events.

1. **Develop an overall positive and relaxed attitude toward food and your body.** When it comes to fueling his body, Dye adheres to the principle that "everything is good in moderation." Dye loves to eat; it's a skill he honed growing up as a typical age-group swimmer who was constantly ravenous. He urges fellow triathletes to focus on functionality and how their body is performing rather than on vanity and the number on the scale or what their body looks like. As Dye, who has never counted calories or restricted his intake, says, "If I need to eat more and I end up weighing two pounds more, so be it. I'm going to do whatever I need to do to perform at my best." Dye also reminds athletes that a triathlon involves three disciplines: swimming, cycling, and running. While losing weight may lead to faster run times, it can result in a loss of power while swimming and biking. "Ask yourself: *How can I go faster?*" urges Dye, "not, *How can I be lighter?*"

2. **For prerace dinners, stick with what you know.** Dye's requirements for prerace meals are very simple. He must like the food, it must be familiar (well tolerated means safe to eat), and it needs to be easy to find when traveling. Pizza fits the bill for dinner the night before a race. Dye aims to finish eating his pre-event dinner by 7:30 to 8:00 pm, but logistics and travel schedules may push dinner to a later time. Nevertheless, Dye eats a substantial amount and stays relaxed about his food intake. "If I stick with what I know and I eat enough, what I eat the night before isn't going to make or break my race," says Dye.

3. **Eat breakfast on race morning.** As recommended by sports nutrition experts, Dye always eats breakfast the morning of a race. A bowl of carb-rich oatmeal (or toast or a muffin) along with a bottle of electrolyte drink (Dye uses First Endurance products) and some caffeine (caffeinated gel

> continued

< continued

or powder or even an energy drink like RedBull) tops off his glycogen and electrolyte stores.

Shorter, high-intensity physical efforts increase the risk that stomach and intestinal problems will occur. "You simply have to train your stomach like any other piece of equipment," says Dye. He gets up three hours before the typical triathlon's early morning start time, and he eats right away. Approximately 20 minutes before the start of the race, he ingests another 200 calories in the form of an energy gel or bar to ward off hunger pangs and to avoid bonking during the race.

4. **Keep on top of electrolytes, too.** Just because you're not undertaking an Ironman doesn't mean hydration and electrolytes (most notably sodium) are unimportant. Get familiar with your sweat rate on training rides and runs and practice replacement strategies accordingly. Dye, a salty sweater, is very conscious of replacing electrolytes on every ride and run he undertakes via the sports drink he relies on. He also consciously uses the salt shaker at mealtimes.

5. **Set yourself up for the run.** Work hard to get in calories (from carbohydrate) on the bike. Dye understands that a shorter-distance endurance race demands high-intensity, all-out effort, under what are frequently hot and humid conditions. Fuel ingested on the bike during a triathlon is of benefit while completing the cycling leg as well as during the run. Along with a bottle of water on the bike, opt for a bottle of sports drink or an electrolyte drink with carbs, also. Energy gels, when consumed with water, are another quick and easy-to-digest option. Dye will often mix an extra energy gel packet into his bottle of electrolyte drink for an energy boost.

Be disciplined about getting enough calories in while on the bike allows many triathletes to drink only (or mostly) water on the run which can help to reduce the risk of gastrointestinal trouble. Plus, due to the shorter nature of shorter-distance endurance endeavors, if you get behind fuel-wise, you won't have time to catch up. As Dye knows well, "If you skip an aid station and don't drink (or lose a bottle on the bike leg), you risk pain on the run."

10

Long-Distance Endurance Events

The past two weeks of racing have been great. A win at Ironman 70.3 New Orleans and a solid 7th place on one of the hardest half-Ironman courses around—Wildflower.

On the bike I aim for about 350 calories per hour: Keep in mind I weigh 165 lbs (75 kg) when thinking of calorie intake.

Started with

- 2 × 24 oz (710 ml) bottles with 350 calories on my bike (200 EFS drink and 150 Carbo Pro and three-fourths scoop of Pre Race powder in each)
- 100 calories of EFS drink in my aero bottle

At Wildflower, because of the long bike, I took an on-course energy drink to make up for the extra 15 minutes of riding.

Source: T. Wurtele, 2012, "Two very different races—same nutrition plan." [Online]. Available: http://team.firstendurance.com/profiles/blogs/two-very-different-races-same-nutrition-plan [April 24, 2013]. Used with permission.

Pursuing endurance-oriented competitions can become addictive. For some, a distance or activity that once seemed impossible or even unimaginable to complete becomes a routine that could (almost) be done while asleep. Seeking new physical conquests and mental challenges, you may be highly motivated to climb the endurance ladder and experience firsthand what it takes to be on the move for longer periods of time. Or conversely, perhaps on a whim with friends or in a moment of foolishness, you signed up and then loudly announced that you're going for the big (in this case, long) one this time—the marathon (26.2 miles, or 42 kilometers of running), Torture 10,000 (10,000 feet, or 3,000 meters, of climbing in 100 miles, or 160 kilometers, of cycling), a full Ironman (2.5 mile/3.9 kilometer swim, 112 mile/180 kilometer cycle, and 26.2 mile/42.2 kilometer run) or some other "see you hours from now at the finish line" escapade.

Whatever your goal, competing in or simply surviving a long-distance event requires that you master drinking and, most likely, eating while on the move. Otherwise, the time that you're out there can pass all too quickly if you're forced to drop out or stop before you've attained your goal, or it will seem that the end will never come as you're reduced to a slow, painful, I'm-never-doing-this-again crawl.

This chapter is for endurance athletes who choose to move up in distance or for those striving to set a new PR in long-distance endurance endeavors and races, such as the following:

Running: half-marathon and marathon races, trail-running adventures or races taking 2 to several hours to complete, relay races of up to a day long with teams of two or more people

Duathlon or triathlon: long-course events, half Ironmans

Cycling: metric century and century rides, especially if hilly, double century rides, road time trials and races lasting 3 hours or longer, mountain bike races lasting 3 hours or longer, or 24-hour races with teams of two or more people

Multisport or adventure racing: off-road triathlons and other multisport races lasting 2 hours or longer, 4- to 8-hour multisport recreational adventures, half- to full-day adventure races, solo efforts in shorter multisport races

Hiking or trekking: 4- to 8-hour continuous hikes, treks, or ascents

Winter sports: half- to full-day snow shoeing outings, backcountry ski outings, or marathon ski races such as the Birkebeiner

Keep in mind that designating these activities as long-range endurance events based on time of exertion or distance is somewhat arbitrary because both criteria are heavily influenced by fitness level and experience—a moderately long effort for a seasoned competitor or extremely fit outdoors enthusiast, for example, could be a daylong activity for a recreational or novice athlete.

There is no substitute for putting in the distance or hours of training required for preparing physically and mentally to succeed at these long-distance challenges. You must also prepare your gastrointestinal (digestive) tract to absorb and digest fluids and fuel during exercise. In other words, it's not enough to know how to run, bike, cycle, ski, row, swim, or climb. Long-distance races also require that you master drinking and refueling while on the move to avoid being forced to slow down, or even drop out because of dehydration, glycogen depletion, or bonking. You must train your brain so that you drink and eat when you have no appetite, under unpleasant conditions, when things are going well (why bother, what could go wrong?), and when they're not (when stomach distress hits you, for example).

Don't look for shortcuts—none exist. Practicing with drinks, foods, and equipment will help you determine which fluids, foods, and equipment work best for you and will bring about progress. Drinking and eating on the move become automatic on race day only if you practice beforehand. Be consistent and stick with what you know, but also be willing to try something new when an old standby or favorite is no longer working. If you're thinking of tackling ultralength challenges (see chapter 11), you first need to establish smart drinking and refueling habits in long-distance endeavors and races.

Be prepared for a lot of trial and error. Experiment under different environmental conditions and take the time to determine and practice the techniques you need to master. Research and determine beforehand which, if any, fluids and foods will be provided along the course. Athletes who struggle with sensitive stomachs and other digestive problems in particular are advised to learn beforehand which sports drink will be served during a race or organized event. They can then train with that product or, if they will have access to water, carry their own acceptable premeasured powdered sports drink in baggies and reconstitute it along the way.

Self-supported challenges mean that you alone are responsible for the logistics of meeting your fluid and energy needs. Adventures and races involving friends and teammates add an additional layer of commitment. All team members must take seriously the responsibility to adequately hydrate and refuel. In other words, pick your teammates and adventure partners wisely.

Carbohydrate loading before long-distance pursuits is an invaluable tool to explore and practice with. In addition, some athletes may want to experiment with using branched-chain amino acids, caffeine, or electrolyte (salt) tablets during prolonged exercise. (See chapter 5 for review, because these strategies require experimentation in training long before the actual competition.) For many endurance athletes, long-distance events and races also serve as training bouts or stepping stones for ultradistance challenges, and thus provide excellent opportunities to practice and hone refueling strategies.

Despite the long distances involved, the reality is that some endurance enthusiasts don't manage to accomplish the recommended hours or miles of training. They undertake endurance challenges that exercise scientists would categorize as being beyond what they have physiologically prepared for. If this is your situation, paying attention to your nutrition needs before, and especially during, the event or race is even more critical for finishing (and avoiding becoming ill or injured in the process). Being underprepared, coupled with making poor decisions about fluid and fuel needs during long-distance races, is disastrous, and it can endanger your life.

Pre-Event Nutrition Game Plan

Your job beforehand is to respect the nutrition aspect of long-distance endurance competitions and eat in a way that prepares you physically and mentally for the challenge that lies ahead. In simple language, you must start a long-distance race or event adequately hydrated and well fueled. If you've trained properly and eaten a normal diet the few days leading up to the race or event, you can expect to store roughly 2,000 calories of glycogen (between muscles and the liver), or enough fuel for approximately 90 to 120 minutes of vigorous activity or a few hours at a moderate intensity or pace.

Because working muscles rely heavily on carbohydrate as fuel during these distance endeavors, as well as on the efficient breakdown of fat (which depends in part on the body having sufficient carbohydrate available; see chapter 2 to review), enhancing or boosting glycogen stores by carbohydrate loading makes sense. This practice reduces the chance that you will deplete your muscle glycogen stores and hit the wall before reaching the finish line.

Keep in mind that for male athletes, carbohydrate loading doesn't translate into eating enormous quantities of extra food, nor does it mean filling up on high-fat foods. To enter the race or event feeling fresh and well rested, you'll want to taper your training as the day of the event approaches. Because you'll be expending less energy in training than normal, you won't require massive amounts of extra calories to boost your carbohydrate intake. Rather, men should aim to consume about 70 percent of their daily calories as carbohydrate-rich food (8 to 10 grams of carbohydrate per kilogram of body weight). Some athletes find it easiest simply to add a serving or two of a high-carbohydrate beverage (see chapter 5 for examples). Female athletes, on the other hand, need to consume carbohydrate at a level of around 12 grams per kilogram of body weight to achieve a similar performance advantage from carbohydrate loading. From a practical standpoint, the only way for female endurance athletes to do this is to consume extra food (an additional 700 calories a day) for 3 to 4 days leading up to their endurance event.

Because you rely on your body not only to perform in long-distance races and activities, but to get you safely back home or to the finish line, you need to know how to prevent bonking (hypoglycemia, or a too-low blood sugar level) and hyponatremia (low blood sodium level). Learn what measures to take beforehand to reduce your risk. (See chapter 14 for an in-depth discussion of hyponatremia.)

Last, endurance athletes must be aware of the risks of using nonsteroidal anti-inflammatory drugs (NSAIDs), such as ibuprofen and naproxen sodium, during long-distance activities and races. Combined with dehydration, taking NSAIDs during prolonged exercise can increase your risk of kidney problems as well as predispose you to hyponatremia. You'll need to pay particular attention to your fluid intake before and during the event or race if you choose to take NSAIDs.

A Few Days in Advance

The main goal is to successfully carbohydrate-load. Ideally, you have found a carbohydrate-loading routine that works for you by experimenting before long training efforts. Understandably, depending on your performance goals and the time of year (or where you are in your season), you may not be able to taper your training fully before every long-distance race or event that you undertake. Boosting carbohydrate intake, however, is helpful, and it becomes more and more essential as you ask your body to perform vigorously past 90 minutes.

As long as you fill up on carbohydrate and not fat, don't be alarmed if you feel bloated or temporarily gain a couple of pounds in the days leading up to your event or race. Your body stores a considerable amount of water as it stows away carbohydrate as muscle glycogen. This extra water will help delay dehydration during the event or race.

Drink plenty of familiar, well-tolerated beverages such as water, fruit juice, sports drinks, and low-fat milk with your meals and snacks. Having beverages along with food helps your body hold on to the fluid longer. To avoid increasing the risk of hyponatremia, avoid the urge to drink too much plain water, especially during the day and evening before the event. Always monitor your urine color. It should be pale yellow, not clear like water.

To further decrease the risk of hyponatremia, maintain or increase your salt intake leading up to races in which you'll be continuously moving for 3 hours (at moderate to high intensity) or longer. An adequate intake of sodium is particularly important if you'll be competing in hot and humid conditions and when the weather will be warmer than what you normally train in. Add table salt to foods or eat your favorite salty foods, like soup, tomato juice, canned vegetables, canned chili, salted pretzels, and pickles.

Female endurance athletes, back-of-the-packers (a slower pace often means more opportunities to drink and thus overhydrate), undertrained athletes (sweat losses of sodium are greater), athletes troubled with cramping, and those not acclimated to the heat need to be particularly mindful of getting adequate sodium. If you've had problems with hyponatremia or dealing with the heat in the past or have a health problem such as high blood pressure, speak with your physician before taking salt (or electrolyte) tablets in the days leading up to (or during) a long-distance event or race.

If your competition involves travel and meals eaten away from home, be sure to take with you any special or favorite food items that you simply can't do without. Make smart food choices a priority on travel days because all-day travel and poor nutrition is a double whammy for even a highly trained athlete. Prepare by bringing foods that travel well and by stocking up on energy bars and powdered meal-replacement products. Consider using a high-carbohydrate beverage or meal-replacement product to supplement your carbohydrate needs if time-zone changes or your travel schedule will interfere with your regular eating habits. As much as you can control it, don't try new foods or change your eating habits in the week leading up to a long-distance event or race.

Now is the time to review your nutrition game plan for the day of the race. Early in the week, make sure that you have enough of all nutrition essentials that you plan to consume during the event or race, such as sports drinks, energy gels and bars, and, if appropriate, foods and electrolyte (salt) tablets that have previously passed the test in training. Double-check that any equipment that you plan to use, such as hip packs or bum bags, bladder hydration systems, and gel flasks, is in good working order. Gather and prepare your sports foods and equipment (as well as a recovery drink or bar and food for afterward) no later than the night before. If feasible, fill drink bottles (or another hydration system) the night before so that you can just grab them in the morning (and so that during warm weather you can freeze bottles beforehand).

Pre-Event Dinner

When it comes to eating the night before a long-distance race, rest assured that no magical or preferred prerace dinner exists. The only rule is to stick with familiar foods that you enjoy. This is not the time to be adventurous because you want to avoid making late-night trips to the bathroom. Although you most likely know to feature carbohydrate-rich foods like pasta, rice, and potatoes, keep in mind that endurance athletes have competed successfully after eating all kinds of foods, including pizza, steak, and Mexican food! (For carbohydrate-rich meal ideas, see chapter 4.)

Stuffing yourself with carbohydrate isn't necessary at this time. In other words, don't feel obligated to get your money's worth at the traditional prerace pasta feed. (Serious competitors, in fact, may do well to avoid eating in public places with crowds.) Don't be afraid to include reasonable-sized portions of meat or other protein-rich foods as well as some fat at this meal. These foods have staying power and can help you sleep through the night. Most athletes do fine having a glass of wine or a beer if it's part of their regular routine. Eat at a reasonable time for you, consume appropriate-sized portions, and know that eating again before bedtime (for example, a carbohydrate-rich snack such as milk and cereal or an energy bar) is more productive than stuffing yourself now.

Some athletes become consumed with having the perfect prerace meal or eating exactly the same thing each time. Keep your stress level in check by becoming comfortable with eating a variety of foods at prerace meals, especially if you travel to races; otherwise, you waste precious mental energy that compromises your performance. The goal is to be open-minded and flexible, which translates into being able to eat as many different foods as possible. If you firmly believe that certain foods will enhance your performance, by all means, eat them!

Finally, remind yourself that your success the next day hinges on numerous factors, and that this last supper is only one of them. Focus your mental energy on how you plan to fuel yourself *during* the event or race. What you do (or don't do) the next day, when you're on the move for several hours, has a much greater effect on your stamina, your morale, and ultimately the outcome, than worrying about eating the perfect meal the night before.

Continue to drink plenty of familiar, well-tolerated fluids, but don't overdo it by drinking bottle after bottle of plain water or other sodium-free beverages.

Morning of the Event

Plan to eat a carbohydrate-rich breakfast a few hours before the start of your endeavor or race, especially for a late-morning or midday start. Although you may be able to skip breakfast and do well in shorter-range events and races, the odds aren't in your favor as you move up in distance. If you don't eat breakfast, how many waking hours, as well as total hours, will have passed since you last ate? What will happen if the start is delayed?

Eating breakfast helps settle your stomach and ward off hunger pangs as you wait for the race to begin. (Many athletes find that they feel satisfied longer by eating earlier and including higher-fat foods like peanut butter or cheese.) More important, eating breakfast refills your liver glycogen stores (which can be almost gone by morning), which are critical for maintaining a stable blood sugar level during prolonged exercise. These carbohydrate reserves help to power hardworking muscles and fuel your brain so that you can make wise decisions while on the move. If you're simply too nervous to eat on race morning, drink your breakfast in the form of a breakfast shake or meal-replacement product. (As a last resort, eat a substantial late-night snack before going to bed.) No concrete recommendations exist; however, most people do well by consuming .5 grams of carbohydrate (2 calories) per pound of body weight (1 gram or 4 calories per kilogram) if they eat 1 hour before their event (for example, a canned liquid meal or energy bar that provides 100 to 300 calories) or up to 2.0 grams of carbohydrate per pound 4 hours before (for example, a substantial breakfast that holds you).

Keep in mind that liquid foods clear the stomach faster than solid foods do. If coffee or tea is part of your usual preexercise routine, go with it. Most athletes do best sticking with what they know (and ideally have confirmed by experimenting before long training efforts). If in doubt, leave it out.

Continue to hydrate with plenty of water or a familiar sports drink up to 2 hours before the start. Doing so will give you time to urinate any excess. Drink another cup of water or a sports drink 5 to 15 minutes before the start. For athletes who consume an energy gel before the start of a prolonged event, this is also the time (as close to the actual time of the start of the activity) to consume a packet with a few gulps of water.

Before you leave home or for the race, double-check that you have all your nutrition essentials: sports foods, equipment (bottle carriers, bladders, and so on), and recovery foods and beverages for afterward. Set up any transition areas or refueling stations as permitted and make certain that every person who needs to be familiar with the nutrition game plan (teammates, friends, support crew) knows this information.

During the Event

Your job throughout your long-distance event or race is to assess and monitor your fluid, carbohydrate, and electrolyte needs. In other words, give your most important piece of equipment, your body, what it needs so that it doesn't prematurely limit you or knock you totally out of the race.

The general guidelines that follow are a consensus of scientifically supported recommendations made by credible sports nutrition and exercise science experts, including the American College of Sports Medicine, the Academy of Nutrition and Dietetics, and the Australian Institute of Sport.

Guidelines for Fluid, Fuel, and Electrolyte Consumption During Long-Distance Events

Fluid
- Drink early and often: Take in 2 to 8 ounces (60 to 240 ml) every 15 to 20 minutes of prolonged exercise, starting immediately from the onset (fluid needs are highly individual and depend on a variety of factors, and they are best determined in training efforts beforehand).
- Do not rely solely on plain water (low in sodium) throughout an entire long-distance event or race to replace sweat losses.
- Properly formulated sports (electrolyte replacement) drinks are the easiest way to meet fluid and energy (carbohydrate) needs simultaneously. If they are available, soda or fruit juice may be an option, depending on the activity or intensity level.
- You must drink to match your fluid losses to avoid potentially dangerous situations—underhydration leads to dehydration, which increases the risk of heat illness, and overhydration leads to hyponatremia, which can be fatal.
- Glycerol users must still replace fluid losses as much as possible by drinking water and fluid-replacement drinks throughout the event or race.
- Despite not feeling as thirsty in cold-weather adventures and races or wanting to avoid making stops for bathroom breaks, make hydration a priority.

Fuel
- Consuming supplemental carbohydrate during prolonged vigorous exercise lasting longer than 90 continuous minutes preserves glycogen stores and allows you to extend the distance traveled at the desired pace.
- The general recommendation for efforts 2 to 3 hours long is to consume 25 to 60 grams of carbohydrate (100 to 250 calories from rapidly oxidized carbohydrate like glucose or maltodextrin) per hour of activity after the first hour. For efforts longer

than 2.5 hours, consume up to 90 grams of carbohydrate per hour. Use a combination of carbohydrate types that are absorbed through different mechanisms (e.g., glucose or maltodextrins combined with fructose in a 2:1 ratio).

- Meet carbohydrate needs with properly formulated sports drinks, energy gels, and other easily digested, well-absorbed, and well-tolerated carbohydrate sources (glucose tablets, sport chews and blocks, candy, soda) as well as with well-tolerated solid forms such as energy bars and other carbohydrate-rich foods.
- Waiting too long to refuel, which increases the likelihood that dehydration will occur, adds to the risk of experiencing gastrointestinal problems (cramping, vomiting, or diarrhea).

Electrolytes
- Being mindful of sodium intake before prolonged exercise lasting longer than 3 continuous hours, matching fluid intake (drinking) to fluid losses (sweating and urination) during exercise, and consuming a properly formulated sports drink that includes sodium will be adequate for preventing hyponatremia in most exercisers and athletes.
- Female endurance athletes, those at the back of the pack, undertrained athletes, athletes who have troubles with cramping, and those not acclimated to the heat or who have experienced difficulties dealing with the heat in the past are at higher risk of developing hyponatremia during or following prolonged exercise.
- Some people will require or benefit from ingesting additional sodium during prolonged exercise (for example, table salt, salty beverages and foods, and salt tablets).
- Use caution when consuming electrolyte (salt) tablets because stomach distress, vomiting, and diarrhea can occur if you use them improperly (take them with too little fluid) or take them in a dehydrated state. No firm guidelines exist, so you must experiment to determine how best to meet your individual sodium needs.
- Consider weight gain during prolonged exercise as a warning sign that you are overconsuming fluid, thereby increasing the risk of hyponatremia.

Sports-Specific Recommendations

Every sports discipline presents unique challenges for hydrating and refueling while on the move. Watch and learn from experienced veterans and practice at every opportunity. Being foolish or lazy about nutrition needs during a race undermines, and can even negate, your prerace hard work and preparation.

Runners

Water stations in marathons are akin to pit stops in auto racing. Don't even think about bypassing them, especially the early stations. Your running pace will determine which water stops to key in on, because you need to drink water or a sports drink every 15 to 20 minutes (aim for 2 to 8 ounces depending on your individual needs). Don't wait until you feel thirsty—once you're dehydrated, you won't catch up. Don't be afraid to drink plain water, but don't rely solely on it throughout the entire race. Sports drinks are undoubtedly the easiest way to meet fluid, carbohydrate, and electrolyte needs simultaneously.

Drink the water offered along the course; don't pour it over your head. Although a quick dousing may temporarily cool you off, pouring water over your head instead of drinking it doesn't help you stay hydrated. Would you drive your overheated car to the gas station, pull up to the water hose, open the hood of the car, and then spray the water on the overheated engine?

Go with gels. Easy to ingest while running, energy gels are best taken with 4 to 6 ounces (118 to 180 ml) of water (not a sports drink) to reduce the risk of stomach upset. Plan to ingest a packet right before an aid station where water is available. Most gels supply 20 to 25 grams of carbohydrate (80 to 100 calories) per packet. If you plan on carrying more than one energy gel packet with you, use one of the convenient palm-sized flasks that clip to the waistband of your running shorts. These refillable flasks can carry and dispense as desired up to five servings (packets) of gel. Runners who plan to take longer than 4 hours to complete a marathon may consider wearing a waist pack instead for toting energy gels or other well-tolerated solid foods, such as energy bars.

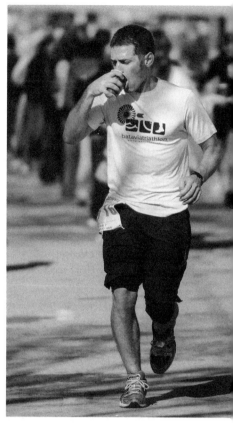

Take advantage of aid stations to stay on top of your fluid needs and to consume much-needed carbohydrate.

If you're fast enough that you've earned the privilege of picking up water bottles at aid stations designated for elite marathoners, use your imagination and decorate your bottles. You want them to be easy to spot and easy to grab. Don't panic if a bottle is not where you planned it to be. Slow down slightly to try to spot it, but don't waste too much time. Remind yourself that you can get plenty of water or sports drinks along the course. Start grabbing cups of fluid immediately and slow down if necessary to be sure that you consume enough.

During off-road endeavors, set your watch and drink on a preplanned schedule, every 15 to 20 minutes. You may forget to drink in trail races because varying terrain and extreme weather conditions can cause time to pass differently. If you're familiar with what's coming up, planning is easier. If you're a novice or the course is new to you, ask experienced runners. If you find that you don't drink enough when using a bladder system or a traditional waist-belt bottle carrier, switch to a handheld bottle carrier.

Don't underestimate your energy needs during self-supported adventures and races. If aid stations are limited or nonexistent, prepare and place drop bags beforehand or enlist the help of family, friends, or teammates to resupply you along the way. (If you're on your own during longer training efforts, plan a loop course that brings you past a central resupply point.)

Cyclists and Mountain Bikers

Keep your thinking cap on. As a cyclist, you walk a finer line than most endurance athletes do when it comes to staying on top of your nutrition needs during prolonged efforts. Cyclists' fluid and fuel needs are some of the highest among endurance athletes because of the distance and duration of endurance cycling events. Despite knowing this, cyclists often find themselves caught off guard. The seemingly rapid onset of muscle glycogen depletion that forces you to slow your pace dramatically (referred to as bonking by cyclists) is a prime example.

Keep in mind that rapid evaporation of sweat can give you the false sense that you're losing only minimal amounts of fluid. The windchill factor that occurs during cycling may prevent you from feeling warm or overheated, which can delay or mask the feeling that you need to drink. On top of that, your body weight is supported while cycling, so you don't receive any feedback from ankles or legs being traumatized by pounding. Drafting and coasting allow you to continue to perform at a good pace. In other words, you can easily ignore or underestimate your nutrition needs because you won't feel poorly until it's too late. Anticipate your needs and adhere to a plan.

Be realistic about your fluid losses (urine and sweat) and your fluid intake while on the bike. Ingesting 16 to 20 ounces (480 to 590 ml) of fluid per hour during prolonged riding is reasonable for most cyclists under normal conditions. Riding in extreme conditions, such as heat and wind or high humidity, further increases your fluid needs. Your stomach should cooperate and be able to tolerate up to a quart (32 ounces, or 950 milliliters, for male riders, less for smaller female athletes) an hour, so aim for two small or one and a half large bottles per hour in extreme conditions. If drinking colder liquids doesn't make you feel nauseated (because of delayed emptying from the stomach), it can help cool you down and provide a needed boost on a ride in extreme conditions. (Add ice to bottles or freeze half a bottle of water or sports drink the night before and top it off immediately before you get on the bike.)

Keep up with your energy needs while on the bike. Continuously replenish the carbohydrate that you burn. By eating breakfast and topping off liver and muscle glycogen stores, most riders can perform well for the first 1.5 to 2 hours of cycling (for example, the first 30 miles, or 48 kilometers, of a century ride), relying only on an electrolyte replacement drink. If you expect to cycle longer than 2 hours, plan to refuel while on the bike. To extend your glycogen stores, begin to eat as soon as the event or race starts. Don't wait until you bonk or until your blood sugar bottoms out to try to remedy the situation.

Your calorie needs will vary tremendously depending on a multitude of variables, such as road surface, terrain, weather, wind resistance, speed or intensity, and your fitness level. Figure on about 30 calories per mile (~19 calories per kilometer) as a rule. Keep in mind that your estimated calorie needs increase dramatically as your speed increases (see table 10.1).

Road Races   Depending on the distance and specifics of each race, you may be carrying most of your own food (in jersey pockets) and drink. In longer pro-amateur races (lasting 4 hours or longer), racers often have food and water distributed to them as they roll through designated feed zones set up on one side of the road.

Stay with foods that you are used to eating as much as possible. Eat after cresting a hill, not shortly before a substantial climb or while climbing. Eat when you're at the end of a pace line, not in the middle or while pulling.

Sports drinks remain the most effective choice for meeting fluid needs, plus they do triple duty by also supplying carbohydrate and electrolytes

TABLE 10.1   Estimated Energy Needs for Cyclists

Average speed (miles per hour)	Calories required per kg of body weight per hour	50 kg (110 lb) cyclist	60 kg (132 lb) cyclist	70 kg (154 lb) cyclist	80 kg (176 lb) cyclist	85 kg (187 lb) cyclist
12	5.6	280	336	392	448	476
13	6.2	310	372	434	496	527
14	6.8	340	408	476	544	578
15	7.4	370	444	518	592	629
16	8.1	405	486	567	648	689
17	8.9	445	534	623	712	757
18	9.8	490	588	686	784	833
19	10.7	535	642	749	856	909
20	11.8	590	708	826	944	1,003
21	12.9	645	774	903	1,032	1,097
23	15.5	775	930	1,085	1,240	1,318

Weight in kilograms = weight in pounds divided by 2.2.

Select your average speed over the duration of the *entire* ride (do not calculate average speed based solely on riding downhill, riding uphill, or riding with a tailwind). Example: A 70-kilogram rider who averages 18 miles (30 km) per hour and completes a century ride in 5.5 hours would require about 3,773 calories or 650 to 700 calories an hour (9.8 cal/kg/hr × 70 kg × 5.5 hours = 3,773 calories divided by 5.5 hours = 686 calories per hour).

Adapted from S.I. Barr and J. Hughes, n.d., "Meeting caloric requirements." [Online]. Available: http://ultracycling.com/sections/articles/nutrition/calories.php [April 25, 2013].

(sodium). If the sweet taste deters you from drinking enough during extended races, carry an extra bottle of plain water and drink alternately from it or use energy gels (begin with one packet taken with a few gulps of water about every 30 to 45 minutes).

Organized and Self-Supported Rides Wearing a bladder hydration system allows you to carry a large volume of fluid without worrying about the need to stop and possibly lose your group. Be sure to choose a model designed specifically for cyclists.

Always carry something with you, such as prepackaged powdered drink mix and a snack (for example, energy bars or a peanut butter sandwich), in case you don't like what is offered at rest stops or need to refuel before or after a scheduled rest stop. What you take with you will determine how you carry it—jersey pocket, backpack, or taped to your bike. Eating on the bike is even more of a necessity if you are a slower rider because of the longer time that you spend riding.

Stopping to enjoy a real lunch break can provide a psychological boost. Just don't gorge yourself, because doing so will divert even more blood away from working muscles to your digestive tract. (Organized rides often offer a boxed lunch that you can buy beforehand.) Save your big meal for after the ride.

Recreational riders may choose to stop and eat at organized rest stops provided during century rides and other daylong events. Foods typically provided include fruit (often apples, oranges, and bananas), energy bars, energy gels, granola bars, bagels, peanut butter sandwiches, cookies, and mini candy bars. During longer rides, you might find potatoes, sandwich fixings, and ice cream bars.

Experienced professional endurance racers suggest this no-fail formula for a 150- to 160-pound (68 to 73 kg) cyclist who is attempting to finish a hilly century ride in approximately 5 hours: Start with a hydration pack full of water, one bottle of electrolyte replacement drink, and one bottle of a high-calorie drink, like Spiz (500 calories in 16 to 20 ounces, or 480 to 590 milliliters). Carry baggies containing premeasured powder and refill your bottles at every rest stop or along the way as needed. Consume 500 calories or one bottle of your high-energy drink per hour religiously right from the start.

Mountain Bike Rides and Races Set up a drinking schedule and stick to it. Keep it simple. Because you can easily lose track of time when you're undertaking a serious personal effort, especially when it involves traversing challenging terrain and negotiating descents, set your watch to remind you to drink every 15 minutes. Take advantage of any opportunity that you have to down a few sips. Drink during easy ascents, for example, when you tend to sit more upright and can more easily steady the bike with one hand.

Depending on the length of the ride or race and the available support, carry extra sports drink powder with you in premeasured amounts. Stop and mix up more as needed. Establish good habits now before you venture into ultralength rides. Develop a feel for where your water bottle is on your bike so that you don't have to take your eyes off the trail when reaching for it.

Keep your hands free by using a bladder hydration system. From a safety standpoint, a bladder system is superior because your hand will be off the handlebars for only a split second while you grab the drinking tube. Clean your bladder system promptly if you put a drink containing carbohydrate into it. These drinks promote the growth of bacteria and mold, especially in hot weather. To avoid having to do time-consuming cleanups, put only water in the bladder and make the sports drink in your bottles two or three times more concentrated. Then alternate drinking between the two.

Fuel up on real food. Over the long haul, real food is more fulfilling than energy bars and gels. Supplement the calories in your electrolyte replacement drink by eating easy-to-carry finger foods (toss them in your jersey pockets) that go down easily, such as raisins, grapes, small baked potatoes (eaten cold), and fig bars. Stick with foods that have worked for you on training rides. During longer races in which you rely primarily on liquid calories from concentrated drinks, snack on real food for a psychological boost.

In 24-hour mountain bike racing, make food an important part of the experience. Get together with your teammates, figure out what everyone wants, and then shop for it together. On the bike, rely on a sports drink and water. Off the bike, refuel with real food. The key to a strong finish is to drink a recovery beverage (for example, a high-carbohydrate or meal-replacement product) immediately after completing each leg to support your body's efforts to replenish muscle glycogen stores. Follow up with a small meal within an hour of getting off the bike.

Triathletes

During a long-distance triathlon, aim to replace 30 to 50 percent of the calories that you expend. For most triathletes, this translates into a starting point of 200 to 300 calories per hour (some elite athletes can train themselves to absorb more). Most of these calories (70 to 75 percent) should come from carbohydrate—sports drinks, energy gels, chews, blocks, bars, and other solid foods that are well tolerated. Consuming items that provide small amounts of protein or fat during half Ironmans can also help sustain you over the long haul.

Swim Because urinating isn't a problem on this segment, hydrate right up to the start of the race. In ocean swims, you'll inevitably swallow some salt water, so be prepared for a burning sensation in your throat. If you swallow enough salt water, your tongue will swell and you may begin the bike ride feeling sick to your stomach. Some triathletes even suffer from seasickness during choppy open water swims. The best plan of attack to minimize the effects of a choppy sea is to wear earplugs to combat nausea and to master bilateral breathing (to both sides).

Bike Become one with your bike. Triathletes spend the longest amount of time in a race on their bikes. This means you need to be proficient at eating and drinking on your bike at your intended race pace. During a race, control or slow your pace slightly when you are ready to rehydrate and refuel. Keeping a sleek aerodynamic bike on the road can be challenging as you juggle food and water bottles, especially in windy conditions. If stomach problems have hindered you during the run in previous races, review what you do on the bike. Don't overload your stomach by trying to do everything at once—consuming carbohydrate-rich gels plus bars and a high-calorie, protein-containing sports drink may be more than your body can handle. This suggestion may be especially relevant for female triathletes who attempt to adhere to fueling "rules." You also can try backing off from eating during the last half hour on the bike.

Run Gastrointestinal distress, such as nausea and bloating, is common during the running segment. The jostling nature of running and the progressive dehydration associated with several hours of continuous exercise slow the absorption of fluid and nutrients from the stomach. Recognize that an inability to urinate during the running segment is a red flag indicating that you've become too dehydrated. Slow or stop when you approach aid stations to ensure that you actually consume some fluid, rather than just pouring it on yourself or the ground.

If vomiting ensues during the run, think of it as wiping the slate clean. Slow or stop, regroup, and start over with your rehydrating and refueling efforts. An episode of vomiting is definitely a temporary setback, but you can rebound after you start to absorb the fluid and calories that you need. Sometimes chewing solid food, such as an energy bar or a banana, can help settle a queasy stomach and provide a much-needed mental lift. Some athletes find that chewing on a calcium tablet helps.

Transitions Relax and take your time as you make the transitions both onto the bike and into the run. Have your transition area set up in a logical, organized manner so that you can't possibly exit without your nutrition essentials. If you're wearing a bike jersey or a sports pack to carry food while on the bike, for example, put it on top of your unbuckled helmet or across your bike seat. Obviously, you want to prepare bike jerseys and packs beforehand, as well as any bike food holders, such as bento boxes and gel flasks, that you need during the race.

Always keep an extra water bottle handy in the transition area to drink from as you head out on the run. Take advantage of your slower pace as you make the transition into running by using it as an opportunity to refuel. As mentioned before, you may feel better by getting fuel in at the start of the run (for example, by drinking a sports drink) than by cramming food down during the latter stages of the bike portion. (To simulate race conditions, practice your transitions by racing against a friend during training.)

Marathon Skiers

Drink early in ski marathon races, ideally within the first 15 minutes. Choose an electrolyte replacement drink to meet your fluid and carbohydrate needs. You may not feel as thirsty while competing in cold weather or you may want to avoid making pit stops, but keeping on top of your fluid needs remains a priority.

Advances in technology have produced bladder hydration systems with tubes and valves that are less likely to freeze up in cold temperatures, but these systems aren't foolproof. If you've experienced problems before or expect extreme temperatures, wear a water-bottle carrier (with an insulated 16-ounce, or 480-milliliter, water bottle or larger) strapped around your waist instead.

Refuel at every feed station. Cross-country skiing uses the body's entire muscle mass, so energy (caloric) needs are extremely high. You can generally expect a feed every 10 to 15 kilometers in most ski marathon races. Be prepared to slow down to obtain a cup of fluid because volunteers may not be trained to deliver feeds by running alongside you. Save the sports drink that you are toting for between feeds and during rough patches when you need an energy boost. Slower skiers may need to stop and refill their bottles at feed stations or wear a bladder system that allows them to carry more fluid. Drinks and foods typically available at feeding stations include sports drinks, water, hot chocolate, soup, orange slices, energy bars and gels, cookies, and brownies.

Carry energy gels as backup fuel. Store them in the pockets of your water-bottle carrier or tape a packet to the front of your jersey or the inside of your arm (on top of your jersey). Choose a place on your body that you can easily reach. Consuming energy gels with water is best, so time your intake with a feeding station.

Be aware of the signs of bonking. You may feel unusually cold and experience shivering, or you may simply run out of energy. Two warning signs that trouble is just around the corner are experiencing hunger pangs and having overwhelming negative thoughts. Recognize that your brain needs fuel immediately. Consume carbohydrate-rich drinks and foods as soon as possible and pay attention to your hydration and fuel needs for the rest of the race. Two situations that may boost your normal energy needs are hilly courses and extreme weather.

Adventure Racers and Off-Road Multisport Adventurers

Know where your next drink is coming from. Whether it's an off-road multisport adventure or a one-day sprint adventure race, adequate fluid intake is paramount for survival and success. Experiment with bladders, waist belts, or water-bottle holsters that attach to the daisy chains on the front of a pack's shoulder strap. Keep in mind the ruggedness of the terrain. A bladder system that becomes punctured won't be of much use.

In single-day races, determine how frequently you will pass through staging areas, which in turn will determine how much fluid you need to carry with you on each leg. Figure on a minimum of one water bottle (20 ounces, or 590 milliliters) per person per hour, depending on the activity and the weather. (In self-supported situations, always use iodine tablets or other safety measures to purify water found along the way.)

Drink a sports drink in addition to plain water. The electrolytes that these drinks contain will help prevent muscle cramps and hyponatremia and will stimulate you to keep drinking. The carbohydrate provided by sports drinks will fuel your brain as well as your muscles. This attribute is a definite advantage during adventures and races that hinge on navigation skills or the ability to decipher mysterious challenges or special tests.

Don't wait until you feel thirsty to drink. Watch for the telltale signs of dehydration: headache, nausea, loss of appetite, personality change (loss of interest in bantering or answering questions), infrequent urination (dark color), clumsiness, lack of energy, and inability to tolerate heat or cold. Dehydration increases your risk for heat exhaustion, heat stroke, and hypothermia, all of which can prevent you (and your group or team) from finishing, especially during longer ventures. Stop before dehydration progresses too far. In severe cases, stop, seek shade, and try to rehydrate by sipping small amounts of water or other fluids as tolerated.

Have a plan for refueling. Lack of appetite is the norm during daylong adventures and races. Just because you're hot, sweaty, dehydrated, fatigued, sleep deprived, covered with mud, possibly well off course, and not the least bit hungry, you still must replenish your limited glycogen stores. In single-day ventures, sports drinks, energy gels and bars, and any other carbohydrate-rich foods (bananas, fig bars, breakfast and granola bars, Pop-Tarts, bagels, sandwiches, and so on) that you find appealing and have access to should do the trick.

Additional Recommendations for All Long-Distance Endurance Athletes

Whatever your discipline, you already should have experimented in training (long before the actual event or race) to discover and build a repertoire of acceptable food, drinks, and any other supplements that you can use to meet your fluid, energy, and electrolyte needs during long-distance races. You should have determined the basics—what and how much you need to eat and drink and when you need to eat and drink it—and put your strategies to the test in various weather conditions at your intended race pace or intensity. Following are some additional considerations to guide your nutrition choices during your event.

- Keep in mind that as your pace or intensity increases, blood flow to the digestive tract falls, which makes it harder to digest and absorb food items you take in. In addition, your ability to consume and absorb calories when running (because of significant jostling of the stomach) is far less (by as much as 50 percent) than when cycling. Rely on simple, readily available carbohydrate sources during high-intensity (closer to your $\dot{V}O_2$max) efforts or when you need a rapid energy boost. Choose electrolyte replacement drinks, energy gels, sport chews and blocks (take with water), glucose tablets, and if tolerated, non-diet soda or juice. During moderately paced longer efforts, add solid foods and high-calorie liquid drinks to boost your calorie intake and your spirits.

- Refuel frequently rather than eating a large quantity of food at any one time, since this diverts blood away from hard-working muscles. Spread out and consume hourly energy needs over 15- to 20-minute increments. In other words, don't try to cram it all down on the hour mark. The best sports drinks, high-calorie liquid drinks, energy gels, and energy bars for you are the ones that go down and stay down.

- Watch for signs of hitting the wall and bonking, and take steps to prevent them. Hitting the wall means that you essentially have depleted your body's reserves of muscle glycogen. Your legs (and other major muscle groups) have gone on strike, even though you may have been consuming adequate fluids and calories. Inadequate training preparation, improper pacing, and general fatigue all can contribute to this phenomenon. You will often be able to continue to the finish, albeit not with the desired performance.

  Bonking, when the body completely shuts down due to a severe drop in blood sugar, is a much more serious situation. The glycogen stored in the liver, as well as that stored in muscles, is essentially gone. Muscles and, more important, your brain are not receiving sufficient fuel. If left untreated, you may become increasingly irritable, confused, and disoriented. You could find you have to sit or lie down; in a severe case, you possibly could pass out and even lapse into a coma. Stop whatever activity you were engaged in and boost your blood sugar quickly by consuming whatever readily absorbable carbohydrate is available, such as sports drinks, soda, fruit juice, glucose tablets, or energy gels, chews, or blocks. Seek medical attention if necessary.

  The best way to avoid hitting the wall or bonking is to create a calorie buffer. Liquid calories in the form of electrolyte replacement drinks and high-energy liquid food products are favored because they tend to be well tolerated and require less effort to get down than do solid foods. Large male endurance athletes often have to consciously work to consume enough calories (as much as 500 calories per hour of prolonged cycling, for example, compared to 300 calories per hour for smaller female athletes) to stay in energy balance.

- The less fit you are, the fewer shortcuts you can take. Knowing what you can survive on while still performing well comes with experience.

If you are less fit or less efficient (a novice rider or trail runner, for example), you must drink and eat on a regular schedule. Set your watch or bike computer and train yourself to drink every 15 to 20 minutes and refuel every 30 to 60 minutes to keep pace with the energy that you're expending.

Team Up to Work on Fluid and Fuel

In races and events in which you rely on others to finish (relay and adventure races, for example) or to provide safety and companionship (treks and ski adventures), be certain that all group members take seriously the responsibility to hydrate and fuel themselves. In other words, pick teammates and adventure partners wisely! It's one thing if you are on your own. You harm only yourself if you don't drink and eat as required. If you're part of a group or team, however, you must be willing to force it down.

1. Make a nutrition game plan together beforehand. Don't wait until you're far from home or falling off race pace to discover that the food and drinks you're lugging around and counting on to get the group to the finish line are not acceptable or well tolerated. Discuss food likes, dislikes, and allergies, if any, first and then plan accordingly.

2. Food can make or break the experience. Besides supplying calories, carbohydrate, and electrolytes, food consumed during long group adventures and relay races provides a mental boost and improves morale—at least, it should. Include fun foods and, as much as feasible, a wide variety of real foods with varying tastes and flavors (especially salty foods, since so many sports foods are sweet tasting) so that something always looks appealing.

3. Divvy up the goods. All members of any group or racing team should carry fluids and some essential foods in their pockets, bum bags, or backpacks for convenience and, more important, in case they become separated from the group. Be sure that everyone in the group is eating and drinking. Share fluids and food as needed.

4. Keep an eye on teammates. Obviously, you need to be responsible for staying on top of your personal fluid and fuel needs, but you also must monitor teammates. In adventure races, for example, the first team to cross the finish line together wins. Teams that lose a member because of illness, fatigue, injury, or a team disagreement are disqualified. Dehydration, depleted muscle glycogen reserves, or a too low blood sugar level will make the endeavor or race seem even harder than it is. Be particularly sensitive to mood swings and personality changes; a friend or teammate in trouble may become extremely quiet or irritable and argumentative.

Postevent Recovery Plan

Do yourself a big favor. Shorten the time it takes to recover from a long-distance race or endeavor by supporting your body's efforts to replenish depleted muscle glycogen stores. You may tend to let down after you've completed a challenging goal; however, train yourself to take advantage of the first 30 minutes (the carbohydrate window) after crossing the finish line. Concentrate on quickly consuming fluids and carbohydrate, especially if you have another race in a few days or the following weekend. Not only will you feel more energetic the rest of the day, your muscles will experience less muscle damage and feel less sore in the following days.

Be prepared: Anticipate that you won't feel hungry following prolonged exercise. Begin by drinking carbohydrate-rich beverages, such as sports drinks, fruit juice, milk shakes, smoothies, lemonade, soda, and high-carbohydrate or meal-replacement beverages. Ease in carbohydrate-rich foods as soon as you can. If feasible, include a small amount of protein (10 to 20 grams) within this same window to prompt muscle repair. (At the very least, eat a well-balanced meal that includes lean, quality protein within 2 hours.)

Don't wait until you reach home (or for your appetite to return) to begin replenishing glycogen reserves. Postrace activities and long car rides home use up valuable time. Get in the habit of packing a recovery drink (powder to mix with water or a canned supplemental beverage) and drinking it within 30 minutes of finishing.

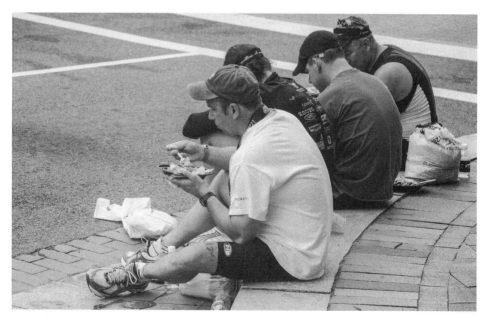

Veteran competitors of long-distance endurance endeavors understand the value of beginning their nutritional recovery immediately after crossing the finish line.

Be mindful over the first few hours following prolonged exercise to avoid rehydrating solely with plain water, especially if you're consuming little, if any, sodium-containing foods. By overdrinking plain water (often in an attempt to feel better because you believe that you're very dehydrated or assume that you must be following prolonged efforts), you may induce hyponatremia (too-low blood sodium level). Rehydrate instead with a sports (electrolyte replacement) drink or other salty fluids, such as soup or broth.

Drinking alcohol can impede your recovery by hampering your efforts to rehydrate (as a diuretic, alcohol causes the body to lose fluid) and by interfering with the body's ability to replenish depleted glycogen reserves. Your best bet is to make rehydrating with nonalcoholic beverages your first priority. Beyond that, realize that following a strenuous physical effort, your body may not be able to tolerate or process alcohol as well as it normally does, so indulge in moderation.

As soon as possible, jot down detailed notes on the success of your nutrition game plan, including prerace meals—what worked, what didn't, and what you want to do differently next time.

Counteract weight loss resulting from heavy training and competitive demands with a recovery period. Many endurance athletes lose a substantial amount of body fat while meeting the high energy demands of training for long-distance events. Give your body a full chance to recuperate, including restoring a modest amount of weight (if necessary), before jumping back into your full training program. (Some serious-minded athletes will have to consciously eat in a manner that promotes regaining lost weight.)

Eating smart and indulging within reason (including higher-fat foods and other fun foods) will help you avoid becoming run-down or susceptible to injuries. It's also part of taking what may be a much-needed mental break. This interlude will allow you to return to an ambitious training schedule and healthy eating habits with renewed motivation.

LEARNING FROM THE BEST: RACING A MARATHON

Deena Kastor, a three-time Olympian (winning a bronze in the 2004 Olympic women's marathon) and the fastest female American marathoner of all time (2:19:36, a 5:20 pace) is still running. In fact, the newly turned masters runner and mother of a 2-year-old is running strongly, easily winning her first masters race (a 1:12:57 half-marathon). Throughout her career, Kastor always emphasized finding a balance as the key to her success. In her words, don't be too obsessive in any one direction, don't get in a rut, and don't be afraid to be creative. Read on to find out how she applies this mind-set to decisions about food and nutrition when undertaking a marathon.

Practice makes progress. Kastor empathizes with fellow runners on the challenges of drinking while running at race pace. She recounts that early on, she needed a couple of months to become comfortable with grabbing a water bottle while running. Kastor says that marathoners shouldn't shy away from drink stops even if they feel foolish or are flustered on race day. She shares that one year during the prestigious London Marathon, she saw the elite runners' fluid station almost too late and literally banged her leg on the table as she grabbed her drink.

Focus on getting in needed carbohydrate—no one cares if the drink splashes onto your face or even into your eyes. "All runners have fumbled through an aid station or two at some point," says Kastor. During a race, the most important thing is to stay conscious of your timing. Replicating what she does during her long training runs, she hydrates and refuels with a sports drink every 20 minutes, right from the race's onset.

If need be, readjust your attitude about drinking and refueling during a race. Kastor, for example, doesn't view a marathon as 26.2 miles (42 km) long. Rather, a marathon is eight water-bottle stations long. She finds that counting down the aid stations is an easy and effective way to break up a marathon and make it more manageable. "I tell myself that each drink I get down brings me that much closer to the finish line."

Because the long training efforts leading up to race day are so critical, Kastor strongly encourages runners to make a conscious effort to start out long runs well fueled and to concentrate on taking in enough energy and fluids along the way. "Otherwise," she stresses, "going the distance has little purpose. Instead of getting stronger, you're only getting out of energy (caloric) balance and overstressing your body."

When the more popular sports drinks didn't settle well, leaving her feeling bloated, Kastor didn't ignore the science. She continued to experiment until she found one that she could tolerate. Instead of becoming discouraged and disgruntled, Kastor coaches runners to make a game out of finding an acceptable sports drink. "Conduct a taste test in which everyone in the family, even the kids, can get involved," she says. Not fast enough for personal bottles at the elite athlete's table? Not a problem. "Your system can and will adapt if you stick with it, so learn what drink will be available on race day and give yourself plenty of time to get used to it."

Make prerace meals count. Kastor's joyful attitude toward food continues right up to the race. "The night before, I find the best Italian restaurant in town and I dine with my closest supporters," she says, "including toasting them with a glass of wine." She focuses on getting in carbohydrate along with some easily digested protein. She doesn't gorge, however, or overdo it. Her favorite prerace meal? Pasta with her favorite sauce (pesto) and fish.

Far more important to Kastor is what and how much she eats on race morning. "This is the only time during the year that I count calories," she says. Adamant about being in energy balance to start the race, she consumes 400 to 500 carbohydrate-rich calories (a bagel, banana, and a sports drink) to replace the energy that her body burned overnight.

If perfection is your goal, be perfect at achieving balance. For Kastor, it's simple. "What runners need to succeed in the marathon is what all humans need to stay healthy and enjoy life—exercise, food, and rest," she shares. She continues to be dismayed by athletes who ruin this art of perfection by ignoring the need for quality fuel and choosing instead to fear food, rigidly restrict what they eat, or allow their training to dominate their family life. Kastor, who professes never to have suffered from prerace anxiety, coaches athletes to make decisions while training that will lead to standing on the starting line confident and eager to race. "That process includes showing up healthy, strong, and well fueled," she states.

11

Ultraendurance Events

We will have most normal foods seen at ultrarunning events along with the extras Across The Years is famous for. Previous years' meals have included M&M pancakes, French toast, grilled cheese, quesadillas, spring rolls, sushi, lasagna, pizza, and chicken cordon bleu. We can make food on demand and help you prepare your food; simply ask our aid station and they will do everything they can to accommodate your needs.

Source: Race information for Across The Years 72, 48, 24 Hour Footraces. [Online]. Available: www.aravaiparunning.com/acrosstheyears/race-information/race-information [April 25, 2013].

Perhaps you've spent a lifetime pushing the limits. So, why would you stop when it comes to sports? Or perhaps you're driven, even just once, to conquer something that only a select group of hardy souls before you has accomplished. The world of ultraendurance sports continues to expand, and opportunities to push the physical and mental boundaries of human endurance appear limitless. For our purposes, ultraendurance includes races that traditionally have served as the longest contests within a particular sport, such as the Ironman within the triathlon world, as well as all types of endurance events that can take up to 24 hours to complete.

This chapter is a must-read for endurance athletes who are considering moving up to or who are new to ultralength challenges, as well as veterans striving to PR in a traditional ultraendurance endeavor or race, such as the following:

Running: traditional and trail 50-mile (80 km), 100K, and 100-mile (160 km) races and 24-hour runs; specialty road and off-road ultras like the Comrades Marathon (90K), Death Valley Marathon (135 miles, or 217 kilometers), and Pikes Peak Marathon (elevation gain of 7,815 feet, or 2,382 meters, topping out at 14,110 feet, or 4,299 meters)

Duathlon, triathlon, or multisport races: traditional Ironman races, double Ironman, or other daylong extreme multisport adventures, such as the Powerman Zofingen long-distance duathlon (Switzerland, 10K run, 150K bike, and 30K run)

Cycling: organized rides (courses), brevets, and randonnees (up to 400 kilometers), especially if unsupported or ridden solo, as well as road races taking 10 to 24 hours or more, extreme off-road rides and races such as the Leadville Trail 100 mountain bike race and the 24 Hours of Moab ridden solo

Adventure racing: 24-hour races (courses), 30-hour races (courses), 1-day extremes

Hiking, trekking, winter sport adventures: sustained daylong (up to 30 hours) efforts and ascents, especially if fast packing or self-sufficient, alpine-style climbing, or solo undertakings

What's the biggest difference as you move up from long distance to ultraendurance-length events? Basically, you go slower and eat more—a lot more. If you don't, you won't finish or meet your time goal. An Ironman triathlon, for example, is a swimming, cycling, running, eating, and drinking contest. No matter how much training you've put in or how accomplished you are in the first three, the last two components will likely determine your success on race day. World champion and Hawaii Ironman winner Karen Smyers contends that her first Hawaii Ironman victory was half due to accomplishing the right training and half due to making the right nutrition decisions on race day. In the same vein, although her training during the following year indicated that she was in better physical condition to defend her title, she readily acknowledges that she was fortunate to rally and finish third after making one error in her drinking regimen during the bike segment.

Obviously, you can't complete an ultra without doing the proper training. It's not possible to just show up and drink and eat your way to the finish. Nutrition, however, is the area in which many ultraendurance enthusiasts can improve the most, especially those athletes who are underprepared for the challenge ahead, are approaching their limits, or are novice racers. As an ultraendurance athlete, you need to balance your nutrition awareness and knowledge against your training. Ignorance, laziness, or excessive focus on training details will doom you on race day. Bending basic rules of physiology and taking nutrition shortcuts has far greater potential to be disastrous (even fatal) during ultras than in other endurance-oriented competitions. Successfully completing (and especially racing) ultraendurance challenges takes extreme willpower, a mastery of all disciplines involved—including drinking and eating while on the move—and a little luck.

Pre-Event Nutrition Game Plan

To be a successful ultraendurance athlete, you must be willing to experiment, practice, and hone nutrition strategies, as much as is feasible, during training efforts and shorter events before attempting an ultralength race. During prolonged physical efforts, the dangers of renal shutdown or kidney failure, hypoglycemia, heat illness, a low blood sodium level (hyponatremia), and hypothermia (cold-induced problems) are very real. That's why credible ultra competitions typically require athletes to prequalify or, at the very least, to submit a resume of prior ultraendurance experience. It's simple—you won't finish, and you could even end up in the hospital, if you haven't learned to respect the nutrition aspect of ultraendurance challenges.

All ultraendurance athletes face, to some degree or another, a myriad of nutrition-related challenges that affect their ability to be successful:

- Managing precompetition stress and anxiety—the most likely cause of nausea, vomiting, and diarrhea before the start—to prevent under-fueling caused by limiting or avoiding pre-event meals

- Handling the logistics of hydrating, refueling, and meeting electrolyte needs when on the move, including answering questions such as the following: What's available? How can I supply, carry, or access it? What goes down and stays down at race-day (or event-day) pace?

- Minimizing gastrointestinal distress, such as nausea, bloating, cramps, vomiting, and diarrhea, during the endeavor or race

- Meeting the mental challenge of continuing to eat and drink when appetite is lacking, when feeling poorly, and during the latter stages of ultraendurance efforts

- Coping with flavor fatigue

- Dealing with personality changes and "brain fog" (loss of good judgment)

- Managing increased risk of kidney failure, hypoglycemia, and hyponatremia

- Dealing with varied, changing, and often extreme environmental conditions, which increase the risk for heat illness, altitude sickness, and hypothermia

- Contending with the effects of increasing fatigue, little or no sleep, and having to exercise through the night

- Solving problems on the go or in a constantly shifting situation (for example, what worked last time may not work this time); determining when to try something new and what to try

- Experiencing situations for the first time during the actual event or race (because, for example, it isn't possible to replicate the last 30 miles of a 100-mile ultra run, or last 48 of 160 kilometers, in training)

- Relying on and effectively communicating with others, such as volunteers, teammates, support crews, and pacers

For ultraendurance athletes, practice does not make perfect; however, it is the only road to follow to make progress. Practice during training and in shorter competitive efforts needs to include the following: preparing the digestive tract to handle and process fluids and foods during exercise; building a repertoire of acceptable drinks and foods to rely on to meet fluid, energy, and electrolyte needs; and experimenting with techniques (carbohydrate loading and prerace meals), supplements, and gear to find what best suits their needs. For serious Ironman competitors, practice may even mean simulating race conditions around transitions by racing against a friend during training.

Essentially, as an ultraendurance athlete, your practice hinges on building the mental discipline to do what you have to do when it doesn't seem necessary (when things are going well) and when you don't feel like doing it (when things are going poorly).

You can learn more about which nutrition-related situations to anticipate or what to experiment with by reading about ultras and talking with more experienced ultraendurance athletes. The information in chapter 10, Long-Distance Endurance Events, serves as a foundation or jumping-off point for moving on to the heightened nutrition concerns and recommendations covered in this chapter, so if you haven't already done so, read and digest chapter 10 now. To pick up invaluable insight before attempting your own ultra, observe longer races and serve as a pacer or as part of an athlete's support crew. To keep up with the vast array of available gear and nutrition options, observe races and visit specialty sports shops and ultra-focused websites.

Every ultra athlete has different requirements that he or she needs to determine well before the day of the endeavor. At a minimum, these include determining personal fluid requirements; choosing how to preload glycogen stores, meet energy needs, and prevent hyponatremia; and testing the effects of consuming electrolyte (salt) tablets, glycerol, caffeine, or other supplements before or during prolonged exercise. Based on science alone, for example, hyperhydrating with glycerol would appear to be beneficial. The incidence of gastrointestinal complaints is so high among ultraendurance athletes (particularly runners and triathletes), however, that the potential bloating, nausea, and abdominal distress associated with glycerol use may only further complicate your situation. The same goes for ingesting caffeine or using salt tablets—how much, when, and what form might work for you? What are the potential drawbacks and risks? (See chapter 5 for a review of supplements.) To determine how best to meet your requirements, gather as much information as you can about the options available to you and then use training bouts and other prolonged efforts, preferably in conditions similar to what you expect on race day, as dress rehearsals.

Being successful in ultra adventures and races will inevitably involve a lot of trial and error. Remember the caveat that every athlete, in the end, is an experiment of one. Also, despite the science, some things simply cannot be produced or replicated in a lab or, for that matter, in training or during shorter efforts. Simulating the last third of a 100-mile ultra run, for example, just can't be done. In the end, you just have to jump in and try it. Experience plays a large role in being a successful ultraendurance athlete. Knowing your body—what works, what doesn't, and what to try next—is truly what builds the necessary self-confidence and mental discipline to complete ultralength challenges.

During the Event

Your job, from a nutrition standpoint, is to hydrate and refuel in a manner that is smart and safe and, if you're racing, helps you maintain your desired pace as long as possible. A mantra worth remembering is "Eat before you're hungry; drink before you're thirsty." Keep in mind that meeting fluid, electrolyte, and energy needs during prolonged exercise is a twofold process—digestion and absorption. As an ultra racer, in particular, you must be prepared to slow down immediately when your digestive system isn't cooperating, regardless of your time or pacing goals. Ignoring or trying to push through gastrointestinal problems increases the likelihood that you won't finish.

Most ultraendurance athletes recognize the need to figure out what they can eat or digest while on the move. It's essential to know what will go down and stay down. Although some digestion, the physical and chemical breakdown of food, occurs in the stomach, ingested fluids and foods must empty from the stomach into the small intestine, where digestion of the three energy-giving nutrients (carbohydrate, fat, and protein) really gets going. The small intestine is also where these nutrients are absorbed, with water being reabsorbed or conserved by the colon or large intestine. Eventually, all absorbed nutrients end up in the blood, where they pass through the liver en route to being transported elsewhere in the body.

Simply figuring out beverages and foods that you can drink and eat during prolonged exercise isn't enough, however, nor is consuming them only when it's convenient or when you feel like it. The critical factor is the total time that it takes for any drink or food consumed during exercise to actually become available as fuel for muscle and brain cells. Your blood sugar level, for example, can bottom out during prolonged exercise if you exceed the stomach's capacity to absorb fluids that are providing supplemental carbohydrate. A sports drink that remains sloshing around in your stomach for a half hour, for example, doesn't help supply glucose to brain cells that are running on fumes.

In other words, to effectively supplement your body's limited internal glycogen stores during prolonged exercise, you will need to take into account the rate of digestion and absorption of what you consume. It's been observed that some extraordinary fit elite male endurance athletes have trained their bodies to be able to process as much as 500 carbohydrate calories per hour. Sports scientists had theorized that 280 carbohydrate calories (about 70 grams of carbohydrate) was the maximum amount that the body could successfully process in an hour. Recent research indicates that absorption increases, however, when multiple carbohydrate sources (sports drinks containing glucose or maltodextrins and fructose in a 2:1 ratio, for example) are ingested. The updated guideline for athletes going longer than 2.5 hours is to aim for 70 to 90 grams of ingested carbohydrate per hour of prolonged exercise. To maximize your performance in ultras, carbohydrate supplementation needs to begin right from the start and occur at regular intervals (to maximize absorption), not after you have depleted your internal glycogen stores. Otherwise, you create a deficit that you can never overcome.

Athletes can burn 400 to 500 calories or more each hour during an ultra adventure or race. Even lean athletes have enough energy stored as fat to sustain days of exercise, albeit conducted at a much reduced intensity (50 percent of VO_2max or less). Due to the constraints of digestion and absorption rates, however, our bodies are limited at fulfilling the hour-to-hour demand for carbohydrate, especially at the rate needed for sustaining the faster paces and harder efforts associated with ultra racing. On top of that, the specific sport also has an effect. An athlete can generally consume more calories per hour cycling (as much as 500 calories per hour), for example, than they can while running (perhaps 200 calories per hour). Hence, your ability to correctly pace yourself on race day is crucial to preserving internal muscle glycogen stores, as is the need to maximize these stores through adequate training and carbohydrate loading before you begin racing (see chapters 2 and 4 for a review).

To delay the onset of fatigue during ultraendurance efforts, commit right from the start to consuming carbohydrate-rich drinks and foods at regular intervals. Nevertheless, during the latter stages of ultra races when internal glycogen stores are depleted, the body increasingly relies on outside sources of glucose. Thus, the delivery of carbohydrate has to occur at a much faster rate to meet the body's fuel needs. The bottom line: If you don't drink and eat early on, you won't be around later on. And if you are around later on, you'll need to pay even closer attention to how often you eat and drink.

Fight Off Flavor Fatigue

The phenomenon of becoming increasingly turned off or repulsed during prolonged exercise by the first taste (sometimes even the mere thought or sight) of previously well-tolerated and well-liked foods is known as flavor fatigue. Getting the item down becomes increasingly difficult, and often times, impossible. This makes it even harder for you to meet your body's fluid and fuel needs. To combat flavor fatigue, train with and always have available various flavors of your preferred drinks, gels, chews, and bars. Alternate flavors frequently. Don't be caught empty handed when an old standby loses its favored status (if you're on the move long enough, it will) and seems inedible to you.

As time passes, most ultra athletes also will complain about the increasing sweetness of what they're consuming (especially sports foods), so anticipate this happening and prepare ahead of time. Include bland and especially salty-flavored options—such as tomato juice, peanut butter or cheese and crackers, small potatoes and hard-boiled eggs eaten with salt, jerky, whatever—even if those foods typically don't appeal to you during shorter events. As time goes on and the miles pile up, the goal is to find at least one item (in a drop bag, at an aid station, or in a turnaround or feed bag, for example) that is appealing to you at any given point. Although feeding zones are not always or entirely under your control, your chances are far better when you have a wide variety of foods to choose from.

Eat Real Food

Some athletes can get the job done during an ultra by relying solely on rehydrating sports drinks (about 14 grams of carbohydrate and 50 calories per 8 ounces, or 240 milliliters) and energy gels (20 to 25 grams of carbohydrate and 80 to 100 calories per packet), along with perhaps an energy bar or two. As the hours pass, however, most athletes will need more than just sports foods to meet their fluid and fuel needs. This is particularly true during the latter stages, when an ultra athlete needs to consume more carbohydrate at a faster rate as their body relies more and more heavily on outside fuel sources.

The easiest way to get in substantial calories is to drink more concentrated (higher-calorie) beverages and sports drinks, like Ultra Fuel and Carboplex sustained energy formula, and to rely on liquid meal-replacement products, like Ensure or Boost. Every endurance athlete knows (or soon figures out) that drinking much-needed calories requires substantially less mental and physical energy than trying to eat them. Use training efforts under various environmental conditions to find a drink that doesn't make you feel nauseated after just a few hours. (See table 5.2 in chapter 5.) Lean toward liquid food any time blood flow to the digestive tract tends to be low or compromised, such as when running or cycling intensely.

As an ultra adventure progresses past 10 hours or so, don't be surprised, however, to find it increasingly difficult to meet your fuel needs with just sports foods. During periods of moderately paced activity, such as while trekking, cycling moderately, or walking during an ultra run, blood flow to the digestive tract is greater (provided you've stayed up with your fluid needs). This is a reasonable time to try easily digested carbohydrate-rich solid foods, like fruit, bagels, fig bars, and energy bars, since you have a good chance of being able to tolerate them. Eating other solid foods (beyond the typical cookies and candy offered at aid stations) can be another real option for some athletes. Pizza, potato chips, milk shakes, even cheeseburgers, in fact, may be what truly save your race.

These protein-rich, higher-fat items, as well as any other similar real food that you can tolerate during prolonged exercise, are digested more slowly than all-carbohydrate foods like energy gels and standard rehydrating sports drinks. Solid foods empty from the stomach more slowly and take longer to be broken down (especially fat), so their absorption takes place over a longer period. You benefit from feeling full longer and from experiencing less queasiness and fewer hunger pangs. Plus, at the slower paces and lower intensity levels (50 to 60 percent of $\dot{V}O_2max$) necessitated by ultra distances, your body has enough time during the actual race to access and use the energy supplied by dietary fats ingested during the race. (Keep in mind that your body will be forced to use protein for fuel if carbohydrate or overall calories are insufficient to meet energy needs.)

What may be most important of all, though, is that eating real food helps to combat the "brain fog" associated with prolonged exercise. Over the long haul, solid foods can be comforting and can provide an invaluable morale boost. Remember, in the latter stages of an ultra, no calorie is a bad calorie!

Avoid Too Little and Too Much

Getting the drinking and eating parts of ultras just right on race day is part science and part art. Dehydration, depleted glycogen stores, and precipitously low blood sugar levels that cause fainting are all related to getting in too little fluid and fuel at the right time; obviously, they do nothing to enhance your performance. Ingesting too much, however, can slow you down almost as quickly and can be just as likely to keep you from crossing the finish line.

Remember that your body can handle and process only a limited amount of calories (particularly from those all-important carbohydrate sources) each hour. Forcing down additional food in the hope of topping off or getting ahead of calorie needs—say, in the early stages of an event to avoid having to eat later when it's less convenient or during the bike portion of an Ironman to try to prevent digestive problems during the run—typically backfires. Instead of having more calories available for fuel, you can turn your stomach into a whirling blender, especially if you will be running. Ingesting too much, most of which then sits in your stomach, will at the very least cause bloating, perhaps even nausea, and it slows the emptying and absorption rate of everything else that you consume. It also greatly increases your chance of vomiting, which means that you don't get any benefit from what you ingested.

Hypertonic, or highly concentrated, carbohydrate-based drinks (above the 5 to 10 percent carbohydrate concentration of standard rehydrating sports drinks), like juice, soda, and most caffeinated energy drinks, are also more likely than not to cause trouble. These beverages take longer to empty the stomach, setting the stage for potential digestive problems. Fructose in the amounts found in juice also is known to be less well tolerated during exercise than are other sugars. (Diluting by at least half with water may be helpful if you want to keep these drinks as options.) Many athletes, nevertheless, report having no problems with concentrated drinks. A smart strategy is to opt for a sports drinks supplying complex carbohydrate, such as malto-dextrins (long chains of carbohydrate that take longer to be broken down into individual glucose molecules), which boost the drink's calories and, in general, are very well tolerated.

Getting behind on fluid (water) can make whatever you ingest seem like it's too much. This is because dehydration slows the rate at which food empties the stomach into the small intestines. There, digestion and absorption is also slowed, which further delays the time it takes for nutrients to actually reach and fuel muscle cells. Athletes tend to mistakenly blame nausea, vomiting, and other digestive concerns on whatever they just ate or drank. Washing down energy gels with a sports drink rather than taking with water to properly dilute them; consuming too much of a concentrated, higher-calorie liquid food (drinks with sugar content above 10 percent, for example, or those containing both protein and carbohydrate) and too little actual water; or trying to do too much at once, such as consuming energy gels, a concentrated higher-energy drink, and energy bars or other solid food in a short period of time can cause athletes to feel they've have consumed too much and to subsequently develop digestive problems. Because eating on the bike is relatively easy, or at least easier than during other activities, road cyclists and Ironman triathletes during the bike leg need to be particularly aware of not overdoing it.

In terms of fluid requirements, athletes vary widely in how much they need to drink during ultraendurance endeavors. The weather, as well as your fitness level, can cause you at the same event or race to need a vastly different amount from one year to the next. As a general rule, however, most athletes will need between one-half and two 20-ounce (590 ml) bottles per hour. This is a lot of fluid to process without feeling queasy.

Dehydration and heat illness are the most common reasons for not finishing an ultra event. Kidney failure, or renal shutdown, is another serious consequence of failing to match fluid losses. Myoglobin, a protein material released into the bloodstream from injured muscle tissue, normally is cleared by the kidneys (causing urine to appear brownish in color). Without adequate hydration, however, myoglobin accumulates and clogs the kidney's filtering system, leading to partial or total shutdown. The participant guide for the Western States Endurance Run (100 miles), for example, cautions that two Western States runners have required a series of dialysis treatments and that others have been hospitalized for several days with IV fluids to correct partial renal shutdown. If not treated promptly, renal shutdown can permanently damage your kidneys.

Again, an important and limiting factor on performance is how much fluid the stomach can comfortably handle and how quickly it empties, with the consensus among sports scientists being a norm of 1 quart (1 liter) per hour. Your body will not be able to keep up, however, if you haven't practiced drinking this much (or more to meet your personal needs) during training efforts. Remember—the oft-given recommendation to drink 20 to 40 ounces (590 to 1180 ml) an hour or 4 to 8 ounces (120 to 240 ml) every 15 minutes, right from the start, is simply a general guideline. If you're considering an ultralength event, you must be very knowledgeable about your personal fluid needs.

Constantly monitor your body during prolonged efforts. Assess your ability to urinate and sweat and look for signs of hyponatremia, such as fluid retention (see chapter 14 for a thorough review of hyponatremia). Drink at a reasonable pace to match your sweat losses as closely as possible. Staying hydrated can be particularly challenging in certain situations. Due to limited resources and extreme conditions, daylong self-supported adventure racers, climbers, and trekkers, for example, may need to focus on drinking the largest quantity of fluid that they comfortably can handle on every available occasion to minimize fluid losses.

Two indicators will tell you how well you are hydrating during prolonged exercise: your weight and the color and frequency of your urine. A drop in weight from your pre-event or race weight is a clear sign that you are dehydrated. Some competitions, ultra runs in particular, require athletes to be weighed before the race. Weight and other vital signs are monitored throughout the race, and medical personnel use this information to decide whether to allow an athlete to continue. The goal is to stay within 3 pounds (1 kg or a little more) of your pre-event or race weight during the entire time that you're on the move. In terms of urinating, you should feel the need to go at least once every 2 hours, and your urine should be pale colored.

Gaining significant weight during prolonged exercise (more than 3 percent of preexercise weight) is just as dangerous. This circumstance indicates that your system is not processing fluids as fast as you are taking them in, increasing your risk for hyponatremia. Keeping the proper balance between fluid and electrolytes, particularly sodium, is crucial to maintaining a proper weight, avoiding cramps, and most important, getting back home or to the finish line safely. The only way to determine what amount of fluid and salt is right for you is to experiment in training. Most ultra athletes, in general, need at least 500 to 700 milligrams of sodium per hour (and for comparison, probably 20 to 50 milligrams of potassium). Every athlete is different. Be aware that your personal needs will vary depending on how well trained you are to perform in heat on the day of the event or race.

Factors That Can Contribute to Gastrointestinal Distress

Endurance and ultraendurance athletes often are quick to blame the last item they ate or drank for any gastrointestinal (GI) distress they suffer during an adventure or race. This is a possibility; however, a multitude of factors are involved, and any one of them or a combination of factors may be the true culprit behind common GI complaints of bloating, belching, heartburn, nausea, vomiting, slow stomach emptying, flatulence, cramps, and diarrhea. Consider just changing one thing at a time to help pinpoint what is an effective change and what isn't.

- Prerace nutrition (including prehydration routine)
- Underlying or undiagnosed medical conditions
- Emotional stress, including everyday stress or race-day stress, especially if it induces changes in bathroom habits
- Weakened digestive system due to lack of fitness, overtraining, or an unhealthy lifestyle
- Use of medications before or during (nonsteroidal anti-inflammatory drugs, for example)
- Placement or fit of sports equipment (fuel belts, waist packs, and so on)
- Disturbance of abdominal wall muscles (starting out too fast relative to ability and training, accelerated breathing from improperly sustained pace above comfortable pace, for example)
- Navigating steep descents too rapidly or with poor form (stride shocks have negative repercussions on digestive system) or eating before long descents
- Failure to slow pace early on to resolve or work through a GI problem (divert blood flow from working muscles in order to improve blood flow to digestive tract)
- Heat intolerance (weather related), overheating in general
- Effects of exercising at altitude, acute mountain sickness
- Taking in too much caffeine
- Taking in too many calories, especially too quickly
- Solid foods—eating foods you think you should eat, instead of those that appeal to you at the time; not chewing solid foods adequately; or in ultraendurance events, eating too few solid foods
- Taking in too much fluid

> continued

< continued

- Incorrect electrolyte content or faulty overall composition of drinks (too many ingredients, too acidic, carbonation)
- Inappropriate use of salt or electrolyte tablets
- Low blood sodium level (due to overdrinking or failing to consume enough sodium to match sweat losses)
- Dehydration or taking in too little fluid
- Taking in too many foods or drinks with concentrated carbohydrate (sugar) or too much fat (fatty foods), especially too much at one time
- Taking in sugar alcohols (i.e., xylitol) through items consumed

Mind Your Sodium

If you're going to be an ultraendurance athlete, you must take seriously the increased risk of hyponatremia, particularly during ultras undertaken in the heat. (See chapters 4 and 14 for more details.) Again, the best way to prevent this potentially fatal fluid–electrolyte imbalance during prolonged exercise is to use a two-pronged approach. First, constantly monitor your body and adjust your fluid intake to your losses (sweat and urine) on that day. Second, don't restrict your fluid intake during the race and do increase your sodium intake before and during prolonged exercise by ingesting salty foods and sports drinks that contain sodium. If you are gaining weight during the race or are plagued by a sloshing stomach, you need to temporarily stop drinking and slow down or stop to allow your body to adjust its fluid status. This is accomplished by getting rid of the excess fluid through urination. After that, you need to mindfully consume fluids with electrolytes or high-sodium foods.

Recognize that juice and cola drinks supply fluid but little or no sodium, thereby increasing your risk of hyponatremia. Some popular sports drinks made specifically for endurance athletes also contain little or no sodium, because you are expected to customize your sodium intake by ingesting salt through foods or by taking electrolyte or salt tablets. Know beforehand the sodium content of the drinks, gels, bars, and other foods that you rely heavily on.

No clear-cut guidelines exist for ingesting sodium during prolonged exercise—500 to 700 milligrams an hour is only a general recommendation. Don't overdo it. Salt tablets can irritate the lining of the stomach and induce vomiting, so take them with at least 6 ounces (180 ml) of water. (If you have a health problem, check with your doctor beforehand about using salt tablets during prolonged exercise.) Some athletes do better with ingesting salt directly (with water, of course), such as from the small salt packets typically found at fast-food restaurants or salty foods.

Protect Your Brain

Usually the first thing to go for an ultraendurance athlete is good judgment. Although persistence is required during ultras, zoning out and operating on autopilot is not an indefinitely sustainable state. Stopping to rest and to feed the brain is oftentimes what an athlete needs to do to get to the finish line faster, or even to continue, for that matter. Dips in blood sugar can leave you feeling overwhelmed, convinced that you are failing to make progress, and questioning your ability to continue.

If your blood sugar bottoms out, reach for readily absorbable, quick-energy carbohydrate sources such as energy gels, soda, juice, sports drinks, glucose tablets, or sugary candy. Slow your pace, walk, or stop altogether to give your body a chance to absorb the necessary carbohydrate. Your blood sugar level usually will stabilize within 15 minutes unless you're severely depleted. Seek or ask for medical attention if necessary. Heed slurred speech, blurred vision, and excessive confusion, crying, or irritability as serious warning signs that you need to do a much better job at keeping up with your energy needs.

Remember, the first half of an ultra is mostly physical. The second half is mostly mental. When you hit a tough patch, rely on strategies that have worked in the past, but, at the same time, be willing to try something new. Successfully finishing an ultralength challenge hinges on your ability to solve problems and keep yourself moving. Trust your training and give it a chance to come through. When you least feel like eating or drinking is when you most likely need to do so. The bottom line is that before making any drastic decisions, such as whether to continue or not, feed your brain.

Finally, if you choose to use nonsteroidal anti-inflammatory drugs (NSAIDs; for example, Advil, Nuprin, Aleve, and Actron) during an endurance competition, be aware of the risks. Although acute kidney failure is rare, be extremely cautious when using NSAIDs, especially while exercising in the heat. Taking NSAIDs during prolonged exercise when also dealing with severe heat stress or dehydration magnifies the potential for kidney problems and may contribute to the development of hyponatremia. Pay particular attention to your fluid needs before and during the event to minimize these risks. Taking NSAIDs may also upset your stomach.

Ultraendurance athletes often take Tums, Rolaids, or Imodium before or throughout prolonged exercise to prevent or minimize gastrointestinal problems. Again, no formal guidelines exist. Just remember that more is not necessarily better.

Sports-Specific Recommendations

Focusing solely on running, cycling, or putting one foot in front of the other during an ultralength challenge is simply not enough. Being competitive, achieving a personal best, or just making it across the finish line requires that you master the nutrition challenges inherent in ultras.

Ultra Runners

A 100-mile race is a running, drinking, and eating contest. You can't leave your nutrition game plan up to chance.

Know the location and timing of aid stations and drop points so that you can prepare what to have available and what to carry. This is why it's vital to write down or record your thoughts in some manner following training runs and shorter races and compile a database of what works for you and what doesn't.

Ultra runners make three classic but avoidable mistakes:

1. Not drinking enough early in the race—Don't just tote fluid around; concentrate on drinking it. Most runners carry two sources of fluid—plain water and a rehydrating sports drink (which contains carbohydrate and sodium). Most bottles hold 20 ounces (590 ml), for many runners, the minimum amount of fluid needed per hour. If you often arrive at aid stations with your bottles still full, consider adding handles to your bottles and carrying them as a reminder to drink more often (try this on training runs first). You should be urinating frequently (at least once every 2 hours), and it should be light in color.

2. Not taking in enough calories early—The crucial time to pay attention to nutrition needs is the first 70 percent of the race. You must make smart decisions about your fuel needs (as well as fluid and sodium) during the first 70 miles (112 km), or you won't be around to finish the last 30 (48 km). Forgetting to eat is easy when things are going well or seem under control early on. If you dig yourself into a hole, however, you probably won't be able to recover enough to continue, even if you desperately shovel in calories during the latter stages of the race. All your training will be for naught if you aren't smart about eating early in the race.

3. Not paying enough attention to the need for salt—No clear-cut guidelines or recommendations exist, since the need for sodium varies because of individual sweat rates and the weather. In hot and humid conditions, some runners may need as much as 1,000 milligrams (or more) of sodium per hour. Know beforehand the sodium content of the products that you intend to use (check the nutrition labels of energy gels, drinks, and so on) and determine how much you will be getting in the amounts of the foods that you intend to consume. During the race, choose salty foods at aid station stops, such as soup or broth, pretzels, chips, boiled potatoes sprinkled with salt, and so forth. If you plan to carry salt tablets with you, keep in mind that they disintegrate quickly if they contact moisture (sweat, for example), so place them in small plastic bags or other waterproof carriers. Take salt tablets with 6 to 8 ounces (180 to 240 ml) of water, and don't overdo it. Unlike salty foods, salt tablets don't stimulate thirst, so it is possible to ingest too many.

As an ultra runner, you definitely must learn to drink your calories. Few athletes can go the distance on energy gels and water alone. Although gels supply quick energy that goes down easily, they provide only 80 to 100 calories per packet, and most ultra runners need to consume roughly 250 to 500 calories per hour during a 100-mile race. The easiest way to get in substantial calories is by drinking highly concentrated energy drinks and using liquid meal-replacement products like Ensure or Boost. Save caffeinated beverages such as cola and Mountain Dew for when you really need a quick pick-me-up, such as in the later stages of the race.

Supplement with solid foods as tolerated. Realize that nothing will taste good or sound appealing as time passes, so nibble on a variety of foods as you pass through aid stations or meet up with your crew. Typical beverage options at aid stations (besides water) include sports drinks, soda, and possibly hot chocolate and coffee. Foods that you are likely to find include salt replacement foods, such as pretzels, soda crackers, chips, and soup; sweeter foods, such as fruit, energy bars, cookies, candy; and more solid choices such as boiled potatoes and sandwiches. Have your crew stock other foods that you've experimented with on training runs.

Time your eating and drinking so that you can do most of it when you're walking. In ultra runs, this typically means that you'll eat and drink when you're heading uphill. In the same vein, if your crew is meeting you somewhere other than an established aid station, have them meet you at the foot of a hill or mountain rather than at the top.

Your blood sugar can bottom out if you exceed the capacity of your stomach to absorb fluid. This may be the case if you feel uncomfortably full or bloated in your lower abdomen (as if you have two stomachs) or if the fluids that you've been ingesting seem just to sit in your belly and slosh around. In extreme cases, veteran ultra runners report relief by vomiting, which wipes the slate clean so they can start over. If you try this remedy, immediately begin your recovery by sipping on a properly formulated sports drink or broth made from bouillon cubes, not plain water. Remember, you will need fluid, carbohydrate, and sodium to be able to continue—the sooner, the better.

Periodic weigh-ins are a common practice at most 100-mile races. Be prepared to be detained (to drink and eat) or pulled from the race if you can't maintain your weight within an acceptable range (generally within 5 percent of your starting weight). As you attempt to rehydrate, consume sodium-containing sports drinks, soup or broth, and salty foods. The sodium in these items will help you retain the fluid that you consume.

Ironman Triathletes

During the race, aim to replace at least 30 percent of the calories that you're expending, which, for most Ironman triathletes, translates into approximately 2,500 to 5,000 total calories. To stay hydrated and to maintain a stable blood sugar level, most triathletes need roughly 250 to 400 calories per hour. Most of these calories (70 to 75 percent) need to come from carbohydrate—sports drinks, energy gels and bars, and other well-tolerated solid foods. Similar to other ultraendurance athletes, triathletes frequently report that consuming small amounts of protein and fat also is helpful over the long haul.

The goal is to enter the running leg in an energy-neutral state or slightly ahead, certainly not digging out from a calorie deficit that occurred from swimming and biking. Increasing fatigue and dehydration, dwindling glycogen stores, and the

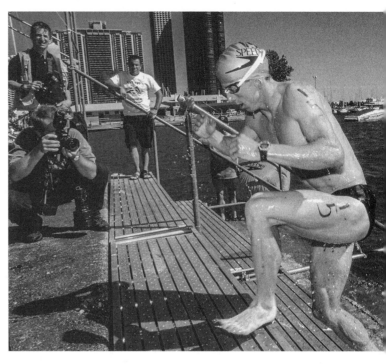

The real challenge of an Ironman competition is to stay hydrated and properly fueled throughout all three endurance disciplines.

likelihood of digestive problems when running all combine to make eating and drinking extremely challenging during the final leg of an Ironman. Ingesting adequate calories just to stay up with the energy needs of running 26.2 miles (42 km) is daunting enough. At this stage in the race, falling behind and needing to dig yourself out of a hole spells disaster.

Swim Because urinating isn't a problem on this segment, hydrate right up to the start of the race. Eating on the swim leg, obviously, is impossible. Due to the nonjostling nature of swimming, however, most triathletes can comfortably tolerate eating and drinking fairly close to the onset of the swim leg. Preload with a final carbohydrate boost (energy gel, chews, or blocks, or a sports drink) 30 to 60 minutes beforehand. You're trying to keep up with or replace at least some of the calories that you will expend during the upcoming swim. Figure about 8 to 10 calories per minute.

Bike Salt water swallowed during ocean swims causes a burning sensation in the throat. If you've swallowed a lot, your tongue will swell and you may begin the bike ride feeling sick to your stomach. Let your stomach, if necessary, calm down a little. Start drinking about 10 minutes out on the bike and take your first substantial infusion of carbohydrate (gel, chews, blocks, or a higher-energy carbohydrate drink) within 20 minutes of starting the bike leg. Be aware, however, that triathletes often get in trouble by drinking or eating too much, too soon, during the bike leg. Blood redirected to the stomach for digestion can interfere with reestablishing blood flow to hardworking leg muscles. Concentrate initially on sipping drinks and hold off on eating anything for the first 20 minutes.

As a triathlete, you spend the largest portion of time in a race cycling, so you absolutely must be proficient at eating and drinking on your bike. During the race, control or slow your pace slightly (or stop entirely if need be) when it's time to rehydrate and refuel. If the race features individual feed bags at the turnaround and yours contains something essential to your race plan, be prepared to stop for it (on the run too). Pack your turnaround bag full of many different foods to increase the chance that at least one item will seem appealing at that point in the race. Try including a treat that you can't get at aid stations on the course.

To stay up with the calories that you're expending and to overcome any calorie deficit that may have occurred during the swim, you need to drink and snack in appropriate amounts at regular intervals (starting early) during the bike segment of an Ironman. Be mindful, however, to avoid overdoing it. Athletes who fear or who have previously experienced significant digestive problems while running often try to get ahead during the bike segment, only to sabotage themselves later. Many triathletes find that they actually do better by getting fuel in at the start of the run (by drinking a sports drink, for example) than by cramming food down during the latter stages of the bike leg. If need be, try backing off from ingesting anything the last 20 to 30 minutes on the bike to give drinks and foods time to empty from your stomach before you begin the run.

When drinking isn't convenient, triathletes tend to not drink enough. Hence, the aero drink bottle was born. Several options exist for when you're on the bike, and this is definitely an area where convenience and optimal race-day nutrition strategies trump aerodynamics. Possible hydration systems include traditional mounted water bottles (on the down tube and seat tube), front mounted aero-bar systems, seat-mounted bottle carriers (for best aero-dynamics, mount a behind-the-saddle system so the middles of the bottles are approximately the same height as the back of your saddle), and bladder hydration systems. Many triathletes find it convenient to horizontally mount a water bottle cage between the aero bars so it rests between their arms.

The aerodynamic drag cost of any of these options (depending on the course, 10 to 20 seconds for every pound of extra weight on the bike in a typical Ironman bike leg) is far outweighed by the penalty of not drinking enough and suffering on the run. Choose the system that works best for you. Insulated water bottles that help keep liquids cold can help athletes consume more fluid. If your setup includes a water bottle on the frame (down tube), remember that, although nice, aero-shaped bottles can't be swapped out at aid stations, so they have little value in long course triathlons. If you opt for a bladder, choose a cycling-specific model.

Be careful of diluting sports drinks too much because doing so also dilutes the amount of sodium that you get. Some triathletes carry bottles of double-strength sports drink and dilute it by alternating with gulps from a water bottle picked up at an aid station. A safe system for novice racers is to start with two bottles—one of your preferred liquid food and one containing a sports drink. You can pick up water and additional sports drinks from aid stations along the course. A popular setup for Ironman racing that maximizes convenience and aerodynamics is two bottles behind the saddle in addition to the aero drink bottle mounted between the aero bars. This setup allows you to refill your aero drink bottle easily by using the rear-mounted bottles. You simply drop the empty bottle at aid stations and grab a full bottle without stopping.

Run Now begins the real challenge of meeting fluid and fuel needs while on the move. Gastrointestinal distress, such as nausea and bloating, is common during the running segment. The jostling nature of running and the progressive dehydration associated with several hours of continuous exercise slow the absorption of fluid and nutrients from the stomach. (Some fluid sloshing around in your stomach is to be expected.) At this point, stick to sports drinks, water, and energy gels, chews, and blocks (and possibly soda) to minimize digestive problems. Take small amounts at regular intervals. Recognize that an inability to urinate during the run is a red flag that you've become too dehydrated. Slow or stop when you approach aid stations to ensure that you consume some fluid, rather than just pouring it on yourself or the ground.

If vomiting ensues during the run, think of it as wiping the slate clean. Slow or stop, regroup, and start over with your rehydrating and refueling efforts. Vomiting is definitely a setback; however, you can rebound once your body starts to absorb the fluid and calories that it requires. Remind yourself that the only way to finish is by replacing, mile by mile, the fluid, calories, and carbohydrate that you need. Chewing solid food, such as an energy bar or a banana, sometimes can help settle a queasy stomach as well as provide a much-needed mental lift. Some athletes find that chewing on a Tums tablet also helps.

Transitions Relax and take your time as you execute the transition both onto the bike and into the run. Set up your transition area in a logical, organized manner so that you can't possibly exit the transition area without your essentials. If you're wearing a bike jersey to carry food while on the bike, for example, put it on top of your unbuckled helmet or across your bike seat. Obviously, you should pack gel flasks, bento boxes, and bike jersey pockets beforehand. Always keep an extra water bottle handy in the transition area to drink from as you head out on the run. Again, rather than overdoing it during the last part of the bike leg, take advantage of your slower pace as you transition into running by using it as an opportunity to refuel.

Monitor your hydration efforts by keeping tabs on your ability to urinate; at least once every 2 hours (every 30 to 50 miles, or 48 to 80 kilometers, on the bike) throughout the race is a rough guideline. If you choose to drink soda (for example, Coca-Cola), consume water with it. You'll dilute the carbohydrate concentration of the soda into a more optimal range that favors absorption. Keep in mind that soft drinks also contain minimal amounts of sodium compared with a typical sports drink, increasing the risk of hyponatremia, especially in susceptible individuals. Some seasoned Ironman triathletes drink Coke from the outset of the run (at every aid station). Others prefer to hold off as long as possible. Reaching for Coke can provide an almost immediate psychological boost; however, in most cases, the lift is only temporary. Be prepared to continue with Coke after you've started drinking it.

Additional Recommendations

The bottom line: When it comes to replacing fluids and electrolytes and keeping up with the fuel needs of the body during ultras, you must develop and follow a plan. You cannot rely solely on thirst or hunger and your memory or good judgment (especially during ultras) to prompt you to refuel. Many interrelated factors conspire to make it extra challenging to get the nutrition piece of ultras just right:

- All exercise reduces blood flow to the digestive system to some degree, especially vigorous exercise (starting around 70 to 75 percent of $\dot{V}O_2$max), and this reduced flow delays the rate at which the stomach empties.

  Train adequately and intelligently to maximize your fitness level and adhere to a proper pace throughout the endeavor, especially during the early stages.

- Dehydration also delays the rate at which the stomach empties, setting the stage for bloating, nausea, and vomiting. Dehydration further compromises the body's fluid and energy balance because it slows the rate of digestion and absorption of all drinks and foods consumed. (Whenever your overall blood volume falls, less blood is available to flow to your digestive system.)

  Right from the start (as much as humanly possible), match your fluid and electrolyte needs with losses on an hour-to-hour basis.

- Activities like running that involve physical jostling (mechanical trauma) of the stomach and other abdominal organs interfere the most with stomach emptying and the rate of digestion and absorption.

  Starting right from the beginning of any ultra, regularly take in small amounts of carbohydrate-rich drinks and foods. Lean toward semiliquid or liquid calorie sources because liquids empty more quickly than solids do.

- Abdominal cramps and diarrhea arise during ultras due to overactivity, including the physical jostling of the lower digestive system (small intestines and the colon). Reduced blood flow to the digestive system makes matters worse.

  You need to have an hourly hydrating and refueling plan that aims to keep up with fluid, electrolyte, and energy needs without overloading the system at any one time.

Stop Reaching for the Water Bottle

Triathletes are needy people. Traditional bike shorts, running attire, and water bottles just don't work for them—especially over the long haul. The logistics of swimming, cycling, and running all in the same event have led to the development of a whole range of specialized equipment and clothing. Aerodynamic hydration systems, in particular, have evolved to meet the needs of the triathlete during a triathlon's cycling leg. Front-mounted to the handlebars or an aero bar, an aerodynamic hydration system offers many benefits during a race:

- Hands can always remain on the handlebars and eyes can remain on the road.
- It enables the rider to take frequent sips instead of big gulps.
- The front-mounted design means no more dropped water bottles from reaching down or behind while riding.
- The translucent container allows fluid levels to be seen at all times, eliminating the guesswork for a refill when approaching an aid station.
- The splash guard prevents spills.
- Bottles or reservoirs are easily refillable while riding.
- It eliminates the extra weight and hassle of carrying and reconstituting a sports drink powder (if using something other than course-supplied drink).
- Cool water (course supplied) added periodically makes the drink more palatable, which encourages more fluid to be consumed.
- The aerodynamic design reduces wind drag.
- Some designs have two separate liquid compartments (each with its own straw), allowing two different fluids to be carried in a single bottle.

Before using a new hydration system in a race, it's a good idea to practice with it. The following tips will help you get the most out of a new system:

- Know the fluid volume of your system and the nutrient data of your sports drink (when reconstituted) in order to mix your drink at the proper carbohydrate concentration. For example, a 28-ounce (828 ml) drinking system can hold 4 ounces (118 ml) of a typical concentrated sports drink and 24 ounces (710 ml) of water. Eight ounces of this mixture will provide about 60 calories and 15 grams of carbohydrate—well within the 6 to 8 percent concentrated carbohydrate range that is recommended during moderate to vigorous exercise.

- Determine beforehand your sweat rate, calorie requirements, and carbohydrate needs while biking (ideally in conditions similar to what is expected on race day). These calculations will help you determine how many times you will need to refill the contents of your bottle during competition.

- Prior to the race, fill one regular water bottle with enough concentrated drink mix for the entire race. Mark the outside of the bottle at 4-ounce increments (or some other predetermined amount).

- When approaching an aid station in a race, add 4 ounces of concentrate to the hydration system. Grab a bottle of water at the station (most races supply the 24-ounce size) and empty it into the hydration system as you ride—you're all set! Additional electrolytes can be added at any time as suits your need. Also, be sure to grab extra bottles of water throughout the race to take with energy gels or solid foods, as necessary.

Postevent Recovery Plan

You really can enhance your recovery if you make smart nutrition choices following an ultra event. Granted, you'll be sore and exhausted no matter what you eat or drink afterward; however, you can lessen somewhat your discomfort and the extent of muscle damage (and rejoin the living sooner) when you make your nutrition needs a priority following prolonged, exhaustive exercise.

Rehydrate with something other than plain water or alcohol. Drinking only plain water, especially if you're not able to get or keep any food down, can induce hyponatremia in the hours and first few days following prolonged exercise. It's crucial to consume electrolyte-containing fluids after ultras for the first few to several days, until your digestive system is fully functioning and your urine is clear and of normal frequency. This means drinking sports drinks, broth, soup, and tomato juice. Eating salty foods, as much as tolerated, will also help your body reestablish its normal fluid–electrolyte balance.

Drinking alcohol following all-out efforts impedes recovery by hampering an athlete's efforts to rehydrate (as a diuretic, alcohol causes the body to lose fluid) and by interfering with the body's ability to replenish glycogen. Beyond that, realize that following an exhaustive physical effort, your body may not be able to tolerate or process alcohol as well as it normally does, so indulge in moderation, if at all.

Do your best to ease nutritious foods in as soon as possible. Liquid calories provided by milk, low-fat milk shakes, fruit smoothies, and meal-replacement drinks (Ensure, Boost, and so on) often are the easiest place to start. (Many ultra athletes anecdotally report being able to tolerate dairy foods, such as milk and ice cream, well after ultras.) Focus on including food rich in high-quality protein (meat, fish, eggs, soy foods, and beans) along with wholesome, complex carbohydrate at all meals for the next several days. This supports glycogen resynthesis and hastens the repair of damaged skeletal muscle. Of course, don't ignore your cravings—you've earned the right to celebrate.

Some degree of muscle necrosis or muscle cell death occurs from participating in ultralength exercise, especially in the leg muscles of runners. This condition is further pronounced in athletes who have become significantly dehydrated or have overexerted themselves. Complete recovery can take months. Eating a well-balanced, nutrient-rich diet supports the recovery process; however, simply eating right is not enough to fix this underlying damage. Don't resume serious training until you have recovered fully on all levels.

To improve the odds of being successful in the future, record your thoughts and observations about your nutrition strategies as soon as possible following an ultra competition. What worked? What didn't work? What do you want to try or remember to do next time? Karen Smyers, former International Triathlon Union World and Hawaii Ironman champion, easily recounted to me the nutrition game plans of her past Hawaii Ironman races. She simply looked up the details in training logbooks that she always kept.

If you were slowed or foiled by digestive issues, particularly intestinal cramps or diarrhea, spend some time thinking objectively about your training and physical preparation. Stomach-related problems are not only about what you did (or didn't) eat and drink before and during an ultralength endeavor. Fitness matters greatly. The fitter you are overall, the greater the blood flow to the stomach and intestines at any given pace or level of exertion. This translates into being able to better handle and process the fluids and foods that you need to consume along the way.

LEARNING FROM THE BEST: TIPS FOR SUPPORT CREWS

Like all good ultra runners, ultra race champions Ann Trason (holder of multiple ultra world records and 13-time women's winner of Western States) and Tim Twietmeyer (5-time winner of the Western States 100) often crewed for other ultra runners when not racing themselves. These accomplished veterans have this advice for you when it's your turn to crew at an ultra run. I put all these tips to good use when I crewed for my husband at the Leadville Trail 100 race in Colorado.

As a support-crew member, make sure to have your own personal stash of food and drinks. Crewing for an ultra athlete is typically an extremely long day, and you don't want to become too hungry. You are the brains behind the operation, and your athlete is depending on you to remain alert. You also want to have fun, and that's a lot easier to do that when you have plenty on hand to eat and drink.

Have the runner write out a plan for you. If the runner won't do that, at least talk to him or her as much as you can about race specifics before the competition. Do this a few days before the event, not the day before. A good ultra runner will want to make your life easy. You need to know, for example, anything unique the runner might need or crave along the way, as well as what he or she must absolutely carry when departing the various aid stations.

Don't bombard your runner with questions as he or she arrives at an aid station. Before the race, have the runner give you a short list of questions that you should always ask. Trason, for example, would have her crew ask whether she wanted more ice in her bottles and whether she thought that she was getting enough salt. Make certain that your runner actually is eating and drinking. Specifically check the runner's bottles, for example, when he or she arrives at the aid station.

Because your runner might not even remember his or her name after 70 miles (112 km), Twietmeyer suggests asking a basic set of questions to draw out important information that the runner might otherwise forget. As a support-crew member, take care of the details as well as the big things. Even simple stuff can bog down a runner late in the race.

Have available as much information as you can about the various drops and aid stations. Write it down so that there is no confusion. Most important, obviously, is to know (and keep track of) the time at which to expect your runner to arrive so that you can be there! Be ready to share information with your runner, such as how far the person has run and the distance to the next aid station. Split times from previous years can be useful to have on hand. If you keep split times of other runners, you can share with your runner how the race is going.

Expect your runner to go through emotional difficulties. Stay positive, be flexible, and work at solving problems as they arise. Always think of yourself as the brains of the operation. Playing games with your runner to keep him or her going is OK. If the runner wants to drop out, for example, tell him or her that dropping is not an option at this point. Reassure the runner that if he or she makes it to the next scheduled place and still wants to drop, you will talk about it then.

12

Multiday and Multileg Endurance Events

The Race Across America (RAAM), widely considered the hardest road cycling race in the world, is an annual 3,000 mile nonstop bike race across the United States. There are no sleep breaks in RAAM, so racers sleep when they want (RAAM soloists average 1 hour per day); however, they're still on the clock and the race doesn't stop. Solo riders eat sugary foods nonstop to replace the 10,000 calories that they burn a day, and for those that don't brush at each pit stop, teeth may decay rapidly.

Source: A. Bland, 2012, "Grueling travel through beautiful places: The madness of extreme races." [Online]. Available: http://blogs.smithsonianmag.com/adventure/2012/05/grueling-travel-through-beautiful-places-the-madness-of-extreme-races/ [April 25, 2013].

Is one day of exertion simply not enough for you? Today, more endurance athletes than ever are asking their bodies to perform beyond 24 hours. Others expect to deliver shorter, all-out performances several days in a row. For example, 60 to 80 hours of nonstop adventure racing is a very long day. Taking part in a weeklong trail-running camp or a cross-state ride, which hopefully includes enjoying yourself and not getting injured, hinges on your body being ready day after day. So, you must be prepared to perform again and again if others are counting on you to complete multiple legs of a relay-type adventure.

These types of endurance endeavors are a real test of your nutrition strengths and weaknesses, as well as your mental discipline. Poor planning and lack of attention to detail, especially on how best to recover from day to day (or leg to leg), quickly become apparent. An otherwise challenging and fun endurance event can dissolve into a slog fest or, worse, a never-ending nightmare. Being smart about what and how you eat and drink during multiday adventures and races is a key component of the ultimate outcome—and it's one of the few factors under your control.

This chapter is for endurance athletes participating in multiday races, such as the following:

Running: road relay races such as Hood to Coast (12-person teams covering 197 miles, or 317 kilometers, from Mount Hood, Oregon, to the Pacific Ocean), cross-state and cross-country runs

Cycling: organized cross-state and cross-country rides, randonnees (400 to 1,200 kilometers), cycling classics, Race Across America solo, tandem, and team qualifiers and races

Adventure racing: expedition-length races (a few days to a week) like the Raid World Championship, solo adventure races (200 kilometers)

Trekking and skiing: climbing trips and expeditions, through-hiking, backcountry trips, and winter hut-to-hut trips

All-endurance sports: organized tours or personal adventures, sports camps, multisport relay-type races (for example, each person is required to perform two or more legs)

The scope of multiday endurance events is tremendous, including everything from a two-day organized ride with supported rest stops to months of being self-sufficient while through-hiking the Appalachian Trail. This chapter provides an overview of the most important nutrition-related principles that come into play. These basic recommendations work well with specific tips and strategies provided elsewhere in part II of the book (see chapters 9 through 11 and 13 through 16).

One of the greatest challenges facing participants in multiday endurance races is knowing when to eat. Many things get in the way—the actual activity (running, cycling, climbing, and so on), maintaining gear and clothing, personal hygiene and tending to injuries (blisters, saddle sores, and so forth), the need to rest or sleep, and, if racing, competitive strategy. Throw into the mix getting lost, spending time connecting with support crews, lost drop bags, misplaced supplies, weather delays, extreme heat or cold, altitude, fickle stomachs, loss of appetite, extreme fatigue, mental apathy, and a host of other unexpected surprises, and you can see how something as basic as eating and drinking can slip off the radar screen. If you neglect to hydrate and fuel yourself during multiday endeavors, however, you will pay a steep price. Although mental toughness, patience, and first-rate problem-solving skills are prerequisites, they do ensure that you will complete your event—your body always has final veto power.

Energy Needs

Before multiday and multileg events and races, your job is fourfold:

1. Start out adequately hydrated by drinking enough of appropriate fluids in the 2 to 3 days leading up to the competition.

2. Start out with an optimum fluid–electrolyte balance by using higher-sodium foods, salting foods to taste, and further increasing your sodium intake for 3 to 5 days beforehand if extreme heat, high humidity, or conditions warmer than what you trained in are expected.

3. Start out well fueled by carbohydrate loading (begin at least 3 days before the event) to ensure maximum muscle glycogen stores.

4. Eat a substantial carbohydrate-rich breakfast 1 to 4 hours beforehand. (Timing is dependent on how important it is for you to start with an empty stomach.)

Once your chosen endurance endeavor begins, your job is to take advantage of any opportunity that arises to rehydrate, refuel, and recover. Make smart use of the time, in other words, any time it makes sense to do so.

Multiple Shorter, Higher-Intensity Efforts

To maintain the faster-paced, higher-intensity efforts required in relay races and events during which you alternate being on and off (cycling pulls or running legs, for example), carbohydrate is burned as fuel almost exclusively. Carbohydrate loading, therefore, is appropriate before these types of events. If your "on time" is 30 minutes or less, you are unlikely to need or benefit from actually eating anything during your pull or leg, since you'll likely be nearing your anaerobic threshold and working hard. Drink once more before you go. For example, drink 5 to 10 ounces (150 to 300 ml) 10 to 20 minutes beforehand or take an energy gel with water 5 to 10 minutes before you go. Consider carrying fluid with you (water or a sports drink, especially during all-out efforts of 45 to 60 minutes) to alleviate dry mouth sensations and to help with heat tolerance. And, remember, you may be able to boost your performance even if all you do is swish your mouth with a carbohydrate-rich sports drink.

What you do nutrition-wise during your off time is much more critical. During short breaks, like 30 to 60 minutes, you must refuel to cover the carbohydrate that you'll burn during the break as well as the carbohydrate that your body will use during your next effort. As a rule, consume 60 grams of carbohydrate per break or during downtime lasting 30 to 60 minutes to keep pace with the body's ability to process or oxidize up to 1 gram per minute of carbohydrate ingested during exercise. Obviously, a 30- to 60-minute break doesn't give you a lot of time for digestion. Liquids and gels are most efficient at this point—4 cups of a sports drink or two gels taken with water supply 60 grams of carbohydrate.

During longer breaks of up to 2 hours, be prepared to consume a liquid-food drink or small amount of well-tolerated carbohydrate-rich food, such as a banana, breakfast bar, or energy bar, in addition to water or a sports drink. You can use real food if desired and available during longer blocks of time off, such as when you have 3 hours or more (runners may need at least 4 hours off). The key is to eat at the start of your break period (and definitely before you collapse and go to sleep), not to do a hundred other things or wait until you feel hungry.

Multiday Events

The biggest danger with multiday rides, runs, treks and tours, cycling classics, sports camps, and climbing expeditions is incomplete recovery—you slowly become glycogen depleted as each day passes and thus become increasingly fatigued. You find yourself less and less capable of responding quickly or of maintaining a desired pace, and, mentally, your commitment and enthusiasm are waning. (Chronic fatigue, of course, can set in as early as day 2 or 3 if you haven't trained adequately with long back-to-back efforts; however, you can't do anything about that now.)

When it comes to eating and drinking, think before, during, and after. To maximize your glycogen stores, fuel up every day before you start with a carbohydrate-rich breakfast. If you'll be pushing the pace or racing (working at moderate to high intensity, above 60 percent of $\dot{V}O_2$max), eat and drink at the earlier end of your acceptable breakfast window so you can start out on an empty stomach and minimize digestive problems. Drink again as near the start time as you can or top off with an energy gel taken with water. If the day is going to be more of a long, slow effort, then it's generally OK to eat closer to the start (say, 2 to 3 hours beforehand) and to include higher-fat foods that take longer to be digested.

During the event or race, you'll need to drink regularly (every 15 to 20 minutes) and refuel (every 30 to 60 minutes) from the onset with the goal of consuming close to 60 grams of carbohydrate per hour. Sports drinks are the rehydrating beverage of choice to replace fluid and electrolytes. Along with sports drinks, a safe approach is to rely on energy gels and well-tolerated carbohydrate snacks during faster-paced efforts. Be prepared with salty foods or electrolyte tablets to help keep pace with your sodium needs. On long, slower days get a mental boost by incorporating plenty of real foods.

The key is to drink and snack regularly as you go, keeping pace with the calories that you're expending. Unless you have planned a break of 4 hours or longer, eating a large amount at any one time, such as a lunchtime meal or a meal during a rest stop, will divert blood away from working muscles when you resume exercising. You will feel lethargic and unresponsive and end the day lamenting how much harder the second half was.

When you finally stop moving for the day, your job isn't over. Consciously take advantage of the carbohydrate window, particularly the immediate 15 to 30 minutes, to maximize glycogen replenishment (see chapter 4 for a review). Ingest a substantial amount of calories from carbohydrate-rich foods and drinks immediately—at least .5 grams of carbohydrate per pound (~1.0 grams per kilogram) of body weight. (Even better, take in .75 grams per pound.) Remember, these are carbohydrate calories, not calories from just anything, so don't count on beer, nacho chips, or candy bars. A meal-replacement beverage or recovery drink with at least 10 grams of protein (see table 5.2) can make the job easier, and the protein ingested along with carbohydrate may help to reduce muscle soreness.

Each evening, eat a high-carbohydrate meal that includes a good source of quality protein (for example, 20 to 30 grams as supplied by 3 to 4 ounces, or 85 to 112 grams, of meat). If need be, eat another carbohydrate-rich snack before bedtime.

Weighing yourself (if feasible) before you start and then again right afterwards can help you quickly ascertain how well you're doing during the race at meeting your fluid needs. Over the next few hours, drink at least 2.5 cups of fluid for every pound (or 1.3 L for every kg) that you are down. If your weight has dropped more than a couple pounds, adjust your drinking plan for subsequent efforts. Pay attention to your sodium intake, too. Losing weight from day to day (especially during endeavors lasting longer than 5 days) and struggling to respond due to sore or "dead" legs are prime signs of chronic glycogen depletion. Your job is to stop the damage that's occurring before it becomes too great to reverse. This means eating more (especially carbohydrate calories), taking more time to recover, or, most likely, doing some of both.

Continuous Efforts

Endurance events such as multiday adventure races or continuous cycling races in which the goal is to keep moving no matter what (especially if you must meet timed cutoff points) present the most complex and challenging nutrition scenarios. How do you consume massive amounts of calories to keep muscles fueled and working while at the same time making sure that this high-calorie infusion doesn't hinder your performance? A few themes become clear.

First, you must refuel on the go at every opportunity, relying on liquid calories as much as possible (and feasible). Liquids are absorbed more efficiently than is solid food, thereby reducing the risk of debilitating digestive problems.

Second, successful multiday endurance athletes consistently report using their training sessions to develop both smart eating habits and the ability to eat constantly. Eating while continuously on the move, in other words, is a learned skill. It requires a lot of mindful practice. Given the wide variation in individual tastes and preferences, the only way to determine what types of food you personally tolerate best is to experiment. This includes discovering how foods perform in various environments, such as hot and cold weather and at altitude, and, of course, how much you can tolerate. Confidence in your ability to cope with the mind-boggling array of conditions and circumstances that you will inevitably confront during a multiday race won't come from a book, a website, or a friend. You develop confidence in your ability only through detailed trial-and-error experimentation.

Third, you must be able to keep separate your nutrition (calorie) and hydration (fluid) needs. Bodies require adequate water and fuel to keep moving continuously. Staying adequately hydrated, however, is the key to everything else you need to have occur (and keep occurring) while on the move. Dehydration disrupts everything: less blood flows to working muscles and to the brain; your ability to tolerate the heat decreases because you are less able to dissipate heat generated by working muscles; less blood flows to the digestive tract, creating a greater risk of digestive problems; absorption and digestion are less efficient, resulting in slower conversion of food into usable energy; and the mechanisms the body uses to regulate and restore normal fluid balance are compromised even further.

Matching the body's need for fluid during continuous endurance exercise is an entirely separate ball game from meeting energy or caloric needs. Relying on a concentrated liquid-food beverage to meet your fluid needs or drinking more of it in an attempt to rehydrate, for example, spells disaster. As with fuel needs, however, the only way to get a handle on what and how much you need to drink to be optimally hydrated is to experiment during training under various conditions.

Salt and Fluid Balance

Sensitive internal balancing mechanisms constantly regulate the total amount of fluid in the body. Your mouth (by sensing thirst), brain (by stimulating you to drink when your blood is too concentrated), and stomach govern your fluid intake, and your brain (by antidiuretic or vasopressin hormone from the pituitary gland) and kidneys are involved in how much fluid is excreted (urinated). Imbalances, such as dehydration and water intoxication (excessive body water) can occur; however, your body works hard to restore itself to normal as promptly as it can. During long-distance, ultra, and multiday endeavors, though, maintaining this delicate balance can be quite difficult. What you do or don't do further complicates the situation.

For decades, endurance athletes undertaking prolonged efforts have been warned about the importance of drinking enough to avoid dehydration. Obviously, avoiding dehydration is a critical piece of the equation if you want to perform at your best. Having too much water on board, known as exercise-associated hyponatremia, however, is just as dangerous for endurance athletes. In fact, it can be life threatening.

Hyponatremia doesn't occur only in athletes who substantially overdrink or overhydrate, especially with plain water, although this is one route. It also occurs in endurance athletes who are drinking modestly more than they need, but whose kidneys can't keep up with excreting (urinating) the excess liquid, which normally occur at rest. The retained water dilutes the level of sodium in the blood. As a defense mechanism, water moves into cells (including brain cells), causing them to swell. This circumstance is particularly problematic in your brain because little room exists to accommodate extra fluid. Thus, changes in mental status, loss of coordination, bizarre

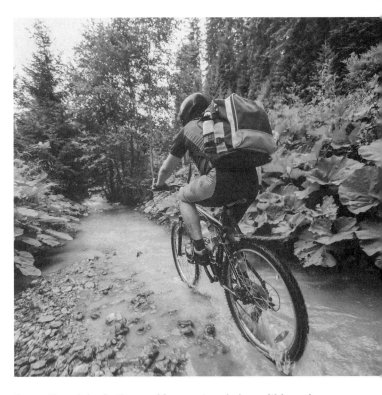

Preventing dehydration and hyponatremia in multiday adventures requires being diligent about replacing both fluid and sodium.

.schock/Fotolia.com

behaviors, seizures, and coma are indicative of advanced hyponatremia.

Weight gain during a prolonged continuous effort is a definite sign that too much fluid is being retained. Using a scale to monitor body weight during multiday events is strongly recommended; unfortunately, it is not always feasible. Drinking primarily a properly formulated sports drink that contains electrolytes (sodium and potassium) is beneficial. Sports drinks alone, however, even in combination with salty foods, are not enough to prevent hyponatremia if you overdrink or exceed your kidney's ability to excrete excess fluid. In other words, taking in sodium during exercise does not make it OK to overdrink.

Following a reasonable eating and drinking plan, even sticking to a tried-and-true schedule, isn't foolproof either. In fact, it can be downright dangerous. Water retention can set in at any time, and you may not be able to determine why it happens. Besides an increase in weight, you (and the crew in supported races) must be alert for other signs of water overload, such as bloating, puffiness at sock or short lines, tightening rings and watchbands, tight or shiny skin, nausea and vomiting, or a prominent forehead headache when descending or traveling over bumpy surfaces.

If you associate bloating with getting too much sodium, you're not alone. This is what athletes have always been told. The universal finding, however, is that the more weight athletes gain during prolonged exercise compared with their starting weight, the lower their blood sodium level is likely to be. Bloated athletes also are much more likely to be hyponatremic.

To further complicate the picture, you can't simply go by your ability to urinate or lack thereof, especially during prolonged continuous exercise. This information isn't always reliable in regard to hydration status. We all know that we stop urinating if we're dehydrated. You also may stop urinating, however, when you are suffering from fluid overload! Urinary shutdown, for example, can occur because of a jammed urinary overflow valve (why this occurs in some people during exercise is not clear) or an inappropriate release of the antidiuretic hormone vasopressin, which stimulates the kidneys to reabsorb or hold on to water.

Bloated athletes, and often those who are vomiting or who've been drinking but not urinating, are fluid overloaded, not dehydrated. These athletes are on their way to becoming hyponatremic, if they're not already there. In this situation, concluding that they should hydrate more until their urine runs clear is incorrect, and it only leads to more problems. The bottom line is always the same: Listen to your body. Bloating is the opposite of dehydration—you have too much water on board. The treatment is to stop drinking (even rehydrating sports drinks) and ingest sodium. Do not resume drinking (unless the fluid is a vehicle to deliver sodium, such as a salty broth) until you have urinated the excess fluid. To give your body the best chance to accomplish this, you most likely will need to slow your pace dramatically or even stop altogether.

Although electrolytes haven't gotten nearly the attention that they deserve, sodium is the other half of the fluid–salt equation. Keeping body fluids (water) and electrolytes (primarily sodium) in balance, especially during prolonged exercise, is what it's really all about. During exercise, water is

Pass the Salt!

Endurance athletes need to consume supplemental salt during prolonged exercise, such as long-distance endeavors, ultras, and events and races lasting longer than a day. Sodium, fortunately, comes in many different forms. Your job is threefold: Know the sodium content of the items that you intend to use (see table), realistically estimate the amount that you will need to consume to meet your personal electrolyte needs, and practice your electrolyte replacement strategies in training under various environmental conditions. (Smart athletes also get heat acclimated and continually work at staying cool during prolonged exercise to reduce their sweat losses.)

Item	Amount	Sodium content
Sport Beans Energizing Jelly Beans, Extreme Sport Beans	1 oz (28 g)	80 mg
Clif Shot Bloks (margarita flavor)	1 oz (3 pieces)	60-70 mg (210 mg)
Sharkies Organic Energy Sports Chews	1.58 oz package (45 g)	110 mg
Energy gel Ultraendurance energy gel	1 packet 1 packet	40–55 mg 200 mg
Typical sports drink	8 oz (240 ml)	70–110 mg
Endurance-type sports drink	8 oz/1 scoop	190–200 mg
Typical meal-replacement beverage	8 oz	130–200 mg
V8/tomato juice	6 oz (170 ml)	420–550 mg
Potato chips	1 oz	150–380 mg
Pretzels (hard, plain, salted)	1 oz	385 mg
Keebler Toast & Peanut Butter sandwich crackers	1 package	300 mg
Table salt	1 pinch (1/8 tsp)	300 mg
Broth	1 cup (from bouillon cube or stock mix)	800–1000+ mg
Nuun tabs	1 tablet in 16 oz (480 ml) of water	360 mg
Gu Electrolyte Brew drink tablets	1 tablet in 16 oz of water	320 mg
Hammer Endurolytes caps/powder	1 capsule or 1 scoop of powder	40 mg
Elete tablytes or add-ins	1 tablet; 1/2 tsp	150 mg/125 mg
Electrolyte Stamina tablets	1 tablet	45 mg
SaltStick Caps (SaltStick Caps Plus)	1 capsule	215 mg (190 mg)
Thermotabs	1 tablet	180 mg
S! Caps (from Succeed!)	1 capsule	341 mg
The Right Stuff	1 pouch in 16 oz of water	1,780 mg
ZYM electrolyte tablets	1 tablet in 16–20 oz (480–590 ml) of water	250–300 mg

lost in many ways—through sweat, expired air, and urine, as well as any time diarrhea, vomiting, or bleeding occurs. Electrolytes are lost by all these routes, too, with the exception of expired air. Sodium is our body's chief extracellular (outside cells) electrolyte. The amount of sodium you lose through sweat and urine depends on your body's preexercise electrolyte stores, your fitness level, and how heat acclimated you are.

Sweat is the major route for the loss of sodium. We also lose some potassium through sweat. Potassium, however, is our body's principal intracellular electrolyte (90 percent of the potassium in the body is stored inside cells). Our bodies actively work to keep potassium within cells. Consequently, potassium is not lost at a rate anywhere near the high rates of sodium loss. Normal sweat rates for endurance athletes can range from .75 to 2 liters per hour, with a rate of 1 liter an hour being common for an acclimated athlete. This rate of sweating means that an athlete also is losing, on average, 800 to 1,300 milligrams of sodium per hour.

Our bodies are extremely sensitive to the concentration of sodium in the blood and in the fluid outside cells. Compensatory mechanisms help the body retain sodium when faced with sodium losses (such as the hormone aldosterone produced by the adrenal glands); however, the body can do only so much. If you keep sweating heavily or long enough without replacing the sodium that's being lost, you will end up with an electrolyte imbalance, such as hyponatremia.

Keep in mind that sodium needs during exercise are not based on the length of time you exercise. Rather, how much sodium is needed depends proportionately on how much fluid you need to consume (ingest per hour) to maintain an adequately hydrated weight. Obviously, your fluid needs vary depending on the weather and your acclimatization to the heat. During exercise, sodium is lost primarily through sweat and urine. The sodium concentration in sweat varies considerably among athletes; during exercise, the sodium concentration of urine is about the same as that of sweat. A loss of 1,000 milligrams of sodium per quart (liter) of sweat is a reasonable average to assume. Note that 1 quart equals 4 cups. On the scale, this means every pound you lose during exercise (due to the loss of body water) is equivalent to 16 ounces or 2 cups of fluid (every kilogram lost is equivalent to a little more than 1 liter).

Before the Event

Give the same time and attention to what, when, and how you're going to eat and drink as you do to your clothing, gear, navigation needs, and other logistical concerns. Remember, a chain is only as strong as its weakest link. If your nutrition game plan falls apart during a multiday endurance adventure, so will you.

Knowledge is power: Know what you are getting into. First, is the event or race supported or unsupported? If supported, what fluids and foods are provided, how often, and in what amounts? What will you need to carry or take with you between aid stations or provided meals? During unsupported ventures, such as randonneuring and backcountry adventures, you are responsible for supplying, carrying, or buying what you need along the way. How will you get the job done? What gear do you need? Will you be relying on others?

Gather beforehand as much information as you can regarding the logistics of hydrating and fueling along the way, so that you know what to expect and plan for. Visit official websites and carefully review participant manuals and any nutrition-related recommendations given by a credible race director or event promoter. Talk to other endurance athletes to gain invaluable insight and practical advice. Lastly, refer to notes that you've kept regarding what has and hasn't worked for you personally during past endurance events.

Have a flexible game plan. You must have a personal nutrition plan built on basic principles that addresses all your needs: fluid, energy (calories), and electrolytes. You can't just duplicate someone else's plan, because what works for a teammate, friend, or highly conditioned elite athlete may not work for you. Practice and become proficient at eating, drinking, and problem solving in shorter events and races before tackling a multiday epic.

Keep in mind that what works on one occasion (or even multiple occasions) may suddenly and mysteriously stop working on another day. Unexpected developments can occur without warning. An upset stomach, for example, is one of the most common problems faced by endurance athletes. This condition can result from a multitude of factors. You often can remedy situations that arise if you stay calm, slow down, and patiently experiment. Your job is to keep trying.

Real problems can arise during a multiday competition when a strong-willed and uncompromising athlete continues to stick with a game plan that is clearly not working. You may continue to force down a set number of calories, for example, despite evidence such as bloating and nausea that your stomach isn't able to keep pace. The mistaken belief is that deviating will be worse than making a change on the fly. In reality, every day (or leg of a relay race) is a balancing act between following your preplanned drinking and eating schedule and listening to your body. You'll need to monitor, interpret, and make adjustments depending on the feedback that your body gives. The bottom line: Approach hydrating and refueling on the move as a flexible work in progress, not as a rigid schedule.

Choose teammates and support people with care. You must trust and rely on the others in your team for an extended period, so give serious thought to assembling that team. Things go much smoother when everyone involved exhibits the same level of commitment, which includes meeting their personal fluid and fuel needs from day to day (or leg to leg.) Take into account the personalities of all those involved and how well they work together—especially when they are fatigued, sleep deprived, or underfueled. Personality issues can make or break your experience. At the very least, they can make the event less enjoyable. From a nutrition standpoint, consider and plan for the needs of the team as a whole. Failing to respect the nutrition component of multiday endeavors doesn't only put you at risk, it can prevent your entire team from finishing and, at its worst, can endanger someone else's life.

If your race or event takes you outside your country, prepare beforehand by researching local resources. Take with you any foodstuffs that you can't do without. If gastrointestinal risks are associated with eating the local cuisine or drinking the water, be extra cautious leading up to a race or once-in-a-lifetime-adventure. Drink only bottled water, pasteurized juice, and soda (without ice). Consider taking extra supplies for the days before you start. Powdered meal-replacement products and dehydrated camping fare come in handy before, as well as during, longer endeavors. You can prepare all these items with bottled or purified water.

Protein-rich foods are particularly challenging to locate in some countries. Besides protein powders and energy bars, be creative and try jerky, pop-top cans of tuna or chicken, string cheese, individually wrapped rounds of hard cheese, peanut butter, and nuts. These foods provide substantial calories and are appealing complements to the array of sweeter-tasting sports foods that athletes typically must rely on.

During the Event

Start from the beginning. Stay on top of your fluid, electrolyte, and fuel needs right from the onset. The best defense against dehydration, glycogen depletion, hyponatremia, and hypoglycemia is prevention: Never allow yourself to become too depleted of anything. If you go too low, you won't come back. Snack at regular intervals and eat at the start of planned breaks. This approach is twofold. It allows you to ingest as much as you reasonably can tolerate, as well as have the maximal time to digest and absorb it, thus reducing the risk of stomach problems.

Divide and conquer. Address hydration, energy, and electrolyte (sodium) needs separately. In other words, don't tie replacing electrolyte losses with meeting your calorie needs. If you can't eat for a while (for whatever reason), for example, you won't get the electrolytes that you counted on, either. Constantly monitor your body. Don't ignore signs such as bloating, mental confusion, or the inability to sweat. For example, you can't become fluid overloaded unless the amount of fluid that you consume exceeds the amount that you lose (through sweat and urine). Drink to thirst and to match your fluid losses, which can vary tremendously depending on your fitness level, sweat rate, and weather conditions.

Stop the bloat. Don't ignore bloating or other signs of having too much water on board. Stop drinking immediately to avoid making the fluid overload worse (unless the fluid is a means to consume salt, such as a salty broth). Ingest salt. Medical experts familiar with endurance exercise suggest using the standard emergency room treatment of at least 300 milligrams of sodium, followed by the same amount 10 to 15 minutes later. Athletes typically report feeling better fairly quickly, within 5 to 20 minutes, if the hyponatremia was mild and caught early enough. As soon as your symptoms abate, slow down on ingesting sodium. You still may not be out of the woods, however, so don't resume drinking until you've urinated the excess fluid. From here on, be extra vigilant about monitoring and meeting both your fluid and sodium needs.

Keep an eye on friends and teammates. Obviously, everyone needs to be responsible for staying on top of their own fluid and fuel needs. At the same time, however, it pays to keep an eye on all group members. In adventure races, for example, the first team to cross the finish line together wins. Teams that lose a member because of illness, fatigue, injury, or a team disagreement are disqualified. Relay races and even personal adventures also can end prematurely if someone is unable to continue or needs medical treatment.

Be sure that everyone is eating and drinking. Dehydration, glycogen depletion, or a low blood sugar level makes whatever you're doing seem even harder than it is. Be particularly sensitive to mood swings; a friend or teammate in trouble may become extremely quiet or irritable and argumentative. Share fluids and food as needed.

Postevent Recovery Plan

Just do it. Accept the fact that you aren't going to feel hungry or want to eat after exhaustive exercise, especially in warm weather or other extreme conditions. Rely on liquid food. Find a carbohydrate-rich recovery drink and have it ready to go. Start drinking it within the first 15 minutes (no later than 30 minutes after you've stopped for the day) to maximize glycogen replenishment. Include some high-quality protein if feasible (in a meal-replacement beverage, for example). At the very least, consume some protein within 2 hours at your next meal.

Replace water, calories, and sodium. After long bouts of exercise, especially multiple days in a row, you will be deficient in all three. Don't just consume large amounts of fluid (water or a sports drink), especially if you can't get or keep other items down, or if you're bloated or have gained weight from your starting weight. The smoothest and most complete recovery requires replacing all three components promptly and consistently—water; sodium in a salty beverage, food, or electrolyte supplement; and at least 200 carbohydrate calories, ideally within the 15- to 30-minute carbohydrate window.

Strategies for Team Efforts

Teamwork, efficiency, and constant communication are crucial to a team's success. During multiday efforts, you, your partner or teammates, or your fellow adventurers must apply the same skills to hydrating and refueling. Serious adventure racers, in particular, need to learn to travel light and fast.

Determine your teammates' or companions' food preferences beforehand (as well as any food allergies), so that you don't end up carrying food that someone doesn't like or can't eat. Assemble food items in one place, check labels, and together make up food bags containing predetermined amounts of calories.

Keep food and fluids near at hand. Easy access is a must. Wear a bladder system or attach water bottles to the outside of your pack. Every athlete also should carry in easy-to-reach pockets their own small stash of quick-energy foods, such as dried fruit, fruit-to-go strips, trail mix, hard candy, chocolate, and energy bars, gels, chews, or blocks. In races, don't waste time taking your own pack off and repacking its contents every time you need to eat. Keep your main stash in an easy-to-reach outer pocket of a teammate's pack.

Keep it simple. Coordinate refueling efforts with the inevitable stops that you'll be making. Serious adventure racing, for example, requires a considerable amount of stopping for navigational purposes. Plan to access more substantial, preassembled team food (packaged in large ziplock bags) at that time while you also make adjustments in clothing and attend to foot problems. If racing, place the food in one person's pack so that accessing it doesn't require a lot of effort or thought when you're in a hurry or feeling the effects of sleep deprivation. Remember, if one person needs to eat to continue, then everybody in the group should refuel.

If you're going to race, learn to eat on the run. Experienced adventure racers will often combine cold water and dehydrated fare in a resealable container (to avoid spending time heating the water) and throw it into someone's pack. After 20 minutes, the concoction is ready to eat. Teammates share by passing the container around and squeezing the contents out of one corner—all while on the move, of course.

Make room for extra powdered sports drink (containing sodium) and electrolyte (salt) tablets. These items are worth their weight in gold during multiday competitions. Adventure racers competing in weeklong races, for example, are required to carry electrolyte tablets because the possibility of consuming only plain water for long periods increases the risk of hyponatremia.

LEARNING FROM THE BEST: CREW-SUPPORTED BIKE RACES AND EVENTS

Long-time cycling enthusiast Kerry Ryan, past RAAM winner (team division) and owner of Action Sports, and Cindy Staiger, a two-time solo finisher and highly sought-after RAAM crew chief who now works as a race official, offer their expertise on crew-supported cycling races.

For the Rider

1. Be selective about who makes your crew team. Choose at least one person you respect more than yourself. Otherwise, you won't have anyone to answer to when the going gets tough. In multiday races, in which you increasingly rely on your crew as time passes, be certain that at least one crew person has considerable nutrition knowledge.

2. Be aware of your personal needs—your typical eating and drinking habits on the bike, what usually works well, what doesn't work—and freely share this information with your crew.

3. Be mentally prepared to drink and eat the calories that you need. If you can't meet your estimated calorie needs successfully in shorter events (for example, a century ride), don't fool yourself into thinking that you can do it for a daylong relay race or multiday race. Establish good habits in shorter rides or races before stepping up to more challenging endeavors.

4. Eat before you get hungry. Devise an hourly refueling schedule and stick to it, whether you feel hungry or not. A stable blood sugar level allows you to think better and stay awake longer. While on the bike, consume liquid calories and small snacks. Solid foods tend to promote sleepiness, so supplement with solid foods only when you're not riding. Avoid eating a large quantity of food at any one time unless you have a substantial rest break or are going to sleep.

5. Drink plenty of water. Stay on top of your hydration status by monitoring your urine output. If you have difficulty urinating or if your urine is dark yellow, you're dehydrated. Urine that is too clear (looks like water) indicates that you're overhydrated. Staiger figures that solo riders need to drink at least one full bottle (12 to 16 ounces, or 360 to 480 milliliters) of plain water per hour, in addition to the high-energy beverages that they are consuming. A rule of thumb is that a rider should be able to urinate a minimum of once every 6 hours.

6. Don't rely on supplements or drugs to improve your performance. The keys to success are training, pacing, eating, and drinking.

7. Go easy on caffeine. Caffeine provides a mental boost and helps you stay awake; however, don't underestimate the additive nature of its mild dehydrating effect during multiday rides and races. Limit your intake, especially during hot weather.

> continued

< continued

8. To avoid the mouth sores commonly experienced in ultraendurance cycling endeavors, which can make eating unbearable, routinely rinse your mouth with a dilute, tepid solution of 1 tablespoon of antiseptic mouthwash stirred into 8 ounces (240 ml) of water.

9. Settle an upset stomach by consuming saltine crackers or sipping ginger ale, bottled seltzer water, or plain water with a small amount of baking soda stirred in.

For the Crew Team

1. Keep a detailed log. A little planning goes a long way, especially when you're in charge of more than one rider. Make extensive notes on each rider as the race unfolds—weather and terrain; speed and distance covered; estimates of calories required and consumed hourly or per leg; fluids and sodium needed and consumed; pit stops; presence or absence of stomach issues, muscle cramps, cravings, and low blood sugar; and any other information that you find useful. Keeping a log helps you anticipate and ward off problems before they become insurmountable.

2. Monitor your rider's calorie intake closely. Aim for your rider to stay ahead of, or at least match, their estimated calorie needs; otherwise, the body begins to break down its muscles to use as fuel. Individual needs vary, but Staiger figures that riders generally need at least 400 calories per hour. Don't focus on overloading your rider with protein. Consuming enough overall calories (from whatever source) is what counts.

3. Think of endurance cycling as cycling with scheduled breaks. Plan breaks carefully to incorporate as much as possible into each stop, especially when crewing for solo endurance cyclists. Establish from the start that the rider is required to eat whenever possible, including while standing up during a rest break.

4. Babysit your rider or riders. A rider's success depends on the ability of his or her crew to take care of the smallest details. For example, keep fluids cold to encourage riders to drink, be certain they start each leg with clean water bottles, and keep plenty of salty foods and electrolyte replacement beverages on hand during hot-weather rides. In multiday events, recognize that 2 to 3 days of around-the-clock cycling may pass before a rider gives up total decision-making control to his or her crew. When the time comes, be prepared to do everything but push the pedals for your rider.

5. Keep your rider or riders happy about their food. Solid normal food helps riders stay properly fueled and mentally satisfied. Expect the unexpected. As the days progress, riders will crave weird foods. Be prepared to get them a small amount of it or a close substitute. If the food they desire goes against your better judgment, convince them to wait until a slightly better time (before going to sleep, for example).

6. Recognize the symptoms of bonking and intervene immediately. Warning signs include lethargy, decreased pedaling cadence or speed, inconsistent thought patterns, shakiness, glazed eyes, and spaced out behavior. Treat a low blood sugar level immediately with liquid foods, such as juice, soda, and energy gels (taken with water). In severe cases, the rider may need 60 minutes or longer to revive sufficiently. Monitor your rider's calorie intake more closely after a bonk.

7. Feed yourself. Your rider's safety and success hinge on your ability to carry out your duties. You may not be able to do anything about getting more sleep, but frequent snacking will help you stay awake and be more alert.

13

Rowing and Open Water Swimming

Ultramarathon swimmer Jamie Patrick's menu for his Swimming California adventure, a 111-mile (180 km), 31-hour charity swim down the Sacramento River from Princeton to Sacramento's Tower Bridge: turkey sandwiches with no dressing or cheese (cut into four manageable bites for ease of eating day or night), salted potato wedges, penne pasta, pretzels, chicken soup, rice balls with scrambled egg, almond milk, dark chocolate, glucose tablets, whey protein, and jelly beans.

Source: S. Munatones, 2011, "Jamie Patrick feeds on swimming California," *The Daily News of Open Water Swimming*. [Online]. Available: http://dailynews.openwaterswimming.com/2011/08/jamie-patrick-feeds-on-swimming.html [April 25, 2013].

It may appear that open water swimmers and rowers have little in common. Open water swimmers, after all, succeed only by getting in the water, whereas rowers must stay out of the water to accomplish their goals. Perhaps you're wondering why advice for oarsmen and women is even included in a sports nutrition book for endurance athletes. Rowers classically take part in races lasting fewer than 8 minutes. And they certainly don't eat and drink during these competitions!

From a physiological standpoint, however, rowing is considered a power–endurance sport. To excel at rowing takes an enormous endurance capacity or the ability to produce energy and endure physical demands placed on the body over a period of time. The energy systems used during traditional sprint rowing races (as well as the long hours of training required for these intense efforts) mimic those in play during other shorter-range endurance activities, such as running a 5K or 10K road race or competing in a 30K cycling time trial.

A 2,000-meter rowing race can be broken down into three parts: the start phase; the middle, or distance, phase; and the finish, or sprint, phase. Sandwiched between a fast start and, ideally, a fast finish (both fueled by anaerobic metabolism) is the middle, or distance, phase. The longest phase of the race, lasting 4 to 6 minutes, this middle phase is fueled by energy produced by the body's aerobic energy system. In fact, the aerobic energy system produces 75 to 80 percent of the metabolic energy used during a rowing race. So, just as a food is grouped with other foods that have similar nutrition profiles (for example, despite being found in the dairy case, eggs are included in the protein foods group, not the dairy group, since they provide virtually no calcium), rowing is categorized as an endurance sport despite its concurrent emphasis on power and technique.

Many opportunities exist if you enjoy competing in open water swimming or rowing. You may be swimming in a pool or in open water, rowing outside (sprints, longer head races, or even marathons), or on an indoor ergometer. Rowathlons (similar to triathlons, but indoor rowing replaces the swimming leg) continue to grow in popularity. And, if you like to swim in open water, you now can strive to be an Olympian. Similar to other endurance athletes, recreational and competitive rowers and open water swimmers require a well-thought-out nutrition game plan on race day.

Rowing

Despite being engaged in one of the most physically demanding of endurance sports, competitive rowers, as a group, often fail to eat in a way that benefits their performance. Competitive rowers commonly are hampered by nutrition misinformation, dehydration, and chronic glycogen depletion due to their high-volume training. Many rowers also struggle with their weight. They either have difficulty in maintaining weight as the season progresses (among male heavyweights, for example), or they engage in unhealthy practices to manage or lose weight (especially among lightweight rowers). As for all endurance athletes, mastering the smart day-to-day eating habits covered in part I of this book sets the nutrition foundation that every serious rower needs.

2,000-Meter Races

In collegiate and international rowing, the standard racing course is a distance of 2,000 meters (2K), requiring an all-out effort lasting approximately 6 to 8 minutes. Rowers, depending on their individual size and fitness level, burn approximately 25 to 35 calories per minute during this intense effort. If rowers go into the race having followed a smart eating plan while training, they should have more than enough glycogen stored in their muscles (up to 400 grams of glycogen, or 1,600 calories) and liver (100 grams or 400 calories) to fuel the anaerobic and aerobic demands placed on working muscles during the race. Rowers, in other words, do not have to carbohydrate-load to superload their muscles with glycogen, as a marathoner or long-distance cyclist would benefit from doing.

Regattas typically last from 2 days to a week, with competitors progressing through heats and semifinals (and possibly repechages) to earn a berth in the finals. Outside the top echelons of the sport, rowers typically compete in more than one race per day. As a rower, your goal on race day, with regard to nutrition, is to show up at each race with adequate muscle glycogen stores to fuel 8 minutes or fewer of intense exercise. Remember, due to the limited availability of oxygen, carbohydrate is the only fuel the body burns during flat-out efforts.

The primary concern is not so much what you eat prerace (for example, what you eat for dinner the night before). Rather, it's about how well you maintain an optimal level of muscle glycogen from day to day. Rowers, especially those overly concerned about or struggling to maintain a desired weight, run the greatest risk of steadily depleting their glycogen stores while preparing for competitions and never allowing their muscles to regain their full potential supply. A rower may then enter a competition with glycogen stores that are unable to sustain an all-out competitive effort. With much of competition day tied up in prerace preparations and the race itself, rowers also need to make recovery nutrition a priority, keeping appropriate high-carbohydrate snacks nearby at all times and committing to consuming something as soon as possible after each race.

Dehydration is a common and often underappreciated foe of competitive rowers. Rowers are at risk due to sweat losses incurred during rowing (even in cold weather) or simply from being outdoors in the sun watching the competition. Dehydration is particularly detrimental to rowers who engage in drastic measures to make weight, such as severely restricting fluids, reducing food intake, and continuing to exercise strenuously in the days leading up to the race. It's simply not possible after the weigh-in to normalize physiology and restore blood volume to its full capacity. A study published in the *Journal of Medicine and Science in Sports and Exercise* ("Rowing Performance, Fluid Balance and Metabolic Function Following Dehydration and Rehydration") simulating these very conditions found that rowers were able to restore only half of their lost blood volume by drinking fluids following their weigh-in. In terms of performance over a 2,000-meter course, rowers who had become dehydrated and then attempted to rehydrate were 15 meters behind. All levels of rowers will benefit from using a sports drink to top off their reserves of fluid, carbohydrate, and sodium, especially those rowers who need to rehydrate after weigh-ins. Consume your preferred sports drink both before and after a race.

Due to the limited weight classifications in the sport of rowing, many rowers find themselves struggling to reach or maintain a weight required for lightweight classification. Internationally, the maximum race weight for lightweight men is 72.5 kilograms, or 160 pounds. At the elite level, the boat (lightweight crew) average, however, cannot exceed 70 kilograms, or about 154 pounds. For women's lightweight events, the weight cutoff is generally 59 kilograms, or 130 pounds. At the women's elite level, however, the boat average must not exceed 57 kilograms, or about 126 pounds.

Further complicating prerace preparations is that lightweight rowers must weigh in before each race, resulting in a less-than-ideal prerace situation. As with all athletes in weight-making sports, lightweight rowers will benefit from partnering with qualified health professionals. Work with a sports medicine physician and a sports dietitian to receive expert individualized advice about establishing an optimal competitive weight with minimal consequences to your health. As the previously mentioned study reveals, a long-term plan to manage body weight that allows a rower to start a race fully hydrated is the best approach.

Head Races, Marathon Rows, and Other Rowing Events

Rowers may compete in venues other than 2,000-meter races, from head races (time trials of 5 to 7 kilometers, or 3 to 4 miles, in length) to marathon rows. Extreme endurance athletes may tackle ultra ocean-rowing challenges, such as rowing across the Atlantic Ocean. As for endurance sports in general, as the duration of the rowing event increases, prerace fueling and what and how you drink and eat during the competition become increasingly critical to your success.

Carbohydrate loading is necessary, for example, if you'll be rowing continuously for 120 minutes or longer at race pace or if you will be rowing several times over a period of several or more hours (see the section One Week in Advance in chapter 4). Rowers, like mountain bikers and Nordic skiers, literally have their hands full during a race, so marathon rowers and ultra rowers can experiment with wearing a hip belt or backpack-style hydration system. Both hold a considerable volume of fluid that is delivered through a flexible drinking tube. Sports drinks, supplying much-needed fluid, carbohydrate, and sodium, are the drink of choice during prolonged races.

All calories are good calories during prolonged exercise, so keep sports foods like energy gels, chews, blocks, and bars (in various flavors to combat flavor fatigue) and other well-tolerated solid foods readily accessible. As the distance (or time spent rowing) increases, food plays an increasingly significant role in helping a rower maintain a positive frame of mind, so it pays to keep a variety of favorites on hand. Athletes involved in extreme rowing challenges, such as the Woodvale Atlantic Rowing Race (more than 2,500 nautical miles, or 4,630 kilometers) will benefit greatly from seeking personalized nutrition advice, including preplanned high-calorie meal plans, from a qualified sports nutrition expert.

As a rower involved in sprint events and head races, your nutrition goals for race day are simple. You want to top off your fluid and fuel (glycogen) reserves as well as correctly time your last meal so that you feel comfortable rowing during the race. Stacey Borgman, half of the winning duo in the B final of an Olympic women's lightweight double sculls race, shares tips on how to get the job done. Borgman founded the first junior recreational rowing program in Lake Oswego, Oregon.

Get Ready Before the Race

No matter how early in the day your race is scheduled, eat something for breakfast. If the race is later in the day, Borgman recommends eating a normal breakfast and, to avoid rowing on a full stomach, eating a light lunch slightly earlier than you normally would. From there, if you get hungry, eat small snacks like fruit, granola bars, or a few nuts, or sip on a sports drink. Energy bars are also good to eat between races or if you're hungry right before a race and want to avoid that full or sluggish feeling.

Establish a Routine After the Race

Get off the water, put your boat up, and get a drink. Borgman made it a habit to carry a sports drink and snacks in her gear bag so that she could get started right away, especially if she was racing again that day.

Nutrition Recommendations for Head Races

Head races can be brutal because of the cold and wind. Keep in mind that you'll be on the water twice as long as the time spent actually racing. You'll be rowing to the starting line or back from the finish line, so you'll be rowing for an hour or more. Expect that you'll also be rowing into the wind in at least one direction! You'll get thirsty and hungry, so plan for it. Borgman requires her athletes to carry in their boat at least a water bottle filled with a sports drink, as well as an energy gel or bar to have after crossing the finish line.

Avoid the Most Common Nutrition Mistakes

From her perspective as a lightweight, Borgman routinely sees rowers who believe that they can stop eating entire food groups to make weight and still keep rowing well. Unhealthy and unsuccessful approaches typically include cutting out all foods with fat or attempting to avoid carbohydrate and eat just protein foods. Borgman stresses balance among carbohydrate, protein, and fat and the need to eat meals that include all three. Eliminating one or two of these elements for any length of time is senseless. Your body isn't going to last. Borgman always relied on real food, not bars and sports drinks, to keep her body going from day to day.

> continued

< continued

Advice for Lightweight and Other Weight-Conscious Rowers

Borgman has this to say about dieting: "To keep your metabolism going, you have to eat! I never was dieting. What I was doing was for my sport, not for the way I looked. I spent 3 months getting down to weight so I could go to the championships! I would always relax in the winter and let my body go back to its natural weight. I've watched a lot of rowers with potential who never make it because they get caught up in the weight stuff versus the sport itself. Don't do something to look good, like trying to keep at your racing weight year round. Do what is best for your performance."

How to Maintain Weight as the Season Progresses

The number one priority when trying to keep weight on is to keep eating. This doesn't mean, however, that you should fill up on junk. Make sure to eat three or four real meals daily. Eat snacks or mini meals in between. Take in lots of quality protein and wholesome carbohydrate from real foods. Always carry healthy snacks with you. Liquid calories from protein shakes or fruit smoothies and sports drinks can really add up.

Indoor Rowing

The sport of indoor rowing was born in 1981 after the advent of the rowing machine. Today, it attracts millions of competitors worldwide. The blue-ribbon championship race distance is 2,000 meters, with recognized age-group records for this distance as well as a range of other distances. Every winter, national championships take place in the United States, almost every European country, and many other countries throughout the world. A world indoor rowing championship is held every February in Boston (United States).

For those with hardy seats and hands, indoor marathon and ultra rowing races are also available. The individual marathon distance is 42,195 meters, and the half-marathon distance is 21,097 meters. Other events include group or individual 100,000-meter rows, group or individual million-meter rows, group or individual 24-hour rows, and group or individual longest continuous time rows. For individual efforts in the standard distances, records are kept for lightweight (165 pounds or 75 kilograms and under for men; 135 pounds or 61.5 kilograms and under for women) and heavyweight categories. Lightweights must be weighed in no earlier than 2 hours before their race.

Outdoors or inside—it doesn't matter. The longer the rowing challenge, the more you enhance your odds of success by embracing an endurance athlete's nutrition weapons. This includes drinking fluids with all meals and snacks in the day or two leading up to the race, as well as including salty foods (or adding salt to the foods that you eat), carbohydrate-loading prerace, eating breakfast to top off liver glycogen stores, and managing energy and carbohydrate needs (at least 30 to 60 grams per hour) throughout the event by consistently consuming sports drinks, sports foods, or other solid carbohydrate-rich foods as warranted.

Open Water Swimming

As defined by U.S. Masters Swimming, an open water event is a swimming event of any distance conducted in an open body of water, either natural or man-made. Open water swimmers can find themselves in oceans, seas, lakes, rivers, dams, reservoirs, canals, channels, fjords, estuaries, basins, lochs, coves, meres, firths, sounds, straits, bays, and harbors. Open water swimmers face a unique set of challenge. There are no lane lines, walls, or starting blocks, and the elements often play a deciding role in determining the winner. Open water championship races are held at various distances (from 1 mile to 6 or more miles), and a myriad of open water swimming endeavors exist today for adventuresome ultra swimmers. Since 2008, a marathon 10K open water swim has been part of the Olympic Games.

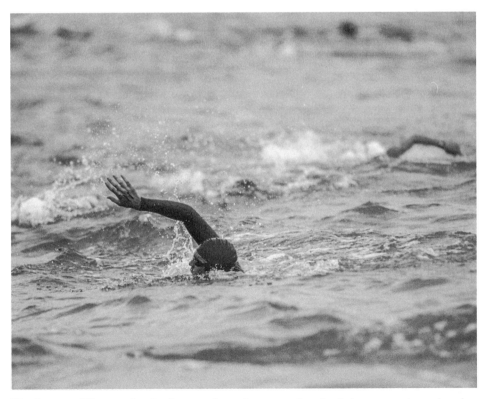

Weather conditions and water temperature play a prominent role in open water swimming endeavors, but hydration and feeding strategies are equally important.

Challenges and Considerations

As an open water swimmer, you face multiple challenges on race day, whether you're aiming to do a half-mile (800 m) lake swim for the first time, cross the English Channel, or win the Olympic 10K Marathon Swim. It's not only about swimming the required distance and maintaining a good pace throughout the swim. You also must withstand the cold or heat for the requisite time, deal with other weather effects (the wind in particular), and choose and implement the proper hydration and feeding-station techniques.

Proper nutrition before and especially during the race is critically important to a swimmer's success. Similar to endurance athletes who race on land, the goal beforehand is to optimize the body's glycogen stores and to hydrate properly. The purpose of feeding during a swim is to supplement the body's other energy sources (glycogen and fat), since it's not feasible (or necessary) to replace in total the calories being burned during the race. The focus is on consuming adequate carbohydrate (a minimum of 30 to 60 grams per hour) in a form and amount the body can easily digest while swimming. Other additions to feeds, such as supplemental protein and electrolytes, are useful only if they don't interfere with this main goal. Appropriately used warm and cold feeds also stabilize a swimmer's core body temperature and help

Common Nutrition Errors Made by Open Water Swimmers

Nutrition goals are twofold for open water swimmers. Optimize carbohydrate storage and hydration prior to competition and sustain carbohydrate delivery and hydration during competition. The following represent significant nutrition-related challenges that open water swimmers must overcome.

Inadequate prerace calories

Overreliance on protein and fat

Underreliance on carbohydrate

Poor recovery and use of recovery time

Neglect of performance-related vitamins and minerals

Failure to strategize and practice feeding

Failure to plan daily food intake

Failure to take advantage of taper

Overreliance on race-day nutrition

Underreliance on training nutrition

Reprinted, by permission, from C. Boudreau, 2008, Fueling for open water: Nutrition strategies for the 10K race with 5K and 7.5K feeding stations. [Online]. Available: www.usaswimming.org/_Rainbow/Documents/b9df2f1a-cf51-411d-b50d-76aaae75b9ae/Nutrition%20Strategies%20for%20Open%20Water.pdf [April 25, 2013].

prevent life-threatening situations of hypo- (too-low body temperature) or hyperthermia (too-high body temperature).

The training for open water swimming events must include opportunities to encounter and master hydration and feeding-station techniques. Simply put—what, when, and how! Efficient feeding requires a plan for identifying the feeder quickly and easily when approaching a feeding station, for example, and using a cup if close enough to the feeder to receive one or, if not, taking a pack or cup from a pole. Open water swimmers also must learn to remain horizontal while feeding and to consume the entire feed as quickly as possible. Training to miss a feed is also an integral part of a smart training program. Last, tactical decisions made during the actual race or endeavor, including what, when, and how to feed, can play a key role in determining the outcome.

Optimal Feeding Strategies

The optimal feeding strategy for any open water race is highly individualized. You must apply sound physiology and nutrition principles within the context of each specific race situation. This means taking into account the distance, location, venue or water type, and feeding opportunities, as well as personal food tolerances and preferences.

If refueling during a long-distance open water race isn't possible, preloading is the next best option. This is accomplished best by eating small meals frequently, rather than stuffing yourself the night before or the morning of the swim. A smart preloading schedule begins the day before and consists of eating three meals and three snacks, including one at bedtime, followed by breakfast on race-day morning.

Triathletes Are From Mars, Open Water Swimmers Are From Venus

The singular topic of the availability of a feeding station at a 10K Swim Across America event serves as a reminder of the fundamental differences between triathletes and open water swimmers. "*A feeding station is available on the course,*" was described in the pre-race information.

For triathletes, this meant that a manned feeding station would provide a variety of sponsored hydration solutions, from popular sports drinks to water. It meant that wide-eyed, happy volunteers would be freely passing out food, from bananas to cookies to gels, to the swimmers as they swam past the feeding station. The feeding station, a necessary requisite and safety measure in the form of a floating pontoon on the course, would have the characteristics of an aid station in a triathlon.

> continued

< continued

At least from the triathlete's experience and perspective, the availability of a feeding station was easy enough to understand. The volunteers and race organization would take care of their feeding needs. There was no need to prepare anything for the 6.2-mile race.

But this was not the perspective of an open water swimmer, who seemed to come from a different planet. "A feeding station is available on the course" subsequently led to a variety of questions:

1. Can our own coach board the floating pontoon?
2. When will our coach have to be onshore in order to be taken to the feeding station?
3. Can I bring my own escort?
4. How many kayakers can I have?
5. Where is the feeding station relative to the straight line tangent between the turn buoys?
6. Can I leave my own hydration and feeds on the pontoon if I do not have a coach?
7. Will there be officials on the pontoon?
8. How many times will we pass the pontoon during the race?
9. How high is the pontoon from the surface of the water?
10. Who will collect our bottles after the race is over?

At least from the open water swimmer's experience and perspective, the availability of a feeding station led to many different questions. They would have to prepare themselves and their coaches to take care of their feeding needs. There was much to prepare in order to successfully complete the 6.2-mile race to the best of their abilities.

To practice feeding during pool works, swimmers can place gel packs in their swimsuits and practice fluid intake during main sets. Opportunities to practice various feeding techniques in open water venues, obviously, are best. Ultraendurance swim endeavors and competitions take considerable planning and preparation, and proper nutrition is critical to the success of such endeavors. Some basic principles that apply to all open water swimmers, especially ultra swimmers, include the following:

- Maximize your taper before long-distance and ultra swims by upping your intake of carbohydrate-rich foods (including supplemental high-carbohydrate drinks at 50 to 70 grams per 8 ounces) and healthy beverages.

- Liquid feeds are better than solid feeds because solids are difficult to chew while swimming. Plus, the digestive system absorbs and digests liquid food faster than solid food.

- To minimize blood sugar fluctuations, feed often—every 15 to 20 minutes.

- The standard feeding schedule is 8 ounces (240 ml) of an electrolyte-and-fluid-recovery drink every 15 minutes. Aim for 20 grams of carbohydrate per feed, or 70 to 80 grams per hour.

- Solid foods, such as cookies, energy bars (precut into small pieces), canned fruit, bananas, and candy, can serve as backup energy and provide a lift during low points in the middle of the race.

- Drop feeds to every 10 to 12 minutes (or less) when feeling poorly. A low blood sugar level can manifest as weakness and a loss of power. If your crew is unaware, yell, "Feed" when you desire quicker feeds.

- Take in enough fluid that you need to urinate at least every hour.

- Maltodextrin tends to be a better carbohydrate source than dextrose and fructose due to a lower osmolality, which is less likely to produce digestive distress.

- If tolerated, augment your carbohydrate-based drink with protein during ultra swims to help mitigate muscle breakdown.

- Take into consideration the water and air temperatures when planning feeds. If you'll be swimming in conditions where both the water and outside air (temperature) are cold, drink warm feeds. Hot water from a thermos can be used to warm feeds. A gel pack mixed with hot water works very well. If both the water and the surrounding air are warm, drink cool feeds. To cool feeds, chill them in advance and keep them on ice in a cooler.

- Extra fluids and feeds, in general, are needed in extreme temperatures for minimizing the risks of dehydration in hot-weather races and hypothermia in cold-water races, when fuel is used more quickly in an attempt to maintain an adequate core body temperature. In warm-weather races, increase feeds to as often as every 6 minutes or double feeds by drinking 1 cup of water along with a cup of a fluid and electrolyte replacement drink.

- Hypothermia can occur in warm water as well as cold water. Early signs include feeling cold (especially along the back), being unable to hold one's fingers together while swimming, and shivering. A trainer or coach on the boat makes the call of when to pull a swimmer from the water. The decision should not be left up to the swimmer. A swimmer in trouble will be unable to swim in a straight line, appear blue, have difficulty speaking, and may seem disoriented. If in doubt, the swimmer should be asked some thought-provoking questions, such as the name of a family member, or be asked to count backward from 20.

- Don't overdo it. Remember, the goal isn't to replace everything you burn. There's a limit to how much the body can process at one time. Feeds need to supply about 30 to 60 grams of carbohydrate per hour of swimming and, ideally, up to 90 grams per hour (from multiple carbohydrate sources) for swimming endeavors lasting longer than 2.5 hours.

- Begin replenishing glycogen stores immediately, especially during the open water swim season. Expect to be tired, achy, and uncomfortable after an open water swim. Speed recovery time by drinking 32 ounces (1 L) of a high-carbohydrate beverage immediately and eating a balanced meal within 2 hours. It's normal for appetite to increase during the few days following a race. Keep essential foods on hand and eat often.

- Pay attention to the science and think for yourself. Don't eat something just because someone who swims faster than you does. Trust what you've figured out about your body and go with what works best for you.

- Feed the crew, because you depend on them always to be alert. An open water swim means a long day on the water for a crew, too, so be certain that plenty of their preferred foods and beverages are on hand.

- Develop a healthy relationship with your weight and body-fat percentage. A few extra pounds and a higher body-fat percentage can be advantageous, providing buoyancy and improving cold water tolerance. Follow a sensible, carbohydrate-rich diet with adequate lean protein and healthy fat, and let your weight fall where it will.

International races present additional challenges. Bring drink mixes and any foods that you plan to use during the race. Prepare your own bottles using powdered mixes and bottled water. If you are without your usual support crew, discuss feeding schedules beforehand with whoever will be in charge of you (in your boat or at feeding stations). To avoid becoming ill before an international race, follow the standard precautions for eating and drinking in a foreign country.

14

Extreme Heat

Exercise in hot, humid conditions can cause dehydration in as little as 30 minutes. Thirst mechanisms don't kick in until an athlete has lost 2 percent of bodyweight as sweat—at this level, sports performance is already impaired.

Source: E. Joy, n.d., "Heat illness," Gatorade Sports Science Institute Sports Medicine Tip Sheet. [Online]. Available: http://ce.gssiweb.com/Article_Detail.aspx?articleID=560 [April 25, 2013].

You're probably familiar with the saying "When the going gets tough, the tough get going." This adage obviously refers to endurance athletes. Who else would be dedicated (or crazy) enough to push their bodies to the limit for a medal or a belt buckle? And I mean to the limits—high altitude, extreme cold, and searing heat.

Often held under mind-boggling conditions, endurance competitions ultimately come down to a battle with Mother Nature. She sets the rules, and anything goes. Be prepared to broil, pant, and freeze, sometimes all in one day. To persevere (or just plain survive), you must be able to handle challenging environmental conditions. Heat, humidity, cold temperatures, and high altitude challenge the fittest of athletes. Whether you want to be competitive in endurance sports or you simply enjoy hiking, mountaineering, or skiing, the following three chapters provide nutrition strategies for dealing with extreme environmental conditions. First, let's take a look at how to beat the heat.

How is it possible to handle temperatures of 90 degrees Fahrenheit (32 °C) or higher without breaking a stride? Thank your body's thermostat—the hypothalamus. Located at the base of the brain, the hypothalamus receives signals from two sets of thermoreceptors. Central receptors sense changes in the temperature of your blood as it circulates through the hypothalamus; peripheral receptors monitor the temperature of your skin and the environment around you. Because the hypothalamus has a predetermined temperature, or set point, that it seeks to maintain, your body must deal quickly with fluctuations in body temperature.

As the body's core temperature rises, the hypothalamus signals sweat glands and blood vessels located in the skin into action. The blood vessels dilate, or open wider, bringing more blood and the heat that it carries to the skin, where the heat can escape to the environment. At the same time, sweat glands produce more sweat. As this moisture evaporates, it pulls heat from the skin.

Extreme heat limits your ability to exercise, especially if you're trying to compete. In hot weather, working muscles and the skin compete for a limited blood supply. Muscles need blood and the oxygen that it carries to keep performing. Your body, however, must divert blood to the skin to take the heat generated by working muscles to the surface to keep you cool. At some point, neither muscles nor the skin receive enough blood flow to function optimally. You can exacerbate the situation by not paying close attention to your fuel and fluid needs.

Performing in Extreme Heat

From a physiological standpoint, our bodies encounter the most severe stress when we exercise in the heat. We must deal with heat gained from a combination of physical exertion and the hot environment. Nevertheless, we still rely primarily on the evaporation of sweat to shed excess heat and remain (relatively) cool. Although sweating is a vital thermoregulatory mechanism for removing heat, it comes at a price. Dehydration results when we fail to take in enough fluid to keep pace with that lost in sweat. An average-size person (110 to 165 pounds, or 50 to 75 kilograms) can lose 1.5 to 2.5 quarts (liters) of sweat per hour, or 2 to 4 percent of their body weight, during an intense effort on a hot, humid day. Fluid losses of as little as 2 percent of body weight (a loss of 3 pounds, for example, for a 150-pound athlete, or 1.4 kilograms for a 68-kilogram athlete) have been shown to impair performance (see table 14.1).

TABLE 14.1   Effects of Dehydration

Bodyweight lost from sweating	Physiological effect
1%–2%	Thirst, some fatigue, minor loss of strength
3%–4%	Reduced maximal aerobic power and endurance, compromised ability to regulate body temperature, increased chance of overheating
5%–6%	Headache, decreased concentration, decreased cardiac output, chills, nausea, faster breathing, rapid pulse
7%–10%	Dizziness, muscle spasms, poor balance, exhaustion, collapse, potential cardiogenic shock, coma

To deliver a cooling effect, sweat must evaporate, not just drip off your body. That's why humid conditions greatly hinder athletic performances—less sweat evaporates off the skin because the air already is saturated with water. Consequently, the risk of heat illness is dramatically increased when we're faced with the dual challenge of exercising in heat and high humidity.

Exercising in hot weather decreases our economy or efficiency. Our bodies use more fuel, in other words, to perform at a particular pace or intensity compared with exercising under cooler conditions. Exercise physiologists estimate that a marathoner who typically runs a marathon in 2.5 hours, for example, will be almost 5 minutes slower over the same distance when the thermometer hits 80 degrees Fahrenheit (27 °C). As you become progressively dehydrated from failing to consume enough fluid to match sweat losses, your blood volume falls and the heart compensates by beating faster. Working muscles receive less blood flow and less oxygen in the heat (as blood is rerouted to the skin for cooling purposes), so they use more muscle glycogen and produce more lactic acid. This adjustment helps to explain why a given effort in the heat leaves you feeling more fatigued and exhausted than undertaking the same effort in cooler weather.

Heat Acclimatization

Bodies acclimatize to heat after approximately 7 to 14 days of training in warm conditions, although how quickly a person adapts and to what extent is highly individual. (Days on which you do not train due to a scheduled

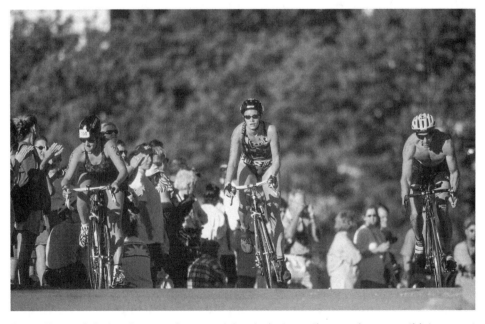

Regardless of their tolerance for exercising in hot weather, endurance athletes must continue to monitor their fluid, carbohydrate, and electrolyte levels throughout the event.

rest day, injury, or illness do not count toward the heat-acclimatization period.) Physiological adaptations that occur prepare the body to better withstand future bouts of exercise undertaken in the heat. Within the first few days, for example, we begin to sweat earlier and at an increased rate. (Remember, sweating is designed to eliminate excess heat and hold down the body's internal temperature, so more blood can flow to working muscles.) Various hormonal messages signal the sweat glands to reabsorb valuable electrolytes such as sodium and chloride. Sweating also triggers the release of other hormones that stimulate the kidneys to excrete less sodium and to reabsorb more water. The body, therefore, is attempting to compensate for fluid and minerals lost through heavy sweating by reducing their losses in urine. Once we're acclimated, the rate at which our muscles use glycogen during exercise in the heat is reduced by as much as 60 percent.

Don't underestimate the effect of making small adjustments when training in the heat, such as wearing light-colored, loose-fitting clothing, seeking out shady training routes, and taking longer rest breaks. While training in the swamplike conditions of a typical Washington, D.C. summer (often 80 degrees Fahrenheit and 85 percent humidity at 6:30 a.m.), I managed with very early morning runs or water-running sessions at the pool. When weather patterns change abruptly or you travel to a warmer climate, reduce your pace and training volume for at least the first few days. If you're competing, lower your expectations of what you can reasonably and safely accomplish.

Dehydration, Hyponatremia, and Heat Illnesses

The dangers of exercising in the heat include severe dehydration, heat cramps, and potentially more serious conditions, such as heat exhaustion, heatstroke, and hyponatremia (blood sodium depletion).

Dehydration

Dehydration, or the loss of body fluid, is the most common problem that plagues athletes, of all ages and abilities, who undertake endurance events in the heat. Besides throwing off the body's ability to regulate core temperature, dehydration also reduces our strength, power, endurance, and aerobic capacity. Many endurance athletes I meet falsely believe that they need to be less careful about replacing fluids as they become acclimated to the heat. In fact, acclimatized athletes need to drink more to offset their body's enhanced sweating response. During endurance exercise, as you become progressively dehydrated, any improved ability to tolerate the heat is negated. Dehydration is also a likely culprit behind the gastrointestinal woes that many marathoners and ultra runners suffer from.

Think of dehydration as a fierce competitor that won't let go. When you become dehydrated during exercise beyond 2 percent of your body weight, your heart rate and body temperature rise and your performance really

---

Meltdown Man

Although many anecdotes relate the travails suffered by those who become dehydrated when exercising in the heat, one of the most highly publicized and horrifying encounters befell Australian Mark Dorrity, often referred to as the Meltdown Man. In the Australian summer of 1988, Mark and a few friends began an 8K run at 2:30 in the afternoon when the ambient temperature was in excess of 38 degrees Celsius (100 °F). In fact, the fun run in which the men were supposed to take part had been postponed from 2:30 until 5:30 in the hope that temperatures would be cooler. Well in the lead near the end of the run, Mr. Dorrity, 28 years old and in good physical condition, suddenly collapsed. He was in such obvious trouble that he was transported directly to a hospital.

On admission, his body temperature was 42 degrees Celsius (107.6 °F). A tracheotomy was immediately done to perform the pulmonary ventilation that his impaired respiratory system could not maintain. Because his immune system was subdued and his blood-clotting mechanisms were impaired by his high body temperature, an opportunistic infection set in, a result of a scrape sustained on his left leg when he initially collapsed. Over the next few days, the muscles of his left leg turned a khaki color and had the stringy texture of overcooked meat. This accelerated rhabdomyolysis (degeneration of skeletal muscle tissue)—overenthusiastically and inaccurately referred to as "meltdown" in the Australian press—caused acute renal failure, requiring months of dialysis. Twenty-seven days after admission, the leg was amputated at the hip. Mark remained comatose for 132 days before regaining consciousness and beginning years of convalescence.

Adapted, by permission, from R. Murray, 1995, "Fluid needs in hot and cold environments," *International Journal of Sport Nutrition* 5(Suppl): S62-S73.

---

begins to suffer. Fluid losses of 3 to 5 percent of body weight can significantly impair performance, and losses of more than 5 percent of body weight are dangerous. There is no way to adapt to dehydration, so don't even try.

Exercise-Associated Hyponatremia

Athletes, especially women, participating in endurance endeavors are at particular risk of developing exercise-associated hyponatremia (EAH), or a blood sodium level below the normal range of 136 to 143 millimoles per liter. EAH can result from losing large amounts of sodium (for example, through prolonged sweating); however, the more likely cause is drinking too much sodium-free (plain water, for example) or low-sodium fluid beyond what your body needs. A drop in blood sodium occurs as a result of replacing the fluid but not the sodium lost through sweating. Essentially, the sodium concentration in your body becomes diluted. EAH can be induced before, during, or following prolonged exercise.

As city marathons became popular around the world in the 1970s and 1980s, the American College of Sports Medicine (ACSM) published its 1975 position statement advocating regular fluid intake during endurance events. The rationale was that this would reduce the risk of heatstroke. During the 1980s and 1990s, however, increasing numbers of endurance athletes experienced EAH. Researchers at the Hawaii Ironman triathlon in the 1990s, for example, found that almost 30 percent of the triathletes who ended up in the medical tent were hyponatremic. More recently, studies from the 2002 Boston Marathon and 2006 London Marathon found that 13 percent and 12.5 percent of finishers, respectively, had asymptomatic hyponatremia.

An international panel of hydration experts at the International EAH Consensus Development Conferences of 2005 and 2007 declared that exertional hyponatremia during exercise is relatively rare. Evidence-based studies predict that probably fewer than 1 in 1,000 finishers of endurance events such as a marathon or triathlon will be affected. Nevertheless, these experts strongly advocated for guidelines promoting drinking "to thirst" rather than the higher volumes recommended by ACSM. In 2007, ACSM revised its position statement advising that fluid intake during exercise should not exceed sweat loss. It's recommended, therefore, that active athletes should monitor body weight changes during training (and if feasible, during competitions) to estimate their sweat losses during a particular exercise activity with respect to the weather conditions.

Although consuming a sports drink during exercise, rather than just plain water, isn't a definitive cure-all for EAH, it's a must for higher-risk athletes. This includes athletes who have more opportunities to drink, such as slower-pace marathoners (those who run or walk for more than 4 hours) and triathletes on the move for longer than 9 hours. Female athletes in general tend to be at higher risk for EAH than male athletes due to a comparatively smaller starting blood volume. Women also are more apt to heed directives about drinking during exercise! Lastly, older adults may be at risk for fluid-electrolyte imbalances due to age-related slower responses by kidneys to water and sodium loads.

If you develop a headache while exercising and become nauseated, lethargic, confused, or disoriented, seek medical attention immediately. Athletes with severe cases of hyponatremia may become unconscious, develop seizures, and even stop breathing or suffer cardiac arrest (see table 14.2). Athletes have died while participating in popular endurance races, such as the Chicago, Marine Corps, and Boston Marathons.

Many ultraendurance events feature weigh-ins at aid stations. If not (and if it's feasible), bring your own bathroom scale. Be alert to signs that you're gaining weight while exercising—a red flag that you're overhydrated and at increased risk for developing EAH. To ward off EAH, consume beverages

TABLE 14.2 Warning Signs of Dehydration and Hyponatremia

Dehydration	Hyponatremia
Early: headache, fatigue, dizziness, nausea, vomiting, dry mouth and eyes, loss of appetite, flushed skin, heat intolerance or exhaustion, dark-colored urine with a strong odor, irritability, muscle cramps, weight loss	Early: feeling bloated, nausea and vomiting, visible bloating (swollen hands and feet, watch or rings feel tight, bloated stomach), dizziness, throbbing headache, rapid weight gain, pale-colored urine (looks like water), cramping
More advanced: difficulty swallowing, clumsiness, abnormal chills, shriveled skin, sunken eyes and dim vision, inability to urinate, delirium, heatstroke	More advanced: restlessness, malaise, apathy, confusion, disorientation, severe fatigue or weakness, respiratory distress, seizure, coma

with sodium (sports drinks and soup or broth, for example) or small amounts of salted snacks, as well as sodium-containing foods at meals and before (and after) prolonged efforts. During ultraendurance competitions, keep track of what you're consuming—calories, fluid, and sodium. The longer the exercise duration, the greater the cumulative effects of slight mismatches between fluid needs and replacement, which can lead to excessive dehydration or dilutional hyponatremia.

Race Day: How to Avoid Both Dehydration and Hyponatremia

Popular endurance events, such as the Boston Marathon, now routinely post hydration guidelines for participants. These race-day tips were developed by the medical directors of four major U.S. marathons—Boston, Chicago, Houston, and the Twin Cities.

Develop your own hydration program using these tips:

- You're unique, so don't copy other runners. Some runners need less fluid than you, while others will need more. Learn your individual hydration needs. Fluid needs vary widely. Slower runners need to be very cautious with their fluid intake, while faster runners may need to drink more to replace higher volume sweat losses.

- Try to match fluid intake to just below weight loss. For example, if you lost 2 pounds (32 oz; 1 kg) during a run, you should try to drink close to 32 ounces (950 ml) but not more during that long run.

- During a marathon, you should lose 2 to 3 pounds (1 to 1.4 kg). If you do not lose weight, you are seven times more likely to get hyponatremia.

> continued

< continued

- Do not overdrink. Weight gain during a run is a sure sign of over-drinking.
- If you are feeling the effects of hot weather, slow your pace. Drinking more fluid will not directly make you less hot or cool you down.
- If you are a slow runner, determine the fluid intake that keeps your weight balanced with a slight 1 percent loss during a long run, or drink when you are thirsty. The rate of sweat and weight loss for the same distance varies according to weather conditions and running speed.
- Keep your urine a pale yellow color like lemonade, neither dark like apple juice (dehydration) nor clear like water (overhydration).
- Recognize the warning signs of dehydration like feeling faint or light-headed while standing or feeling very thirsty or experiencing a rapid heart rate, sunken eyes, dry mouth, or dull headache. Try some fluids to see if you improve.
- Recognize the warning signs of hyponatremia, like experiencing the sensation of water sloshing in your stomach, a severe and worsening headache, wheezy breathing, or feelings of puffiness or bloating in the hands and feet, nausea, or upset stomach. Stop drinking until you begin to urinate and the symptoms resolve.
- If you are not feeling well during or after the race, and simple changes do not make you feel better, seek immediate medical attention.

Reprinted, with permission of American Medical Athletic Association and American Running Association, from "Optimal Hydration: Establishing a Hydration Plan for Marathons" (brochure, 2013 update).

Heat Cramps

If you've suffered from heat cramps or watched someone else do so, you won't soon forget the experience. Severe cramps hit the skeletal muscles most heavily used during exercise. For endurance athletes, that means the abdominal, calf (lower leg), quadriceps (front of the thigh), and hamstring (back of the thigh) muscles. During my first adventure race, our three-person team had to kayak, mountain bike, and trail run while conquering various obstacles along the way. We encountered a hot (over 90 °F, or 32 °C), sunny day in Portland, Oregon. Unfortunately, our star athlete, although blessed with a competitive spirit, was low on physical conditioning and had just stepped off a plane after spending a year in England. An hour in the kayak and two more on the mountain bike didn't seem to faze him, until he hopped off the bike. He collapsed to the ground with severe cramps in both quadriceps. Having survived 2 hours of single-track mountain biking, I was not about to miss the chance to put my running background to good use. With the help of a sports drink and electrolyte tablets, we got him up and running.

We managed to pass more than 10 teams on that final leg and finish among the top 25 teams overall.

You don't have to be dehydrated necessarily to experience heat cramps. A low level of minerals involved in muscle contraction, such as sodium and chloride, is most likely the major cause of heat cramps. You're especially at risk if you sweat heavily for several hours and are rehydrating with plain water only. To prevent heat cramps, acclimate to hot and humid conditions as much as possible, be liberal with the saltshaker in your daily diet, and rely on sports drinks rather than plain water for prolonged, strenuous exercise in the heat. If you do experience a heat-related cramp, ingesting a properly formulated sports drink (with adequate sodium) or any other source of sodium, such as a salty food, can help to resolve the situation.

Heat Exhaustion

Heat exhaustion, or the inability to continue exercising in the heat, results from dehydration. When you suffer from heat exhaustion, your cardiovascular system simply can't meet the simultaneous demands of sending blood to active muscles and to the skin. This situation occurs as your blood volume drops due to the excessive loss of fluid or minerals from sweating. Your body's thermoregulatory mechanisms are still working; however, you can't dissipate heat quickly enough because too little blood (and the heat it carries) is going to the skin.

Signs of heat exhaustion to watch for during exercise include extreme thirst, headache, weakness, dizziness, heat sensations on the head or neck, abdominal cramps, chills, goose bumps, nausea, and vomiting. You also may hyperventilate (breathe rapidly and deeply), act confused, and possibly faint. The risk of suffering heat exhaustion increases when you're exercising at or near maximum capacity, when you're dehydrated, and when you aren't physically fit or haven't yet acclimated to the heat. Athletes suffering from heat exhaustion are advised to immediately stop all activity and seek a cooler environment (get in the shade or an air-conditioned area if available). If you're coherent and conscious, consume fluids, preferably beverages that contain sodium, such as sports drinks, tomato juice, or soup. Force yourself to drink, even if you feel nauseated.

Heatstroke

If left untreated, heat exhaustion can deteriorate into heatstroke, a potentially life-threatening disorder. Characterized by severe hyperthermia or a body temperature that has risen to a dangerously high level (exceeding 104 °F, or 40 °C), heatstroke can damage the central nervous system permanently or can even lead to death. During heatstroke, the body's thermoregulatory mechanisms fail because of excessive heat buildup and dehydration. Symptoms include vomiting, diarrhea, disorientation, convulsions, and unconsciousness. The person may stop sweating altogether, and the skin feels hot and dry. Rapid cooling of the entire body is crucial. This can be accomplished by applying wet towels and fanning the person, applying ice packs, or immersing the person in a cold stream.

Don't be lulled into thinking that heatstroke is a danger on only the hottest days of the year. Incidents of heatstroke have been reported in cool to moderate environments (55 to 82 °F, or 13 to 28 °C). Several factors may increase the risk of heatstroke, including being overweight or in poor physical condition, advanced age, lack of sleep, alcohol or drug use, having a sunburn, not being acclimated to the heat, and previously having suffered a heat injury.

Nutrition Strategies for Beating the Heat

Let's assume that you are physically fit, heat acclimated, well rested, and well fueled for whatever endeavor you choose to undertake in the heat. What else can you do to maximize your chances of performing well? You can work to minimize the risk of both dehydration and hyponatremia in several ways.

Before the Event

- **Know your hourly sweat rate.** Fluid and electrolyte needs of sports-minded people vary widely, depending on a person's genetics as well as the environmental conditions under which the endurance exercise takes place. Cyclists, for example, may not appreciate how much they sweat because of how quickly it evaporates. Aim to determine your hourly sweat rate while training under the same or similar heat and humidity conditions that you expect to encounter during your endeavor.

  Use the following formula to estimate your average hourly sweat rate. Note that pre- and postexercise weights refer to nude body weight. The formula assumes no urine output during the one-hour test bout of exercise. Every pound lost = 16 ounces (480 ml) of fluid.

  Preexercise weight (convert to oz) − postexercise weight (oz) + fluid intake (if any) during 1 hour of exercise (oz) = individual hourly sweat rate (ounces/hour)

- **Practice drinking while on the move during longer training efforts.** The number one priority before undertaking any endurance endeavor, especially one taking place in the heat, is to develop a solid rehydration plan. This requires that you practice during workouts matching as closely as possible the fluid and electrolytes that you're losing by sweating (your hourly sweat rate). Now is the time to develop this fluid plan and to experiment with bladders and other hydration systems to determine which is best for your particular sport or situation. If you're responsible for meeting your own fluid needs (no aid stations), figure out how you are going to carry the fluid that you need or how you will resupply along the way. If race organizers will be supplying the sports drink, find out in advance what brand will be offered on the course so that you can experiment with it during longer training efforts.

- **Pass the saltshaker.** If you're a normal healthy adult, your body has several sophisticated mechanisms for regulating how much sodium you take in and retain, so it's not necessary to make a conscious effort to restrict your intake. When faced with hot weather, especially when making seasonal changes or traveling to an event in a warmer region than you trained in, add salt to the foods that you eat. You also can consume sodium-rich foods such as bouillon, canned soup or beans, cheese, tomato or vegetable juice, pretzels, salted crackers, and other low-fat snack foods. The sodium in these foods (and in sports beverages that are consumed before and during exercise) helps you to retain water and avoid a sodium deficit, as well as boost your drive to drink.

  Even if you're fit and well acclimated to the heat, expect to lose large amounts of sodium and chloride through extensive and repetitive sweating (115 to 700 milligrams of sodium or more per liter of sweat), along with the sodium typically excreted in urine. For some endurance athletes, such as those with high sweat rates like 2.5 liters per hour, this can translate into a substantial sodium loss exceeding 1,500 milligrams per hour during prolonged exercise. Exercise-induced losses of sodium are exacerbated if you consciously follow a low-salt training diet (as in the 2,300 milligrams a day recommended limit for inactive people) and incur persistent sodium losses from prolonged training efforts and competitions.

- **Experiment with electrolytes (salt) tablets and other salty foods.** For those who undertake prolonged endurance efforts or who previously have suffered a heat illness, ingesting salt or electrolyte tablets (which contain primarily sodium) during prolonged exercise may be necessary if sports drinks and salty foods (if available) don't get the job done. You may experience nausea, vomiting, or diarrhea when taking electrolyte tablets, so don't wait until an important race to figure out what works for you. Be sure to carry tablets in a plastic bag or waterproof case because they disintegrate upon contact with moisture, such as sweat.

- **Start out with a full tank.** Common sense should tell you that if you set out to exercise without being adequately hydrated, things will only get worse, especially in the heat. Consciously remind yourself to drink during the day by carrying a water bottle with you (especially during air travel) or leaving one in plain view, such as on your desk. Every time you eat a meal or a snack, make sure to also drink a healthy beverage (see chapter 1). Drinking at regular intervals throughout the day is best, since downing a large volume of fluid at any one time only sends you running to the bathroom.

Don't become anxious and overhydrate (especially by drinking excessive amounts of plain water) in the day or two before the competition. Running to the bathroom hourly or having very pale-colored urine (it looks like water) means you're exceeding your fluid needs. You're also setting yourself up for trouble when you finally do begin to exercise.

If practical, freeze water bottles beforehand or buy an insulated bottle to help keep liquids cool and refreshing. Young athletes dehydrate quickly, especially on warm days, so if you're with kids or teenagers, make sure that each one has their own water bottle or bladder. For ventures into the backcountry, pack a water-filtration device and be certain that you know how to use it.

During the Event

- **Stick to a predetermined drinking plan.** Remember, the goal is to minimize both dehydration and hyponatremia. Dehydration is far more common, however, so plan to drink early and often, about every 15 to 20 minutes. During exercise, our thirst mechanism fails to keep up with our actual fluid needs, so set your watch alarm as a reminder to drink. Water is generally adequate for events lasting 1 hour or less (like a 10K road race), although a sports drink won't do harm and is likely to boost your finishing kick.

  If you'll be on the move for more than 60 minutes at a moderate or faster pace, drink a sports drink with multiple carbohydrate sources and adequate sodium to meet your fluid, carbohydrate, and sodium needs (ideally the same one that you've been training with). Research has shown that athletes who are exercising in the heat and have free access to water replace only one-half to two-thirds of their fluid losses. The flavoring and electrolytes in sports drinks encourage hydration.

  Drinking on a predetermined timeline is mandatory on warm, windy days and hot days with low humidity, since it's easy to forget that you are sweating. And any time that you're with kids or teens, schedule and take frequent mandatory fluid breaks because young athletes can become dehydrated quickly. Young athletes typically do a much better job of rehydrating if a flavored beverage, such as a sports drink, is readily available.

- **Drink to match your fluid losses.** You can't just wing it during endurance races, nor can you simply try to drink as much as you can—you need to drink intelligently. Both severe underdrinking and severe overdrinking are dangerous! Consuming fluids beyond what you're losing as sweat, for example, increases your risk of developing hyponatremia. Simply not drinking at all, however, is not a safe option. You have to know your body and constantly monitor the signals that it sends.

Because endurance athletes can't rely on the perception of thirst alone, you will need to monitor your body weight and the rate at which you are sweating. Pay attention if you find yourself gaining weight (in events with mandatory weight checks, for example), if you feel puffy or are noticeably bloated, or if your rings, watch, or belt become tight. These signs point to the fact that you are likely overhydrating. This scenario is a real risk if you've chosen to drink mostly plain water or have elected to do so in an attempt to deal with intestinal woes. If you're not sweating heavily (as may occur if you are running slowly, for example) and you aren't thirsty, then you need to replace any fluid losses at only a modest rate.

- **Be prepared to carry what you need.** In many endurance events and races, you will be responsible for meeting your own fluid needs most or all the time. Don't let the concern of carrying extra weight prevent you from wearing a bladder or a waist belt that holds a water bottle or two. The benefit of having fluid readily accessible, especially during prolonged endeavors, far exceeds any negative consequences of carrying additional weight in the form of water or powdered sports drink. Drinking at regular intervals promotes sweating, our primary avenue to heat loss. If you can't cool off adequately, your brain will find a way to slow or possibly even completely shut down your body.

  Even in situations in which fluids are provided, such as organized rides, triathlons, and marathons, you may benefit from (or even find it necessary) to carry some of your own. Planned aid stations or rest stops with food and drinks, for example, may not be frequent enough for marathoners and other athletes who sweat heavily or larger athletes with high fluid needs. Be honest with yourself. You will lose far more time being reduced to a crawl or stopping to deal with muscle cramps than you ever will because of being weighed down by a pound of fluid and extra sports drink powder.

- **Consume salty foods and beverages (and possibly electrolyte tablets).** Much of the time, consuming a sports drink during exercise, along with getting enough salt on a daily basis, will be enough for most endurance athletes. Look for salty foods at organized events (soup, cheese, pretzels, pickles, tomato juice) or foods that you can add salt to, such as potatoes or sandwiches. (See Pass the Salt in chapter 12.) If you're participating in prolonged events and plan to be on the move for 4 hours or more and you choose to supplement with electrolyte tablets, don't overdo it. Keep in mind that no definitive guidelines exist. Start by taking one tablet (200 to 350 milligrams of sodium) per hour of exercise and take it with plenty (6 to 8 ounces, or 180 to 240 milliliters) of water. Some athletes may require two tablets per hour during long, hot races, as may athletes participating in multiday events who have access only to plain water.

- **If need be, force yourself to eat.** Be aware that hot conditions and intense or prolonged exercise can doubly suppress your appetite. If you're in for a long day, such as an all-day hike or an adventure race that may stretch even past 24 hours, you most likely will have to force yourself to eat. Eating anything is better than eating nothing, so don't be worried if you survive on the same few foods. Carbohydrate-rich foods, either sports foods like energy bars, chews, blocks, and gels, or real food like fig bars and gumdrops, will work. Basically, anything that goes down and stays down is a winner.

The Beauty of a Bladder Hydration System

Whether you're traveling by foot, bike, ski, snowshoe, or kayak, you need to hydrate or you'll die—figuratively, if not literally. Many of the problems encountered during endurance activities, such as nausea, headaches, heat illness, and altitude sickness, often result from not drinking enough. Bladder hydration systems encourage drinking by making fluids readily accessible. You don't have to come to a stop, miss a step, or tie up your hands as you do when reaching for a water bottle. Bladders also allow you to carry large quantities of fluid comfortably. A 50-ounce (1.5 L) bladder is equal to two large water bottles, and a 70-ounce (2 L) bladder equates to three large bottles. The granddaddy of all bladders can hold 100 ounces (3 L), the equivalent of four large water bottles. Bladder hydration systems come in multiple styles designed specifically for various sports and activities. Worn alone or as part of a pack, sports vest, or hip-mounted belt, a bladder hydration system can efficiently distribute the weight of the fluid without interfering with normal movement. Bladders are available at outdoor and sporting goods stores or specialty shops that cater to cyclists, runners, hikers, and skiers.

Fully insulated bladders help liquids stay cool as temperatures rise, and you can add ice to some models.

Keep a bladder system clean and free from mold and bacteria by rinsing it with warm water following every use. For a more thorough cleaning, use a biodegradable dishwashing detergent and a bottlebrush to clean the tube. You can buy bottlebrushes at a local hardware store or supermarket, or buy a cleaning kit from the manufacturer. To sanitize a bladder, add a teaspoon or two of household bleach to a full bladder. Shake vigorously, and then rinse the bladder and tube well with hot water. Don't overkill potential germs. You can make yourself sick from using too much bleach or not rinsing well enough with hot water. Use a paper towel to dry the inside of the bladder and then prop the sides open with a paper towel or similar item and hang it to air dry. If residual tastes and odors bother you, fill the bladder with water, add 2 teaspoons of baking soda, let it sit over night, and then rinse well and dry.

Postevent Recovery Plan

- **Rehydrate to match your fluid losses.** For one-day events, drink (over the next few hours) at least 2.5 cups of fluid for every pound (~1.5 liters for every kilogram) of body weight that you're down. Don't, however, only consume plain water. Athletes have been known to induce hyponatremia in the hours following prolonged exercise when they avoid or are unable to eat solid food and they're rehydrating by drinking plain water or other low-sodium beverages, like beer. Monitor your ability to urinate and its color—you want it to be pale yellow.

- **Refuel promptly.** Anticipate a decrease or lack of appetite. Drinking the calories (and carbohydrate) that the body requires for refueling is usually easier at this time. Lemonade, fruit juices, milk shakes, yogurt, instant breakfast drinks, fruit smoothies, and complete meal-replacement beverages go down fairly easily. Ease in other carbohydrate-rich foods, such as bananas, bagels, and cereal, as soon as you tolerate them.

  Resist the urge to wait until your appetite returns to eat. You'll miss the valuable window of opportunity (the first 30 minutes) immediately after exercise to jump-start replenishing muscle glycogen and repairing damaged muscle fibers. Refueling promptly is essential for all athletes! Eating solid foods also will help replace other electrolytes lost through sweating (in much smaller amounts than sodium), such as potassium. Potassium-rich foods include juices, fruits, vegetables, milk, and yogurt.

LEARNING FROM THE BEST: PERFORMING IN THE HEAT

Ultra runner Scott Jurek knows how to beat the heat. A seven-straight-time winner of the Western States 100-Mile Endurance Run, he decided to tackle the Badwater Ultramarathon. This 135-mile (217 km) nonstop jaunt from Death Valley to Mount Whitney, California, is run in temperatures reaching 130 degrees Fahrenheit (55 °C). He won on his first attempt, running 24 hours and 36 minutes to break the course record at the time. Jurek, who recently set a new U.S. all-surface record in the 24-Hour Run with 165.7 miles (267 km), has nearly two decades of racing ultras under his belt, and he sports a 2:38 marathon PR. Although you may never literally face the heat of Death Valley, here's his advice on how to do more than merely survive hot-weather endurance endeavors.

Training Priorities for Racing Well in the Heat

You need to do two main things before the start of the race: Figure out your sweat rate (what you lose each hour) and train your digestive tract to handle the large volumes of fluid that will need to be consumed during hot weather. For a sweat test, replicate as closely as possible the conditions that you expect

> continued

< continued

and then see what you've lost after 60 to 90 minutes of exercise. (See How to Estimate Average Hourly Sweat Rate in chapter 4.) Then factor in duration (how long you will be out there), the intensity at which you'll be working, and any extenuating circumstances that further increase fluid losses, such as being at altitude or in high humidity.

No shortcuts exist. You have to figure out what your body needs and then train your digestive tract, which means improving your stomach's emptying rate. As Jurek emphasizes, you can't expect to handle 60 to 70 ounces (1,775 to 2,070 ml) of fluid per hour on race day if you've been drinking only 30 ounces (890 ml) in training.

Day of the Race

Focus on hydrating and getting in enough carbohydrate. Stay on top of it from the beginning. Know what you need to drink each hour and stick with it. Ultraendurance athletes, especially, can't make it up as they go along. Jurek reminds athletes that although they may be able to gut out a marathon in 5 or 6 hours, there's very little wiggle room in longer races. You won't be able to make up for falling behind, especially fuel-wise. It can take hours to come back because of the time it takes the body to absorb and process what it needs. Slow down if necessary so that you can digest what you're taking in.

Some degree of dehydration will occur. Jurek agrees with expert's recommendations, however, that a loss of 2 to 3 percent from preexercise weight is the defining edge. At Badwater, he brought his own scale and monitored his weight throughout the race.

As for carbohydrate, know what you need per hour based on your body weight and then stick to it. Jurek uses the following formula: .7 to 1.0 × body weight in kilograms = grams of carbohydrate per hour. This equates to a minimum of 30 grams per hour for most endurance athletes. Look at the total time or number of hours that you will be competing. Although elite athletes seem not to eat or drink that much when racing marathons, realize that they're out there for little more than 2 hours! In addition, they are extremely fit and, as a result, are burning more fat for fuel. Endurance athletes, especially ultra athletes, need a steady supply of carbohydrate, as much for brain power as for fueling muscles.

Diluting Sports Drinks During Hot Weather

Jurek doesn't believe in diluting sports drinks. He agrees with sports nutrition experts that it's too easy to get behind on carbohydrate and electrolytes since these components go too when a sports drink is diluted. He makes sure that he has both plain water and a sports drink available. If he craves water, then he drinks water and gets his carbohydrate some other way (with energy gels, for example). Jurek also keeps plain water on hand to help ensure that things don't become too concentrated in his stomach from, for example, mixing a concentrated sports drink and gels.

Meeting Electrolyte Needs

Jurek thinks that most serious ultra athletes have learned how important sodium is during prolonged exercise; however, he remains concerned that less experienced or less competitive endurance athletes, or newcomers like marathon runners who are moving up in distance, may not have gotten the message. He stresses the fact that most sports drinks, even if consumed in appropriate quantities, aren't high enough in sodium to meet the needs of marathoners who are going to be on the course for 4 to 8 hours.

As the heat, humidity, or pace picks up, you sweat more, especially if you're not heat acclimated. You can be losing sodium at an extremely high rate. Depending on the race and environmental conditions, Jurek advises the athletes he coaches to boost their sodium intake either by mixing their drinks to be very strong or by using salt tablets.

Tried-and-True Strategies for Competing in the Heat

Jurek's first strategy is to keep his drinks as cold as possible. Second, for any sports drink or food that he plans to use, he always brings a variety of flavors. Third, not eating during a race simply is not an option, so he doesn't overdo anything early in the race (energy gels, for example) that he knows he has to rely on late in the race. If you carry salt tablets, you need to keep them dry. Jurek uses a widget (a small squeezable pill purse); however, you can also use a baggie. Be sure to reseal the baggie completely after each use.

Last, during hot-weather races Jurek advises athletes to keep it simple. He eats less fibrous solid food and opts instead for sports foods like sports drinks and gels and simple foods like potatoes and bananas. The bottom line is that if you don't eat, you'll be forced to go very slowly because of insufficient fuel; as Jurek notes, that's not a fun way to do long races.

15

Extreme Cold

> The production of heat which occurs after eating is referred to as the "thermic effect" of food, or diet-induced thermogenesis. The body must expend energy to process foods you consume, leading to a temporary increase in resting metabolic rate. You can feel warmer 30 to 60 minutes after a meal, in other words, as your body generates about 10 percent more heat than it does on an empty stomach.
>
> Source: Evidence Analysis Library, Academy of Nutrition and Dietetics.

Thanks to year-round sporting opportunities and advances in performance clothing, you may find yourself out in the cold for a long time. Like those who deal with extreme heat and humidity, cold-weather athletes must learn to master the unique challenges of exercising in less than ideal conditions, especially if intending to compete. In cold environments, we must maintain our internal, or core, temperature.

As discussed in chapter 14, the hypothalamus acts as a thermostat to keep your body temperature at acceptable levels. Located at the base of the brain, the hypothalamus receives signals from central receptors, which sense changes in blood temperature, and from peripheral receptors, which monitor the temperature of your skin and the environment.

The body relies on three main mechanisms to avoid excessive cooling: shivering (uncontrolled muscular contractions that can raise the body's resting rate of heat production four to five times), nonshivering thermogenesis (whereby the nervous system increases the body's metabolic rate so as to produce more internal heat), and the vasoconstriction (narrowing) of peripheral blood vessels to prevent unnecessary heat loss. Proper clothing and subcutaneous fat (found just below the skin's surface) also help insulate deep body tissues from the cold.

Performing in Extreme Cold

While exercising in the cold, trouble sets in if you dissipate heat faster than you produce it. Prolonged exercise normally increases the use of free fatty acids for fuel. This process is attenuated in the cold, however, because vaso-constriction impairs blood flow to the subcutaneous fat, the major storage site for free fatty acids. As fatigue sets in, as may occur during prolonged running, swimming, or skiing, muscle activity slows and the body struggles to generate enough internal heat to maintain its temperature. Blood glucose plays an important role in how well you tolerate the cold. Hypoglycemia, or low blood sugar, for example, suppresses shivering. Muscle glycogen also appears to be affected, for example, being used at a somewhat faster rate in cold water than it is in warmer conditions. No matter what activity or sport you're involved in, you withstand the rigors of performing in a cold environment better when you're well hydrated and well fueled.

Cold Acclimatization

Exercising in cold weather may be something that you grin and bear, or it may be an activity that you relish. Although acclimating to the cold is possible, the process is not well understood and it appears to be harder to accomplish than is warm-weather acclimatization. Generally, extremely fit athletes and those with slightly higher body-fat levels tolerate cold-weather exercise most comfortably.

As anyone who lives and trains in the cold can attest, adjusting psycho-logically may be what counts the most. Whether it's because of growing up running in the snowbelt of upstate New York, surviving ice and snowstorms while attending Georgetown University in Washington, D.C. (a city with few snowplows), or tolerating seven winters in Boston and two more in Colorado, I know that I can handle the cold. Over time, you, too, will come to better tolerate the cold if you commit to the adaptation process physically and mentally.

Dehydration and Hypothermia

Performing in the cold brings its own set of challenges. Endurance athletes must be aware of two potential problems that can strike at any time: dehy-dration and hypothermia. Performing at your best while exercising in the cold requires you to be as savvy about fluids and fuel as you are during warmer conditions.

Dehydration

Although many athletes fail to believe it, dehydration hinders cold-weather performances just as it limits exercising in the heat. Have you wondered how you possibly could have to make a pit stop in the middle of a snowstorm?

Blame it on cold-induced diuresis. As you venture out into the cold, your peripheral blood vessels, which carry blood to the skin and other outer regions of the body such as the ears, hands, and feet, constrict to conserve heat and maintain the body's core temperature. This peripheral vasoconstriction causes a rise in blood pressure, including within the kidneys, which induces you to urinate and thereby lose fluid.

You also lose a considerable amount of fluid while breathing as you exercise in the cold. When you inhale, your respiratory passages warm and humidify the cold, dry air that you are taking in. When you exhale moisture-saturated air, you lose water (this why you can see your breath in cold weather). This process can result in a loss of as much as 1 quart of fluid daily. Also, although Jack Frost is nipping at our ears and toes, we don't stop sweating. Any time our body temperature rises sufficiently, sweating occurs. If you tend to overdress for cold-weather exercise, you can sweat profusely, especially during intense efforts. Researchers estimate that if clothing with insulating properties equivalent to four business suits is worn, sweat losses can reach 2 quarts per hour during moderate to heavy exercise in freezing conditions.

Despite the loss of moisture that occurs, athletes often don't consume as much fluid during cold-weather exercise. It's normal to simply not feel as thirsty when exercising in the cold. Suitable drinks may not be readily available, and it can be a struggle to keep them from freezing. And some athletes consciously restrict their fluid intake to avoid the logistical problems or discomfort associated with making pit stops in the cold. It's easy to see why athletes become dehydrated during cold-weather exercise.

Using a Bladder Hydration System in Cold Weather

To keep your hydration system bladder and hose from freezing, wear a layer of clothing on top of it and keep the drinking hose covered until it's time to drink. Drinking small amounts at regular intervals keeps you hydrated and helps keep the contents from freezing. In severe cold, blow air into the tube and force the liquid back into the bladder or experiment with winterizing adaptation kits available from some manufacturers. (See The Beauty of a Bladder Hydration System in chapter 14 for more information on using and caring for a bladder hydration system.)

Hypothermia

Hypothermia, a decrease in core body temperature below 98.6 degrees Fahrenheit (37 °C), occurs when you lose more heat than you produce. Occurring in stages, the warning signs of mild hypothermia include shivering, a red face, and an increase in respiration and heart rate. Often accompanied by dehydration and exhaustion, hypothermia can quickly progress to lethargy, weakness, slurred speech, disorientation, and combative behavior as the core temperature continues to fall. Left untreated, a hypothermic person may stop shivering, become progressively delirious, and lapse into a coma.

You don't have to be scaling the world's tallest mountain in the dead of winter to become hypothermic. Because it can develop in relatively mild temperatures (50 to 65 degrees Fahrenheit, or 10 to 18 degrees Celsius), hypothermia is a real danger any time you exercise in cool or cold weather. Be alert for signs of hypothermia in the following high-risk situations: on windy days, when the weather changes rapidly (in spring and autumn and at high altitudes, for example), in endeavors that involve swimming or passing through water, and during the second half of long races (such as marathons and triathlons), when you generate less heat because of moving at a slower pace, which is further compounded by losing heat through wet clothing (from sweat, rain, or snow).

As long as you're moving, you may be generating enough heat; however, you can still easily get into trouble when you stop. I encountered hypothermia while climbing Mont Blanc, the tallest of the Alps (15,771 feet, or 4,807 meters), on a sunny August morning in relatively light wind conditions. Unfortunately, I don't remember the spectacular views from the top of Italy and France because I was too busy shivering uncontrollably. Caught up in the moment (and not wishing to slow the French guide), we ascended on record pace (5,000 vertical feet, or 1,500 meters, in 4 hours) without stopping to adjust clothing or to eat anything beyond the candy we carried in our pockets. I was in trouble as soon as we reached the summit and I stopped generating heat from kicking steps into the snow with heavy double boots. Fortunately, I'm still around to tell you how to avoid this scenario!

Nutrition Strategies for Beating the Cold

Mom's advice to have a bowl of stick-to-your ribs oatmeal before heading outdoors to play in the snow makes a lot of sense. Not because of the cold temperatures (we can compensate by dressing appropriately), but because

---

Hot Chocolate Smoothie

Here is a rich, thick beverage to drink during cold-weather outings.

4 teaspoons of sugar

4 teaspoons of cocoa powder

4 tablespoons of powdered milk

4 teaspoons of potato starch (used as a thickener; available at your local supermarket or at Asian markets)

At home: Combine all ingredients and place them in a ziplock bag.
On the trail: Place ingredients into an insulated mug, water bottle, or thermos. Add 1 cup of boiling water, stir well, cover, and let stand 5 minutes. Makes one 8-ounce (240 ml) serving.

---

we expend more energy (calories) performing most outdoor activities in winterlike conditions than we do in temperate conditions. The simple act of walking on snow, for example, uses almost twice as much energy as traversing the same route at the same speed on dry ground. We also burn more calories due to the extra weight of heavy boots and winter clothing, which can increase energy needs by 5 to 15 percent. No universally accepted standard exists for figuring caloric needs when exercising in the cold; however, the U.S. Army sets a goal for the average male soldier of 4,500 calories a day.

The ability to think clearly and avoid injury and hypothermia diminishes when you don't consume enough carbohydrate to keep a steady blood sugar level and to replenish glycogen reserves. Look at the scientific basis behind the adage "Never ski tired." (Skiers often lament having ignored their desire to call it a day when they get injured on their last trip down the mountain.) As glycogen in fast-twitch muscle fibers is depleted, muscular strength and, consequently, power, is lost. You rely to a large degree on fast-twitch muscle fibers to correct and control movements while skiing (and during similar activities). The ability to execute perfect telemark turns late in the day, therefore, can ultimately hinge on whether or not you stopped for a midafternoon snack.

Your muscles need carbohydrate, and your brain relies exclusively on glucose (a simple carbohydrate) for fuel. If blood sugar falls below a critical level, your judgment and the ability to perform skilled maneuvers will severely deteriorate, which could result in injury or death. Shivering, the body's attempt to raise core temperature, uses carbohydrate, and severe shivering can deplete glycogen stores. Exercising in cold water also uses muscle glycogen at a somewhat higher rate than does exercising in warm water.

When it comes to providing the calories needed for cold-weather exercise, athletes and experts alike continue to debate the merits of a carbohydrate-rich diet versus a diet higher in fat. This debate likely endures because people who traditionally live in cold regions often appear to favor high-fat (higher-protein) foods. Keep in mind, however, that the relative use of carbohydrate and fat as fuel varies widely among athletes. Factors such as your fitness level and degree of cold acclimatization, the pace or intensity of the exercise, and the severity of the cold may play a role. A fitter, more acclimatized athlete, for example, is able to burn more fat during exercise, an advantage that extends the body's limited glycogen reserves. Studies on energy metabolism in the prolonged cold are limited. The findings suggest, however, that in the cold, both fat and carbohydrate are metabolized at higher rates. The bulk of the calories consumed during cold-weather exercise, however, should still come from carbohydrate-rich foods because the increase in carbohydrate metabolism is substantially larger than the increase in fat metabolism.

To improve cold tolerance, take a look at what you eat and when you eat it. Despite conventional wisdom, a high-carbohydrate diet has been found superior to a high-protein diet in improving cold tolerance, but high-fat and high-carbohydrate diets have essentially the same effect when meals and snacks are consumed every 4 hours. A high-fat diet may be superior, though, when snacks and meals are eaten more frequently, every 2 hours, for example. (Nevertheless, adequate carbohydrate still must be consumed to replace muscle glycogen and prevent excess fatigue.) The best advice that I have for athletes looking to stay out in the cold (especially prolonged adventures that involve overnight stays) is to be in good physical condition, to wear proper clothing, and to eat enough calories (regardless of the source) to maintain a normal body temperature.

Assuming that you're properly clothed, venturing out to play in the cold doesn't increase your requirement for any specific nutrient. Negotiating difficult terrain and carrying the extra weight of a pack and heavy cold-weather clothing, however, does increase calorie needs. It's not unusual to feel less thirsty in cold weather, though, so eating may be logistically difficult or uncomfortable.

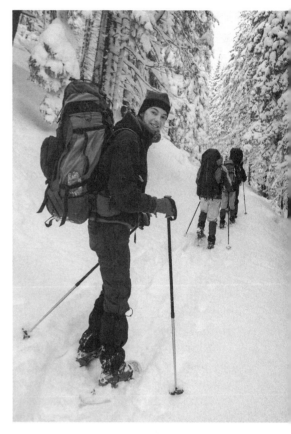

Attending to your increased need for fuel when exercising in the cold improves your performance and enhances your enjoyment.

Kapu/Fotolia.com

Without conscious and deliberate efforts to fulfill fluid and fuel needs, prolonged cold-weather exercise can rapidly deplete carbohydrate reserves to the extent that hypoglycemia (low blood sugar) and hypothermia (low body temperature) occur. The following sections outline how to give yourself the best chance to perform well in the cold.

Before the Event

Respect the added challenges of performing in the cold. As with clothing and gear, planning out your nutritional strategies beforehand really pays off.

Mind Your Iron Reserves

Low iron levels may make you more susceptible to the cold. Researchers found that iron-deficient women were able to produce heat but had difficulty retaining it to maintain their body temperature. Men who suffer from iron deficiency, although not studied, probably respond in a similar manner. Have your serum hemoglobin, hematocrit, and ferritin (stored iron) checked before you take an iron supplement. There is no evidence that you can enhance cold tolerance by taking excess iron if you're not deficient (see the Iron-Deficiency Anemia section in chapter 6 for more information).

Find Fluids and Foods That Work in the Cold

Now is the time to discover that your favorite energy or candy bar turns into an inedible rock when the temperatures dip, not when you're clinging to the side of a cliff or halfway through a bucket-list skiing adventure. Before a cold-weather endeavor, test all your favorite energy-boosting snacks. Do this during outdoor training efforts in the cold, or put the item in the freezer for a few hours and see what happens. If you can't eat it, don't bother packing it.

If you rely on a bladder to carry fluid, choose an insulated one designed for cold-weather activities and choose clothing that allows you to wear it underneath, as close to your body as possible. Experiment with the bladder over a range of temperatures, because the hoses on even the best models can freeze up. If possible, preheat drinks and pour the fluid into an insulated water bottle (even closed-cell foam secured by duct tape will help) or a sturdy thermos in the morning. Remove unnecessary wrappings and packages from food to save time and reduce the weight that you have to carry. To avoid having to remove your mittens or gloves, chop, slice, and dice foods such as energy bars and cheese before you leave home and repackage the bite-sized pieces into plastic food storage bags.

Rise and Dine the Morning of the Event

The mere act of eating temporarily revs up your metabolism and generates heat (although not nearly enough to warrant throwing away the long johns). At the very least, warm and nourishing foods provide a psychological boost. If high in calories, they also will help you meet your anticipated energy needs. If you're heading out for a single, short bout of cold-weather exercise, you don't need to worry as much. Hours of continuous exercise, however, can really boost calorie needs. Depending on body size, pace, pack weight, and terrain, for example, you can expend 3,000 calories (or more) on top of your normal daily energy needs during a 6-hour hike with a full backpack.

Unless you fuel up before setting out, you'll likely dig a big hole by lunchtime, even if you snack along the way. And I don't mean a Starbucks Grande and biscotti. Carbohydrate-rich foods are the fuel of choice for hard-working muscles. Dress up oatmeal, a classic send-off, by stirring in raisins or other dried fruit, brown sugar, honey, or a scoop of peanut butter. If oatmeal isn't high on your favorite foods list (it's not on mine), opt for a peanut butter sandwich or just-add-water products that take only minutes to prepare, such as individual-serving cups of chili, couscous with lentils, mashed potatoes, or grits. My breakfast of choice before a long hike, for example, includes a just-add-water cup of macaroni and cheese (230 calories—71 percent from carbohydrate, 14 percent from protein, and 14 percent from fat). If you're worried about stomach woes, try drinking your calories instead. An ultra-runner friend swears by a couple cans of Ensure before he hits the trail. Instant breakfast and meal-replacement drinks are another option.

During the Event

As is true for exercising in other environments, don't rely on thirst alone to trigger the need for fluid. And always remember that the imperative to maintain core body temperature puts added demand on the body's glycogen stores. To generate heat, you'll need to keep moving, and to keep moving, you need fuel. It's simple—drink and eat at regular intervals to improve your chances of performing well in the cold.

Plan to Drink Early and Often

Dehydration often is coupled with hypoglycemia (low blood sugar), and both compromise your ability to perform in the cold, as well as significantly increase your risk of becoming hypothermic. You must have access to a source of safe, drinkable water or other acceptable fluids. A good rule of thumb is that you need a minimum of 2 quarts (liters) per person for a day-long (6-hour) endeavor. Drink smaller amounts at regular intervals (a few gulps every 15 to 20 minutes) rather than a large amount at lunchtime and then again later in the day. Performing with dehydrated muscles increases the risk that you'll injure yourself, and if you wait to consume a large amount in one sitting, you'll simply urinate out much of the fluid.

Keep fluids from freezing by stashing the container near your body, in a breast pocket in your jacket rather than in your backpack, for example, or strap on a bladder hydration system that you know performs well in the cold. Depending on the activity, instant fruit or sports drinks, herbal teas, apple cider, cocoa, and soup make good choices. (Be aware that tea and coffee provide no calories unless spiked with sugar or honey.) Stay away from alcohol because it causes you to urinate. When you first drink alcohol, you may feel warmer; however, it isn't actually increasing your core temperature. Drinking alcohol, in fact, causes you to lose heat by opening the blood vessels to the skin.

Eating snow is a poor option too. The energy that you expend warming the snow can lower core body temperature enough to induce hypothermia. If you're a winter camper and want to obtain water by melting snow, be prepared to spend two precious commodities—time and fuel. You will have to melt approximately 5 cups of snow to obtain 1 cup of water. Be sure to bring the water to a rolling boil (keep an eye on it; 5 minutes isn't necessary) to kill waterborne microorganisms. If you're on the move, speed up the process by packing snow into your water bottle while the bottle still has some liquid in it. Filter or chemically disinfect any melted snow or water that isn't brought to a rolling boil. Despite your best intentions, in an emergency, eating snow or drinking untreated water may be the only option to ward off dehydration and enable you to keep moving. Look for clean snow or running water free of contaminants from animals or other humans.

Feed the Furnace

Your body generates about 10 percent more heat 30 to 60 minutes after eating than when you have an empty stomach. The energy released during digestion is primarily responsible for this increase in metabolism. Eating, therefore, not only provides fuel but also increases heat production, helping you to feel warmer. Shovel in carbohydrate-rich foods, preferably warm, at regular intervals to keep liver and muscle glycogen reserves full. Include more higher-fat foods the longer you'll be out in the cold to help meet elevated calorie needs and improve cold tolerance. Choose high-calorie foods that pack a lot of wallop, especially if you'll be spending prolonged periods in the cold (like overnight) or are limited in what you can carry. Prepared food items stored in inner pockets soak up body heat and are readily accessible.

Snack or break for mini meals regularly. Don't wait until you're too wet, tired, or cold to think about eating. Make sure that you actually get in the calories. Because I like to travel light and fast while hiking, I often found myself carrying food in my hands for long periods of time, rather than ingesting it as I intended. I now consciously make myself stop and eat. Plan ahead and anticipate the terrain, weather, and any other elements that you likely will encounter.

On longer excursions, such as 4- to 9-day cold-weather excursions, figure on at least 2 pounds (1 kg) of food (precooked weight) per person per day. Don't skimp on protein foods, but don't overdo them, either. Carbohydrate and fat are superior to protein when it comes to providing fuel for muscles and improving cold tolerance. The chief concern when exercising in the cold is to maintain body temperature by eating enough calories, regardless of the source. Bring a small reserve of extra food in case you get lost or the adventure takes longer than expected.

If you're out for hours at a time or temperatures are extreme, you may be able to improve your cold tolerance by snacking on high-fat foods throughout the activity. Aim for a 500-calorie snack every 2 hours. A peanut butter and jelly sandwich made with 2 tablespoons of peanut butter fits the bill, or gorp made with 2 to 3 ounces (60 to 90 g) of peanuts mixed with the same amount of raisins. If you plan to sleep in the cold, eat another 500-calorie snack immediately before retiring to your sleeping bag. You may sleep better, and your extremities (fingers and toes) may stay warmer through the night.

Fuel for Cold-Weather Adventures

Pushing your limits, especially when performing in the cold, means you need to eat high-performance foods to replace calories, carbohydrate, and other key nutrients. Although sports foods like energy bars, chews, and gels certainly fill the bill some of the time, consider the following real foods as you pack for your next cold-weather adventure. Plus, to warm yourself up, consume warm foods with carbohydrate, such as oatmeal, chili, soup, and hot chocolate. The warm food, combined with the thermogenic effect of eating, promotes a more rapid recovery.

Note: The foods that you select will depend on the activity, length of time outside, your personal tastes, and other practical considerations, such as how much you can carry and how long it takes to prepare the item.

Fluids

Fruit juices and drinks, lemonade, apple cider, herbal teas, coffee, cocoa, fluid-replacement (sports) drinks, powdered drink mixes, instant soup packages

Grains

Instant whole-grain cereals (oatmeal, Wheatena), granola (eat hot or cold), instant grits, rice, mashed potatoes, couscous and bulgur, quick-cooking pasta and bean products, instant ramen noodles, bagels, pita bread, tortillas, crackers, cookies (especially fruit filled), rice pudding, breakfast bars

Fruit

Fresh fruit such as apples, oranges, grapes, and so on; dried fruit such as raisins, apricots, banana chips, apples, prunes, dates, pineapple, and cherries; fruit leathers; freeze-dried dessert products

Vegetables

Freshly cut and peeled (packaged and ready to go), dehydrated, or freeze dried

Protein Foods

Peanut butter, nuts, seeds; cured meats such as ham, sausage, and so on; dried meat sticks and jerky; assorted cheese; powdered hummus; powdered eggs; no-cook refried beans; canned or foil packets of turkey, chicken, tuna, and shrimp; prepackaged, freeze-dried, or dehydrated entrees

Milk/Dairy

Powdered milk, cocoa mixes, powdered breakfast drinks, powdered cheese

Snacks

Chocolate, candy bars, cookies, gumdrops, hard candies, licorice, instant pudding, trail mixes

Fats and Oils and Extras

Margarine, butter powder, seasonings, condiments (honey, sugar cubes, and so on)

Adapted from D. Bernadot, 1993, *Sports nutrition: A guide for the professional working with active people,* 2nd ed. (Chicago, IL: American Dietetic Association), by permission of the author.

Postevent Recovery Plan

Rehydrate and refuel promptly after your adventure. Basic recovery rules apply following cold-weather exercise—start rehydrating and refueling by drinking a carbohydrate-rich beverage (with a small amount of protein if you can tolerate it) within 30 minutes of finishing, and eat solid, real food as soon as possible. This habit is particularly important if the next day is another long, intense effort. Trekkers and mountain climbers who drink and eat a quick snack first, rather than waiting until after they've taken care of every other task, fare much better over the long haul.

LEARNING FROM THE BEST: PERFORMING IN THE COLD

Having grown up in Vermont and currently living in Montana, ultra racer Nikki Kimball knows a thing or two about performing in cold-weather conditions. Initially an accomplished country-country ski racer, she has mastered mountain running (three-time member of the U.S. Mountain Running team and 2007 Ultra-Trail du Mont Blanc champion) and ultra running (two top-10 finishes in the 100K World Cup Championships). Kimball, a three-time winner of the Western States 100, specializes in trail ultras. In 2012, she set the women's supported speed record on Vermont's iconic Long Trail, covering 273 miles (439 km) in just 5 days, 7 hours, and 42 minutes. Here, she shares valuable nutrition strategies for thriving in the cold as she recounts her return to ski racing after 12 years away.

Common Nutrition-Related Experiences When Performing in the Cold

In the season's final race, a 50K in the American ski marathon series (the Yellowstone Rendezvous), Kimball admits to poorly managing her nutrition. The day was extremely cold—minus 26 degrees Fahrenheit (−32 °C) when she awoke and a mere 0 degrees Fahrenheit (−18 °C) at the start. The snow, therefore, was very slow. The consequences of cold temperatures in cross-country skiing, especially in racing, are at least twofold as they relate to nutrition. First, you need more calories just to stay warm. Kimball knows that in the extreme cold, she becomes more fatigued from normal prerace activities, such as walking around, waxing skis, and warming up, because her body must expend extra energy just to maintain its core temperature. She also found herself working harder than normal in the beginning of the race because she wanted to get warm. She cautions ski racers that correct pacing is more difficult when you feel driven to attain a more comfortable body temperature. The second factor of extreme cold is that the snow is much slower. You work harder and need more time to cover a given distance. In the Rendezvous, Kimball acknowledges that she did not drink and eat enough, partly because she didn't account for the extra time and effort required for racing in such cold temperatures.

> continued

< continued

Consequences of Nutrition Choices

Fortunately for Kimball (who won with 2:53:26), many experienced marathon ski racers made the same mistakes that she did. She bonked at 47 kilometers; however, she had already passed the lead women, who bonked at 43 kilometers. Had the race been any longer, Kimball says that her former coach (age 48) would have passed her! Despite having a hip replaced 16 months prior, this woman was passing the race leaders in the final 6 kilometers because she handled her pacing and nutrition better than the rest of the field. This race serves as a great example of experience trumping youth and biomechanical health (those with naturally healthy joints) in a sport in which the stars are typically in their 20s and 30s.

Challenges to Fueling While Skiing

Another factor regarding taking in adequate fuel during the cold is the logistics of feeding, especially when ski racing. Kimball, an accomplished ultra runner, finds it comparatively easy to eat in ultra running races because both her hands are free. And she's confident that she can eat without slowing her pace. She admits that she hadn't practiced feeding prior to the ski race. During the Rendezvous, she found it difficult to drink at feed stations with poles in her hands, as well as to feed from the bottle in her hip pack.

Be Committed to Drinking and Eating

Kimball frequently hears runners use the excuse that they don't want to lose time during a race by drinking at aid stations. She finds this ridiculous, since she knows firsthand that the gains made by proper hydration and feeding far exceed any time lost in taking in the required nutrition. Nevertheless, she found herself underfeeding in the ski race because she didn't want to take the time to mess with drinking with poles in her hands! Her message to racers is that if you're concerned about the time that it takes to feed—in running, skiing, or any activity—then practice feeding in training. The logic of passing up feeds to save time is completely flawed. Sufficient fueling is accomplished in seconds, whereas dehydration and bonking will cost you minutes, or even hours, and will increase your risk of dropping from the race.

Fluid Management Tips

The urge to urinate always comes on earlier in the cold, whether you drink or not, so you won't escape making pit stops by not drinking. Kimball advises athletes, particularly female ski racers, to update their cold-weather wardrobe to include technical clothing that is designed to make taking pit stops easier. She also tries to take in fluids that are warm (at least room temperature) because they're easier to drink, thereby encouraging her to drink more. Kimball initially makes her drinks (tea or sports drink) with hot water. She typically relies on an insulated hydration pack, especially during ski outings, because it doesn't bounce up and down with the smooth motion of skiing. At the end of all cold-weather endeavors, she has a thermos filled with a hot drink waiting. She begins immediately to replenish needed calories, and she swears by the boost that a warm beverage gives in helping her to warm up more quickly.

16

High Altitude

Fat absorption may [also] be reduced at extremely high elevations. However, elevations commonly reached by recreational skiers, snowshoers, and backpackers are usually not associated with impaired fat or protein or carbohydrate absorption.

Source: E.W. Askew, n.d., Nutrition at high altitude. [Online]. Available: www.wms.org/news/altitude.asp [April 25, 2013].

If your favorite endurance activity or competitive endeavor has lost its challenge, try doing it at altitude. Dealing with rapidly changing weather and less oxygen to draw on for physical efforts, coupled with having a headache, queasy stomach, and a lack of appetite, can make things far more interesting. Mother Nature may rule when it comes to the weather; however, you can stay in the game by acclimatizing, drinking adequate fluid, and making wise food choices.

Altitude Acclimatization

If you travel too quickly to higher elevations, you may develop a headache, suffer from general malaise, experience difficulty breathing, become nauseated (even vomit), lose your appetite, and have trouble sleeping. Welcome to the world of acute mountain sickness (AMS), also known as altitude sickness. Experts estimate that 6.5 percent of men and 22 percent of women will suffer from this malady when traveling above 6,000 feet (~1,800 m). The underlying mechanism remains unclear; however, carbon dioxide accumulating in tissues and fluid seeping into the brain are likely culprits as your body adjusts to less oxygen than it is accustomed to. Why women tend to suffer more from AMS than men do also remains unclear.

What else is happening as we gasp for air and our exercising muscles scream for oxygen? We breathe more rapidly, initially, in an attempt to extract more oxygen from the air. Our plasma volume (the watery portion of blood) drops so as to increase the concentration of red blood cells (oxygen carriers) in blood, and the heart kicks into overdrive to deliver more blood, and thus more oxygen, to active muscles.

The percentage of oxygen in the air (20.93 percent), by the way, remains constant regardless of the altitude. Atmospheric (barometric) pressure is what varies—decreasing as we ascend, thus decreasing the partial pressure of oxygen in the bloodstream. This substantially reduced pressure gradient between blood oxygen and the oxygen in active tissues hinders the transfer of oxygen from the blood to the tissues. The decrease in oxygen to working muscles impairs aerobic capacity and translates into reduced performances during endurance exercise.

If you stay long enough at high altitudes, at least 10 days, the body begins to acclimate and make more permanent adjustments. Plasma volume expands, and muscles begin to extract more oxygen from the blood, thus reducing the workload on the heart. If you stay even longer (4 to 8 weeks), you'll end up with more red blood cells, which will really help you compensate for the thinner air.

Dehydration and Glycogen Depletion

Dehydration and glycogen depletion remain common nemeses at higher elevations. In addition to sweat losses (which athletes at altitude tend to be less aware of), the air holds little water (especially cold air), increasing the amount of water that is lost during respiration. The rate of water lost at altitude through breathing is, in fact, about twice that for the same activity at sea level. A diminished thirst response in cold conditions further compounds the situation, making it easier for athletes to become dehydrated.

Exercising at altitude, particularly for extended periods at high altitude (9,000 feet, or 2,700 meters, and above), also influences the body's metabolic response. At acute exposure to high altitude, the body's basal metabolic rate, or the energy needed for maintaining the basic processes that support life, jumps as much as 30 percent. You need more calories simply to maintain lean mass and overall body weight (about 30 to 35 calories per pound, or 65 to 75 calories per kilogram, of body weight). You need even more energy to fuel high-intensity exercise efforts, such as carrying a heavy pack up a steep grade, as compared to doing the same work at sea level. You also need extra energy just to maintain your core body temperature.

A shift takes place within exercising muscles, too. At altitude, exercising muscles appear to rely less on fat and even more heavily on carbohydrate (glucose) than they already do at lower elevations. The increased reliance may be advantageous because working muscles use carbohydrate more efficiently (meaning less oxygen is required for converting them to energy) than they do fat. Carbohydrate metabolism contributes relatively more to carbon dioxide production than either protein or fat. This increase in carbon dioxide production leads to faster breathing rate, which means an increase in the amount of oxygen being delivered to the blood. Remember, anything that fights altitude-induced hypoxia (when less oxygen gets delivered to body tissues) and brings more oxygen to muscles, the heart, and the brain is a good thing. Fortunately, carbohydrate-rich foods also seem to be more palatable at altitude than protein and high-fat foods.

If you spend several days to a few months above 14,000 feet (4,300 m), expect to lose some weight. As you go higher and stay longer, it becomes more difficult to maintain a daily balance between calories consumed and calories expended. As you acclimate, you can initially lose a few pounds of fluid. Your appetite may decrease as well, especially if you suffer from AMS, and your food intake may be low for several days. If your adventure involves a lot of physical activity, you will, of course, expend a substantial amount of calories. To fuel your daily activity level, as well as replenish glycogen adequately, aim to ingest 30 to 35 calories per pound of body weight daily. Fortunately, you may be able to avoid losing significant weight (at least up to an altitude of 16,500 feet, or 5,000 meters) by having access to a variety of tasty foods. Researchers followed eight healthy Caucasian males at the Italian Research Laboratory in Nepal (16,650 feet, or 5,050 meters) to test this theory. After one month in comfortable surroundings with a wide choice of palatable foods available, the men did not experience significant changes in weight, body-fat percentage, circumference of their arms or legs (measures of muscle mass), or their performances on strength and vertical-jumping tests.

Overall, the digestibility and absorption of nutrients do not appear to contribute to weight loss except for at extreme altitude (above 23,000 feet, or 7,000 meters), in which case the digestive tract may lose some of its absorptive capacity. At that altitude, of course, you may experience a few other problems, too! Weight loss following prolonged exposure to altitude is simply the result of losing body fat and muscle mass. The cause is a combination of taking in too few calories—because of physical discomfort, lack of appetite, and limited food choices—and to expending more calories, in part due to an elevated resting metabolic rate.

A sizable portion of altitude-related weight loss, up to 70 percent, is the loss of lean muscle mass. In elite mountain climbers, researchers have documented losses over a 2-month period at altitudes above 18,000 feet (5,500 m) that decreased the thigh cross-sectional area by 15 percent. Detraining may partially cause the loss of muscle. Athletes who arrive in top condition can lose muscle due to a relative lack of exercise while acclimating, recovering from hard days, and waiting out weather delays. Acute hypoxia (lack of oxygen), on the other hand, may directly affect protein metabolism by decreasing the body's ability to synthesize new proteins.

Nutrition Strategies for Handling High Altitude

Athletes exercising at 6,000 feet (1,830 m) or above should focus on three primary areas—energy balance, carbohydrate, and hydration. The nutrition bottom line is that those who do best at altitude are those who drink and eat the most, and doing that basically takes a good deal of discipline and mental fortitude. On a trip to Kilimanjaro, Africa's tallest peak (19,341 feet, or 5,895 meters), I could tell which group members were experiencing AMS just from their lack of mealtime conversation! Underfueling (especially during multiday endeavors), whatever the cause, doesn't only put you at risk, it threatens your companions' enjoyment and safety, too.

The key factor in reducing the negative effects of altitude and optimizing performance, as summarized in the 2012 International Olympic Committee consensus statement on thermoregulatory and altitude challenges for high-level athletes, however, is to arrive early to acclimatize. At moderate altitude, most athletes acclimatize within 2 weeks. To minimize AMS effects, arrive at least 2 weeks before a competitive event, or if that's not possible, compete within 24 hours of your arrival. On hikes and expeditions during which you plan to spend the night, ascend slowly, in stages. A good rule to follow above 10,000 feet (3,000 m) is to climb only 1,000 feet (300 m) per day. To limit weight loss (remember, it's primarily muscle that you lose), bring a variety of palatable foods and try to limit the time spent at extreme altitude.

Before the Event

Undertaking endurance challenges at high elevations demands that you be mentally ready and physically prepared. Boost your training efforts and your confidence going in by eating smart in advance.

Eat Iron-Rich Foods and Supplement as Necessary

If you live and train at moderate altitudes (3,000 to 8,000 feet, or 900 to 2,400 meters), be sure to consume plenty of iron-rich foods regularly. Red meat and dark poultry are excellent sources of iron, while fortified breakfast cereals, dark leafy greens, legumes (dried beans and peas), dried fruit, and prune juice are good choices. You want to take advantage of the body's desire to build new red blood cells. Iron is a crucial component of hemoglobin (housed in red blood cells), the prime carrier of oxygen in blood. Female athletes, in particular, must pay attention to their iron status while training at altitude. The need for supplementation can be determined easily though routine blood tests (see the section titled Monitoring Your Iron Status in chapter 6).

Explore the Merits of Vitamin E

Vitamin E, a powerful antioxidant, helps keep cell membranes healthy. Without enough of it, red blood cells and muscle cells are destroyed more rapidly by oxidative damage from free radical molecules. Exercise raises the need for vitamin E, and exercise at high altitude probably raises it even more. Eat a training diet rich in whole-grain products, wheat germ, vegetable oils, green leafy vegetables, nuts and seeds, liver, and eggs (yolks) to ensure an adequate intake of vitamin E. Supplementation may help protect against chronic oxidative damage to membranes during intense, prolonged exercise (at high altitude, for example), although not all scientists agree and no firm recommendations exist currently. A suggested reasonable daily dose for endurance athletes at sea level is 100 to 200 IU per day. Vitamin E has low toxicity (the tolerable upper intake level is 1,500 IU daily); however, some people report flulike symptoms when taking more than 400 IU daily for prolonged periods.

Plan Ahead and Bring What You Need

Any time that you travel with others, especially as part of a prearranged or supported trekking trip, the time to speak up about nutrition needs and concerns is before you go. You should inquire about the planned menu ahead of time anyway, rather than complaining about the food (or lack of it) after the trip is underway. Vegetarians and those who have special concerns or issues, such as food allergies or gluten intolerance, must make requests and develop an alternative plan ahead of time.

Experiment and Determine What Works Up High

Use short adventures and forays to altitude to become comfortable with a variety of foods and drinks that will be essential during longer or more involved outings. You can't go wrong with items that are premade and crush-proof and that require no cooking. (For expeditions, never underestimate the importance of the cook.) Practice eating and drinking at altitude under various conditions and line up a reliable hydration system. Anticipate that your tastes will change as you go higher. Talk to experienced old-timers and heed their advice. They may suggest particular foods that you wouldn't normally choose or identify foods that would be best to leave behind. To enhance appetites and to boost group morale, have all group members bring (within reason) some of their favorite treats to enjoy, as well as to share with friends and fellow adventurers met along the way.

Play It Safe

For the last few days (even the entire week) before an altitude adventure, play it safe and eat familiar foods that you tolerate well and enjoy. Now is not the time to be adventurous. Working hard at altitude will quickly exacerbate the dehydration and feelings of weakness related to having the runs or not being able to eat. Being ill, in addition, makes AMS even worse.

Going to high altitude (for treks and adventure races, for example) often means traveling to a non-Westernized country. Staying healthy is particularly challenging. Do not sample the local street cuisine beforehand. No matter how good it looks, do not eat salads, raw vegetables, fruit that you can't peel, or ice cream. Make sure that drinks you order do not contain ice; request the can or bottle. Stick to dining at the better hotels and restaurants that cater to tourists, or (if reasonable) bring your own prepackaged foods.

During the Event

Don't waste your hard work and time spent preplanning the hike by becoming lazy about nutrition once you hit the trail. Food is what gets you to the top and, even more important, what gets you back down.

Drink on a Schedule

Exercising in cold, dry air, common in winter and always at altitude, increases the rate at which the body loses water, so your fluid intake must increase to match this loss. Based on my experience, the recommended guidelines hold true, so don't be surprised if you require double the amount of fluid that you do normally. By the time you reach 10,000 feet (3,000 m), for example, you may need to drink 4 quarts (~4 L) or more per day. Set a watch alarm, if necessary, as a reminder to drink. Alternatively, put a group member in charge of scheduling predetermined breaks.

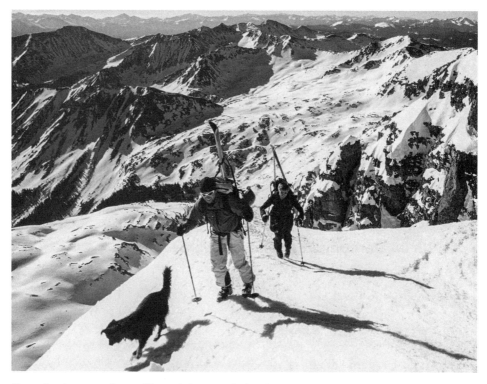

Expect a decreased appetite and changes in food tastes when exercising at higher elevations. Be mentally prepared to eat anyway.

Brand X Pictures

Sports drinks do triple duty by providing calories in the form of carbohydrate as well as fluid and electrolytes. Other good choices besides plain water include instant-mix fruit drinks, reconstituted powdered milk, meal-replacement drinks, hot chocolate, tea loaded with honey or sugar, and soup. Avoid alcohol completely, since it exacerbates dehydration and feelings of nausea. The oft-repeated advice that urine is pale yellow when you're well hydrated holds true at any elevation.

Ignore a Lack of Appetite

Feelings of nausea or lack of appetite don't let you off the hook. With less oxygen going to the brain and to the stomach, you should expect to feel as if you don't want to eat during the first few days as you acclimatize, as well as during extended stays at high altitude. Active muscles, unfortunately, can't wait that long. Food is fuel, so the more you eat, the more you'll be able to do. Besides, you'll feel better and enjoy the experience more. It's your job to keep yourself adequately fueled. Eating during endurance endeavors at altitude can require as much willpower as continuing to put one foot in front of the other.

Don't worry about eating exactly the right thing. At high altitude, in particular, all calories are good calories! Just be sure to bring a variety of appetizing foods with you because your tastes will change as you go higher. Bring several flavors of gels and energy bars to ward off flavor fatigue. Foods that you love at home are typically the easiest to make yourself eat when you're up high.

Keep in mind that sweeter-tasting foods, in particular, can become undesirable at altitude. I was caught off guard by the complete lack of appetite I experienced as I hiked up to the 15,000-foot (4,500 m) camp on Kilimanjaro. Although I was partial to sweeter-tasting red-colored sports drinks at sea level, I couldn't look at my favorite drink at altitude, never mind stomach it. Finding a canister of lemon-lime powdered sports drink in the bottom of my pack saved the trip. (Butterfinger candy bars and Tanzanian potato chips helped me reach a new high, too.) Eat small, frequent meals to keep your energy up and to help combat nausea.

Load Up on Carbohydrate and Eat Some Fat

Fill up on carbohydrate-rich foods (ideally at least 60 percent of the calories you take in) because they require significantly less oxygen to be metabolized, and they are generally better tolerated at altitude than high-fat foods. If you don't constantly replenish your liver and muscle glycogen stores by eating foods rich in carbohydrate (bread, cereal, rice, pasta, fruit, powdered milk, sports drinks, candy, and sugar, for example), you'll end up exhausted and less able to tolerate the effects of being at altitude. On top of that, your body will be forced to use valuable protein reserves (from muscles and internal organs) as energy instead. In addition to sports drinks and energy bars, gels, and chews, keep portable carbohydrate-rich items handy to snack on, such as bagels, pita bread, instant pudding, fresh and dried fruit, carrot sticks, pretzels, gorp, low-fat granola, breakfast bars, Pop-Tarts, fig bars, and candy.

That said, don't be surprised if you crave and can tolerate fattier foods, such as nuts, cheese, pepperoni, sausage, chocolate, and peanut butter. These foods represent the best way to consume calories quickly. Adding oil, margarine, or butter to foods is another efficient (and often necessary) way to boost calories. Relatively lightweight and easy to carry, high-carbohydrate or meal-replacement drink powders (some provide as many as 200 calories and 30 grams of protein per cup) can be a real lifesaver.

Cook Simple Fare While on the Trail

Preparing even routine foods at altitude can be tedious, so get everyone in the group to pitch in. Don't weigh yourself down with foods that take a long time to cook, such as dried beans, brown rice, and elbow or shell pasta. Concentrate on refueling with quicker-cooking foods, like instant mashed potatoes, couscous, thin pastas, low-fat ramen noodles, quick-cooking rice, dehydrated foods, and freeze-dried foods. Be sure to estimate how many cups of hot water and fuel will be needed for preparing these items. To save time and energy, pack entire meals together ahead of time and label them with the dates that you intend to eat them. Soak dehydrated foods in an extra water bottle during the day to shorten their cooking time.

Don't worry about preparing gourmet fare. That's not the goal. A simple spice kit can perk up otherwise ordinary fare. You could, of course, carry a bigger pack and bring the entire contents of your kitchen with you. I observed a woman at base camp at 10,000 feet (3,000 m) on Mount Rainier, for example, who brought a fresh lemon and a large kitchen knife to slice it just so she could flavor her drinking water!

Postevent Recovery Plan

Refuel promptly. As with all physically challenging and prolonged bouts of exercise, take advantage of the carbohydrate window and begin refueling as soon as possible. Anticipate a decrease in appetite by initially drinking the calories and carbohydrate that you need to replace. Refueling promptly after each day's walk is particularly essential for through-hikers, those on expeditions, and other athletes involved in multiday adventures and races at altitude. Those able to finish, and finish strongly, are almost always those who paid attention to their fluid and fuel needs from the very first day.

LEARNING FROM THE BEST: PERFORMING AT ALTITUDE

Max King knows how to race with great success on every running surface imaginable. He's run 8:30 in the steeplechase, represented the United States multiple times in the cross country world championships, won a mountain running world championship (2011), and captured five straight 21K XTERRA Trail Run national championships. A blazing course-record victory of 5:24:58 (a per-mile pace of 6:42) at the 50th running of the venerable JFK 50-mile (80 km) in Maryland and a win in his first 100K, the Ultra Race of Champions 100K in Charlottesville, Virginia, garnered Max *Trail Runner Magazine's* 2012 Trail Runner of the Year award.

Freshly back from winning El Cruce Columbia, a three-day stage race in Chile that winds through the Andes, where he outran the best European trail runners, King shared the following tips for handling the altitude during endurance events and races.

Hydration Rules at Altitude

Max's game plan is to keep his nutrition routine the same when competing at higher altitudes. He recognizes that dehydration happens at a faster rate at altitude, so fluid management is a priority. He rarely loses his appetite or acceptance of sweet-tasting sports foods. When it has happened, he attributes it to dehydration rather than to the particular item. He recommends using race fuels based primarily on a maltodextrin formula, like Hammer Gel, to keep sweetness issues to a minimum.

Get the Fuel In

Max's fueling and hydration regimen is based on time rather than mileage. In general, the effort being put in at high altitude is the same as that in lower altitude endeavors; however, the pace will be considerably slower at high altitude. This equates to needing more calories and fluid per mile at higher altitudes, but the formula he relies on to calculate what he requires remains constant over time. "I used to think I could get through a 50K with one gel," he says. "Turns out that if I start taking gel and electrolytes, maybe even more than I really need, I'll feel a lot better and run a lot faster with fuel on board." Max, who is 5 feet, 6 inches (168 cm) tall and weighs 135 pounds (61 kg), needs approximately 400 calories and at least 400 milligrams of sodium an hour.

Max shares that he made a lot of mistakes when he started out by simply not taking in enough fuel or electrolytes during ultras. "It was really difficult and took a long time to learn just how much fuel and electrolytes I needed in order to run well and not bonk," he says. "I started with one gel during a 50K race. Then I moved up to three gels and a couple of electrolyte tablets, and I still bonked. I then started taking gel at 1 hour 15 minutes into the race, way before I really needed it. From that point, it's a gel every 30 minutes, plus an electrolyte tablet every 30 minutes, and I finally had a breakout race where I was running strong to the finish." He concedes that it took a few more years to figure out that the same plan wasn't going to work for efforts longer than 35 miles (56 km). "During a 50 miler, I use that plan up to the 3.5-hour mark [his usual time in a 50K race]," explains Max. "I then double the gels but keep the electrolytes the same. This seems to work for now."

> continued

< continued

Keep It Simple and Consistent

Max, during races, sticks with what he knows works well for him. He prefers Hammer Gels as his primary fuel, and rehydrates with plain water. He's tinkered with how many gels and electrolytes and how much water he needs over the course of a couple years, and he's always stuck with these components. Just recently, in some longer races, however, he has tried adding Hammer Bars to the mix. Max was pleased to discover, provided that he's well hydrated and capable of digesting solid food, that eating bars prolongs his energy level and helps to satiate the hunger that can be common when relying on gels alone.

Start the Day Right

Max finds it important to eat breakfast on race-day morning, mainly to raise his blood sugar level and satiate his hunger. He, once again, keeps it simple with a bowl of oatmeal or a Hammer Bar or two.

Avoid This Pitfall

In general, Max stresses the perils of starting out inadequately hydrated or not staying hydrated during an event or race at altitude. However, at any altitude, he contends that the biggest trap he sees athletes fall into is experimenting with their nutrition during a race. He reports that the one time he just about lost it in a race was when he thought the Coke looked refreshing on a hot day. That incident taught him to avoid soda, as well as other simple sugars, during an ultra run. "It's true that a race is different than practice; however, races shouldn't be for experimentation," says Max, "That's what training is for. Races are for refining what you do."

APPENDIX A

Measurement Conversion Charts

Energy in Foods

1 kilocalorie (kcal) = 4.18 kilojoules (kJ)

(The kilocalorie is most commonly referred to as "calorie" in nutrition usage.)

grams carbohydrate × 4 kcal/g (16 kJ/g)
+ grams protein × 4 kcal/g (17 kJ/g)
+ grams fat × 9 kcal/g (37 kJ/g)
+ grams alcohol × 7 kcal/g (29 kJ/g)

= total energy (calories or kilojoules) in a serving of food

Converting Information From Food Labels

Examples: 1/2 cup (120 ml) of orange juice = 60 (kilo)calories

60 kcal × 4.18 = 250 kilojoules
1/2 cup (120 ml) of orange juice = 250 kilojoules
250 kilojoules / 4.18 = 60 (kilo)calories

Metric Conversion Made Easy

To change weight in	To	Multiply by
Ounces	Grams	30
Pounds	Kilograms	.45
To change volume in	To	Multiply by
Teaspoons	Milliliters	5
Tablespoons	Milliliters	15
Fluid ounces	Milliliters	30
Cups	Liters	.24
Pints	Liters	.47
Quarts	Liters	.95
Gallons	Liters	3.8

Body Mass Index (BMI)

Imperial Formula

$$BMI = [\text{weight in pounds} / (\text{height in inches})^2] \times 703$$

Metric Formula

$$BMI = \text{weight in kilograms} / (\text{height in meters})^2$$

Food Measurement Conversions: Imperial to Metric

Liquid Volume

Imperial	Metric
1 teaspoon	5 milliliters (ml)
1 tablespoon (3 teaspoons)	15 ml
1 fluid ounce	30 ml
1 cup (8 ounces)	240 ml
2 cups (1 pint)	480 ml
4 cups (1 quart)	.95 liter
4 quarts (1 gallon)	3.8 liters

Weight

Imperial	Metric
1 ounce	28.35 grams
1 pound	454 grams, or .45 kilograms

Food Measurement Conversions: Metric to Imperial

Liquid Volume

Metric	Imperial
1 milliliter (ml)	.034 fluid ounces
5 ml	1 teaspoon
15 ml	1 tablespoon
100 ml	3.4 fluid ounces
240 ml	1 cup
1 liter	34 fluid ounces; 4.2 cups; 1.06 quarts; .26 gallons

Weight

Metric	Imperial
1 gram (1,000 milligrams)	.035 ounces
100 grams	3.5 ounces
500 grams	1.10 pounds
1 pound	.45 kilograms
1 kilogram	2.2 pounds
1 kilogram	35 ounces

Food Measurement Equivalents

Dry Volume

Imperial (US)	Metric	UK/Canada
1 tsp	.986 tsp	1.388 tsp
1 tbsp	.986 tbsp	1.041 tbsp
1 cup	.946 cup	1.041 cup

Length Measurement Equivalents

Metric	Imperial
1 centimeter	.3937 inches
1 inch	2.54 centimeters
1 meter	39.37 inches
1 kilometer	.62 miles
5K	3.1 miles
10K	6.2 miles
25K	15.5 miles
40K	24.8 miles
50K	31 miles
100K	62 miles
150K	93 miles
200K	124 miles
Marathon (official distance)	26.2 miles

Temperature Measurement Equivalents

To convert Fahrenheit to Celsius (Centigrade): subtract 32 and multiply by .6.
To convert Celsius (Centigrade) to Fahrenheit: multiply by 1.8 and add 32.

	Fahrenheit	Celsius
Boiling point of water	212°	100°
Freezing point of water	32°	0°
Normal body temperature	98.6°	37°

APPENDIX B

Facts About Vitamins and Minerals

Vitamin or mineral	Dietary reference intake (DRI) for females/males age 19 to 50	Best food sources	What it does
Thiamin	1.1/1.2 mg/d	Wheat germ, whole-grain breads and cereals, organ meats, lean meats, legumes, fortified grains	Releases energy from carbohydrate; maintains healthy nervous system
Riboflavin	1.1/1.3 mg/d	Milk and dairy products, green leafy vegetables, lean meats, beans, fortified grains	Releases energy from protein, fat, and carbohydrate; promotes healthy skin
Niacin	14/16 mg/d	Lean meats, fish, poultry, legumes, whole grains, fortified grains	Releases energy from protein, fat, and carbohydrate; aids in synthesis of protein, fat, and DNA; promotes healthy skin and nervous system
Vitamin B_6	1.3 mg/d	Liver, lean meats, fish, poultry, legumes, whole grains	Aids in metabolism of protein; synthesis of essential fatty acids; forms hemoglobin and red blood cells
Vitamin B_{12}	2.4 μg/d	Lean meats, poultry, dairy products, eggs, fish	Aids in metabolism of carbohydrate, protein, fat; produces red blood cells; maintains nerve cells
Folate	400 μg/d	Green leafy vegetables, legumes	Aids growth of new cells; forms red blood cells

> continued

Vitamin or mineral	Dietary reference intake (DRI) for females/males age 19 to 50	Best food sources	What it does
Biotin	30 μg/d	Meats, legumes, milk, egg yolk, whole grains	Aids in metabolism of carbohydrate, fat, protein
Pantothenic acid	5 mg/d	Found in variety of foods	Aids in metabolism of carbohydrate, fat, protein
Vitamin C	75/90 mg/d	Citrus fruits, green leafy vegetables, broccoli, peppers, potatoes, berries, kiwi, cantaloupe (rock melon)	Maintains normal connective tissue; enhances iron absorption; serves as antioxidant; helps heal wounds
Vitamin A	700/900 μg/d	Liver, milk, cheese, fortified margarine, carotenoids in plant foods (orange, red, or deep green in color)	Maintains healthy skin, mucous membranes, vision, and immune system; serves as antioxidant
Vitamin D	600 IU/d	Vitamin D–fortified milk and margarine, fattier fish, fish oil, sunlight	Promotes normal bone growth; aids in calcium absorption
Vitamin E	15 mg/d	Vegetable oils, margarine, green leafy vegetables, wheat germ, eggs, whole grains	Serves as antioxidant; helps to form red blood cells
Vitamin K	90/120 μg/d	Liver, eggs, cauliflower, green leafy vegetables	Promotes normal blood clotting
Calcium	1,000 mg/d	Milk, cheese, yogurt, ice cream, legumes, dark green leafy vegetables	Helps in formation of bones and teeth; has role in muscle contractions, nerve impulse transmission, and blood clotting
Phosphorus	700 mg/d	Meat, poultry, fish, eggs, milk, cheese, legumes, whole grains	Aids in metabolism of protein, carbohydrate, and fat; repairs and maintains cells; helps in formation of teeth and bones

Vitamin or mineral	Dietary reference intake (DRI) for females/males age 19 to 50	Best food sources	What it does
Magnesium	320/420 mg/d	Milk, yogurt, legumes, nuts, whole grains, tofu, green vegetables	Aids in metabolism of carbohydrate and protein; aids in neuromuscular contractions
Iron	18/8 mg/d	Organ meats, lean meats, poultry, shellfish, oysters, whole grains, legumes	Aids in formation of hemoglobin and transportation of oxygen in red blood cells
Zinc	8/11 mg/d	Lean meats, fish, poultry, shellfish, oysters, whole grains, legumes	Aids in energy metabolism; synthesizes protein; helps with immune function and wound healing
Copper	900 μg/d	Lean meats, poultry, shellfish, fish, eggs, nuts, beans, whole grains	Is necessary for iron absorption, manufacture of collagen; heals wounds
Fluoride	3/4 mg/d	Milk, egg yolks, water, seafood	Helps form teeth and bones
Selenium	55 μg/d	Meat, fish, poultry, organ meats, seafood, whole grains, and nuts from selenium-rich soil	Serves as component of antioxidant enzymes
Chromium	25/35 μg/d	Organ meats, meats, oysters, cheese, whole grains, beer	Regulates blood sugar; aids normal fat metabolism
Iodine	150 μg/d	Iodized salt, seafood, water	Serves as component of thyroid hormone that helps regulate growth and development rate
Manganese	1.8/2.3 mg/d	Green leafy vegetables, whole grains, nuts, legumes, egg yolks	Aids in synthesis of hemoglobin

> continued

< continued, **Facts About Vitamins and Minerals**

Vitamin or mineral	Dietary reference intake (DRI) for females/males age 19 to 50	Best food sources	What it does
Molybdenum	45 μg/d	Legumes, cereal grains, dark green leafy vegetables	Involved in carbohydrate and fat metabolism
Sodium	Daily need varies based on sweat losses, at least 1,500 mg/d	Table salt; found in virtually all foods, especially processed items	Promotes acid–base balance, fluid balance, nerve impulses, muscle action
Potassium	4,700 mg/d; if high sweat rate, may need more	Fruits and vegetables (bananas, orange juice, potatoes, tomatoes), milk, yogurt, legumes	Promotes fluid balance, acid–base balance, nerve impulses, muscle action, synthesis of protein and glycogen

Note: μg = microgram

APPENDIX C

Eating on the Run

It isn't always possible to fully plan your meals far in advance. But it is possible to make smart choices, even when your time for meal preparation is limited or when you are eating out.

Stock Your Kitchen

Contrary to popular opinion, eating healthy doesn't take a lot of time. What busy athletes don't have time for, however, is pedaling or hoofing it to the grocery store in search of a missing key ingredient. Even worse is arriving home ravenous, looking in the fridge, and realizing that you forgot to go food shopping—again. Keep your pantry, refrigerator, and freezer stocked with nutritious fast food, and you'll find it easy to whip up simple, wholesome meals and snacks.

Grains (Emphasize Whole Grains)

Instant brown or white rice (cooking time: 5 minutes or less)

Pasta (cooking time: 10 minutes; fresh pasta: 3 to 5 minutes)

Other prepackaged quick-cooking pastas and grains: couscous (cooking time: 5 minutes), quinoa (cooking time: 10 to 15 minutes), cracked wheat bulgur, pasta and beans, wheat pilaf, tabbouleh (cooking time: 15 minutes)

Instant stuffing mixes (cooking time: 5 minutes)

Instant cups of polenta, lentils, beans (just add boiling water)

Corn and flour tortillas

Whole-grain breads, bagels, rolls, pita bread, English muffins (most store well in the freezer)

Low-fat crackers (4 grams of fat or less per ounce, or per 28 grams)

Quick-cooking oatmeal, Farina, Wheatena (cooking time: 5 minutes)

Ready-to-eat whole-grain cereals, breakfast bars, granola bars

Pancake mix, whole-grain toaster waffles

Fruits and Vegetables

Potatoes and sweet potatoes (store in a cool, dark area; bake in the microwave)

Instant mashed potato mix (cooking time: 5 minutes)

Frozen or canned vegetables (rinse canned varieties to reduce sodium content)

Prewashed salad from a bag

Mini carrots, prechopped vegetables and fruit (from salad bar)

Canned fruit, such as mandarin oranges and pineapple chunks; frozen berries

Oranges, apples, bananas (store in the fridge to slow ripening)

Dates, raisins, and other dried fruit

Frozen 100 percent juice concentrates and individual-serving juice boxes

Dairy

Low-fat milk (regular or calcium-fortified soy)

Low-fat yogurt (regular or calcium-fortified soy)

Low-fat cheese (including part-skim ricotta and mozzarella, and Parmesan)

Low-fat cottage cheese

Protein Foods

Boneless, skinless chicken breasts (store in the freezer)

Lean ground meat (ground round, sirloin, turkey breast)

Cubed meat for kebabs and stir-fries

Cooked shrimp

Lean deli meats such as turkey, ham, or roast beef

Packets or cans of water-packed tuna, chicken

Edamame (ready to eat or frozen), roasted soy nuts

Canned chili, baked beans, frozen burritos

Canned kidney, pinto, and black beans; chickpeas, vegetarian or nonfat refried beans

Frozen veggie or soy burgers

Tofu

Eggs or egg substitutes (can be stored in the freezer)

Peanut or other nut butters

Healthy Oils and Fats

Soft (tub) or liquid margarine

Oil for cooking and baking—olive, canola, peanut

Low-fat salad dressing

Reduced-calorie mayonnaise

Nuts and seeds

Avocado

Olives

Extras and Fun Foods

Condiments such as mustard, ketchup, salsa, cocktail sauce, soy sauce, vinegar, jelly or jam

Seasonings such as onion and garlic powders, dried herbs

Spaghetti sauce (4 grams of fat or less per 4 ounces, or per 125 grams)

Canned soup

Sports bars

Pretzels, low-fat chips, popcorn

Lower-fat fun foods such as cookies, fig bars, and angel food cake

Tip: Replace perishables, such as milk, yogurt, fresh fruit and vegetables, fresh pasta, and deli meats, weekly. Other staples, especially if unopened, generally keep well for longer.

Dining Out

Dining away from home doesn't mean giving up your high-performance eating habits. Use My Plate as a template for putting together smart, well-balanced meals just as you would at home. By mindfully choosing the restaurant or eatery, you'll have plenty of options. The following list emphasizes higher-carbohydrate, lower-fat selections for those who eat out regularly.

Fast Food

Pizza with vegetarian toppings

Broiled burger or grilled chicken with lettuce and tomato on whole wheat bun

Sandwich, sub, or wrap made with lean meat and vegetables

Chicken and grilled steak fajitas, soft tacos

Bean burrito

Salad bar, entrée salads with grilled chicken or lean red meat and low-calorie dressing served on the side

Hearty soups (feature beans or whole grains)

Baked potato with vegetables and low-fat toppings

Chili with crackers

Bagel or English muffin, lightly buttered or with jam or honey

Waffle or pancakes with syrup

Ready-to-eat cereal (hot or cold) or oatmeal

Low-fat muffins and cookies

Regular and flavored nonfat or low-fat milk

Low-fat milk shake, yogurt, and fruit parfaits

Frozen yogurt or soft-serve ice cream

100 percent fruit juice, fruit cups, fruit salad, bags of sliced apples

Tips: Go easy on extra cheese or meat toppings on pizza, supersized burgers and fries, fried chicken and fish sandwiches, creamy soups, salad dressings, breakfast biscuits, sausage and bacon, tartar sauce, mayonnaise, special sauces, Danish pastries, and soft drinks.

Mexican Cuisine

Gazpacho or bean soup

Red or black beans

Refried beans (made without lard or fat)

Spanish rice

Marinated vegetables

Grilled shrimp and fish

Grilled chicken

Soft plain tortillas

Burritos (not deep fried)

Soft tacos

Fajitas

Enchiladas

Tamales

Pico de gallo

Salsa

Baked tortilla chips

Tips: Go easy on crispy fried tortillas (nachos) and taco shells, quesadillas, chile relleño, tostados, chimichangas, sour cream, cheese, and guacamole, and always ask how the refried beans are prepared. Order à la carte if you can and choose your sides wisely.

Chinese Cuisine

Wonton or hot and sour soup

Steamed rice and vegetables

Steamed dumplings

Stir-fried dishes (chicken, beef, scallops, shrimp, or tofu) loaded with vegetables

Chow mein dishes

Moo goo gai pan

Chicken or beef chop suey

Fortune cookies

Tips: Go easy on fried rice, fried wontons, egg rolls, fried chow mein noodles, spare ribs, sweet and sour dishes, crispy beef, Kung Pao chicken, lemon chicken, General Tso's chicken, and Peking duck.

Italian Cuisine

Minestrone soup

Crudités (raw vegetables)

Bread sticks or plain bread

Pasta with lower-fat sauce (marinara, red clam, white clam)

Meat sauce (rather than meatballs)

Chicken cacciatore or primavera

Spinach or mushroom tortellini

Thick-crust plain or vegetable pizza

Salads with dressings on the side

Italian ice or fresh sorbet

Tips: Go easy on antipasto plates, creamy salad dressings, extra cheese and meat toppings on pizza, alfredo or pesto sauce, Italian sausage, fried calamari, parmigiana dishes, manicotti, lasagna, and butter, margarine, or olive oil served with bread.

Indian Cuisine

Dahl (bean soup)

Naan

Roti (breads)

Basmati rice

Shish kebab

Curries

Tips: Go easy on fried appetizers, samosas, and dishes that load up on cheese or sauces, such as Palak or saag paneer. Ask how sauces are made, because many restaurants add cream (Malai) besides the ghee (clarified butter) and coconut milk normally used.

Classic Western Cuisine

Lentil or bean-based soups and side dishes

Plain bread

Salad with dressing on the side

Steamed vegetables

Baked or mashed potatoes

Brown or wild rice

Stir-fried dishes and kebabs made with lean meats and loaded with vegetables

Barbecued chicken

Pot roast

Turkey with stuffing

Hamburger or garden burger

Filet mignon or sirloin steak

Pork tenderloin

Grilled, broiled, or baked fish or skinless chicken

Fruit

Sorbet or frozen yogurt

Low-fat milk shakes

Tips: Go easy on salads already dressed (for example, Caesar salad); buffalo wings; stuffed potato skins; French fries; onion rings; fried chicken, steak, and shrimp; gravy, tartar sauce, and creamy and buttery sauces; sour cream or butter on baked potatoes; pot pies; grilled cheese and cheese steak sandwiches and patty melts; and New York strip, T-bone, and porterhouse steaks. Watch out for excessively generous serving sizes—split with a friend or request a takeaway bag.

SELECTED RESOURCES

Sports Nutrition Information

Australian Institute of Sport, www.ausport.gov.au/ais/nutrition

Female Athlete Triad Coalition, www.femaleathletetriad.org

Gatorade Sports Science Institute (GSSI), www.gssiweb.com

International Olympic Committee: The IOC Medical Commission, www.olympic.org/medical-commission

Peak Performance, www.pponline.co.uk

SCAN (Sports, Cardiovascular, and Wellness Nutrition), to locate a board-certified sports dietitian, www.scandpg.org

USDA Nutrient Data Laboratory, www.ars.usda.gov/nutrientdata

USOC: Sports Performance, Nutrition, Resources, and Fact Sheets, www.teamusa.org/About-the-USOC/Athlete-Development/Sport-Performance/Nutrition/Resources-and-Fact-Sheets.aspx

Hydration Systems and Related Gear

CamelBak Hydration Systems, 800-767-8725, www.camelbak.com

Mountain Safety Research, 206-505-9500, www.cascadedesigns.com/msr

Nalgene, 800-625-4327, www.nalgene.com

TriSports, 888-293-3934, www.trisports.com/hydsys.html

Ultimate Direction, 800-426-7229, www.ultimatedirection.com

Universal Cycles, 800-936-5156, www.universalcycles.com

Body Image and Disordered Eating

About-Face (tools to resist harmful media messages), www.about-face.org

Eating Disorders: Resources for Recovery (home of Gurze Books), www.bulimia.com

National Eating Disorders Association (NEDA): eating disorders information and referral helpline, 800-931-2237, www.nationaleatingdisorders.org

Food and Exercise Logs

Athlete in Me app, www.athleteinme.com

Check-Off Diet Tracker app (using food group portions), https://itunes.apple.com/us/app/checkoff-diet-tracker/id429083337?mt=8

Lose It! app, www.loseit.com

My Fitness Pal app, www.myfitnesspal.com

My Plate, www.choosemyplate.gov

Planning Meals and Recipes

Busy Cooks (Crock-Pot recipes), http://busycooks.about.com/cs/crockpotrecipes/a/3ingredcrock.htm

Clean Eating magazine (monthly menus and corresponding weekly shopping lists), http://cleaneatingmag.com/Meal-Planning/Meal-Plans.aspx

Eating Well, www.eatingwell.com

Epicurious, www.epicurious.com/recipesmenus

The Food Network (healthy recipe makeover feature), www.foodnetwork.com

The Gluten-Free Girl, www.glutenfreegirl.com

Healthy Appetite with Ellie Krieger, www.foodnetwork.com/healthy-appetite-with-ellie-krieger/index.html

My Plate, www.choosemyplate.gov

Thomas, B.K., and A. Lim. 2011. *The feed zone cookbook: Fast and flavorful food for athletes.* Boulder, CO: VeloPress.

Supplement Information

Consumer Lab, www.consumerlab.com

Informed Choice, www.informed-choice.org

National Center for Drug-Free Sport, 816-474-8655, www.drugfreesport.com

NSF Certified for Sport Program, www.nsfsport.com

Quack watch, www.quackwatch.com

U.S. Anti-Doping Agency (USADA), www.usantidoping.org

World Anti-Doping Agency (WADA), www.wada-ama.org

Vegetarian Nutrition

Larsen-Meyer, E. 2007. *Vegetarian sports nutrition.* Champaign, IL: Human Kinetics.

The Vegetarian Resource Group, www.vrg.org

Vegetarian Dining (around the world), www.vegdining.com

Note: The inclusion of a website does not automatically constitute an endorsement of that site.

BIBLIOGRAPHY

ACOG Committee. 2002. Opinion no. 267. Exercise during pregnancy and the postpartum period. *Obstetrics and Gynecology* 99(1):171–173.

American Celiac Disease Alliance. What is celiac? www.americanceliac.org.

American College of Sports Medicine. 2007. Position stand on exercise and fluid replacement. *Medicine and Science in Sports and Exercise* 39(2):377–390.

American Dietetic Association, Dietitians of Canada, American College of Sports Medicine. 2009. Joint position stand on nutrition and athletic performance. *Medicine and Science in Sports and Exercise* 41(3):709–731.

Anderson, O. Eating practices of the best athletes in the world. www.active.com/running/Articles/Eating_practices_of_the_best_endurance_athletes_in_the_world.htm?page=4e world.

Armstrong, L.E. et al. 1996. Heat and cold illnesses during distance running. American College of Sports Medicine position stand. *Medicine and Science in Sports and Exercise* 28:i–x.

Australian Institute of Sport. 2012. Sport nutrition: AIS sports supplement program fact sheets. www.ais.org.au.

Baker, J. et al. 2005. Effects of indomethacin and celecoxib on renal function in athletes. *Medicine and Science in Sports and Exercise* 37(5):712–717.

Beals, K.A. 2004. *Disordered eating among athletes: A comprehensive guide for health professionals.* Champaign, IL: Human Kinetics.

Benardot, D. et al. 2001. Can vitamin supplements improve sport performance? *Sports Science Exchange Roundtable* 12(3):1–4.

Bergeron, M. 2000. Sodium: The forgotten nutrient. *Sports Science Exchange* 13(3):1–4.

Bergeron, M.F. et al. 2012. International Olympic Committee consensus statement on thermoregulatory and altitude challenges for high-level athletes. *Journal of Sports Medicine* 46:11 770–777.

Borsheim, E. 2005. Enhancing muscle anabolism through nutrient composition and timing of intake. *SCAN's PULSE* 24(3):1–5.

Burke, L.M. 2001. Nutritional needs for exercise in the heat. *Comparative Biochemistry and Physiology—Part A: Molecular & Integrative Physiology* 128(4):735–748.

———. 2012. New guidelines for carbohydrate intakes in sport from the international Olympic committee. *SCAN's Pulse* 31(3):7–11.

Burke, L.M., and V. Deakin, eds. 2010. *Clinical sports nutrition.* Sydney: McGraw-Hill.

Casa, D. et al. 2005. ACSM roundtable series on hydration and physical activity: Consensus statements. *Current Sports Medicine Reports* 4:115–127.

Castellani, W., and A.J. Young. 2012. Health and performance challenges during sports training and competition in cold weather. *British Journal of Sports Medicine* 46:11 788–791.

Chatard, J.C., I. Mujika, C. Guy, and J.R. Lacour. 1999. Anemia and iron deficiency in athletes—practical recommendations for treatment. *Sports Medicine* 27(4):229–240.

Clapp, J.F. 2002. *Exercising through your pregnancy.* Omaha, NE: Addicus.

Coleman, E. 2000. The glycemic index in sport. *SCAN's PULSE* 19(3):1–4.

———. 2004. Does adding protein to a sports drink improve performance? *Sports Medicine Digest* 26(1):10–11.

Cox, G.R. et al. 2002. Effect of different protocols of caffeine intake on metabolism and endurance performance. *Journal of Applied Physiology* 93:990–999.

Doubt, T.J. 1991. Physiology of exercise in the cold. *Sports Medicine* 11:367–381.

Dunford, M., and J.A. Doyle. 2011. *Nutrition for sport and exercise,* 2nd ed. Belmont, CA: Wadsworth.

Eberle, S.G. 2005. Disordered eating + runners: A troublesome combination. *Running Times,* September, 44–50.

Eichner, R.E. 2001. Anemia and blood boosting. *Sports Science Exchange* 14(2):1–4.

———. 2002. Heat stroke in sports: Causes, prevention and treatment. *Sports Science Exchange* 15(3):1–4.

Fallon, K. 2010. Athletes with gastrointestinal disorders. In *Clinical Sports Nutrition,* ed. L. Burke, and V. Deakin. Sydney: McGraw-Hill.

Farquhar, B., and W.L. Kennedy. 1997. Anti-inflammatory drugs, kidney function, and exercise. *Sports Science Exchange* 11(4):1–6.

Gibbs, J.C., N.I. Williams, and J.L. Scheid. 2011. Drive for thinness, energy deficiency and menstrual disturbances: Confirmation in a large population of exercising women. *International Journal of Sport Nutrition and Exercise Metabolism* 21:280–290.

Hargraves, M. 2005. Metabolic factors in fatigue. *Sports Science Exchange* 18(3):1–6.

Helge, J.W. 2000. Adaptation to a fat-rich diet: Effects on endurance performance in humans. *Sports Medicine* 30(5):347–357.

Hew-Butler, T. et al. 2008. Statement of the second international exercise-associated hyponatremia consensus development conference, New Zealand, 2007. *Clinical Journal of Sports Medicine* 18(2):111–121.

Hopkinson, R., and J. Lock. 2004. Athletics, perfectionism and disordered eating. *Eating and Weight Disorders* 9:99–106.

Hsieh, M. 2004. Recommendations for treatment of hyponatremia at endurance events. *Sports Medicine* 34:231–238.

IOC Medical Committee Working Group Women in Sport. 2006. Position stand on the female athlete triad. http://multimedia.olympic.org/pdf/en_report_917.pdf.

Jeukendrup, A.E. 2007. Carbohydrate supplementation during exercise. Does it help? How much is too much? *Sports Science Exchange* 106(20):1–6.

———. 2010. Carbohydrate and exercise performance: The role of multiple transportable carbohydrates. *Current Opinion in Clinical Nutrition and Metabolic Care* 13(4):452–457.

———. 2011. Nutrition for endurance sports: Marathon, triathlon, and road cycling. *Journal of Sports Science* 29(1):S91–99.

Jeukendrup, A.E., W.H. Saris, and J.M. Wagenmakers. 1998a. Fat metabolism during exercise: A review (part I). *International Journal of Sports Medicine* 19:231–244.

———. 1998b. Fat metabolism during exercise: A review (part II). *International Journal of Sports Medicine* 19:293–302.

Jeukendrup, A.E., and M. Gleeson. 2004. *Sport nutrition: An introduction to energy production and performance.* Champaign, IL: Human Kinetics.

Joy, E. 2012. Is the pill the answer for patients with the female athlete triad? *Current Sports Medicine Reports* 11(2):54–55.

Lambert, E.V. et al. 2001. High-fat diet versus habitual diet prior to carbohydrate loading: Effects of exercise metabolism and cycling performance. *International Journal of Sport Nutrition and Exercise Metabolism* 11(2):209–225.

Lambert, E.V., and J.H. Goedecke. 2003. The role of dietary macronutrients in optimizing endurance performance. *Current Sport Medicine Reports* 2(4):194–201.

Levis, S. et al. 2011. Soy isoflavones in the prevention of menopausal bone loss and menopausal symptoms: A randomized, double blind trial. *Archives of Internal Medicine* 171(5):1363–1369.

Littlefield, K. et al. 2006. Athletes with eating disorders. *The Remuda Review* 5(1):2–11.

Loosli, A.R., and J.S. Rudd. 1998. Meatless diets in female athletes: A red flag. *The Physician and Sportsmedicine* 26:45–48.

Lowery, L.M. 2004. Dietary fat and sports nutrition: A primer. *Journal of Sport Science* 3:106–117.

Manore, M.M., L.C. Kam, A.B. Loucks, and International Association of Athletics Federations. 2007. The female athlete triad: Components, nutrition issues, and health consequences. *Journal of Sports Science* 25(S1):S61–71.

Manore, M., N. Meyer, and J. Thompson. 2009. *Sport nutrition for health and performance.* Champaign, IL: Human Kinetics.

Maughan, R., and S.M. Shirreffs. 2010. Exercise in hot environments: From basic concepts to field applications. *Scandinavian Journal of Medicine & Science in Sports* 20(3):40–47.

McArdle, W., F.I. Katch, and V.L. Katch. 2009. *Sports and exercise nutrition,* 3rd ed. United States: Lippincott Williams & Wilkins.

Medicine and Science for Women in Sport group of Sports Medicine Australia. Women, menopause and sport: How does menopause affect the sport woman? *Women in Sport:* fact sheet no. 4.

Messina, V., R. Mangels, and M. Messina. 2004. *The dietitian's guide to vegetarian diets,* 2nd ed. Boston: Jones & Bartlett.

Meyer, N.L., and S. Parker-Simmons. 2006. In preparation for Torino 2006: Dietary needs of winter sport athletes. *SCAN's PULSE* 25(1):1–6.

Murray, R. 1995. Fluid needs in hot and cold environments. *International Journal of Sport Nutrition* 5:S62–S73.

Nattiv, A., A.B. Loucks, M.M. Manore, C.F. Sanborn, J. Sundgot-Borgen, and M.P. Warren. 2007. The American College of Sports Medicine position stand: The female athlete triad. *Medicine and Science in Sports and Exercise* 39(10):1867-1882.

Nieman, D.C. 2008. Immunonutrition support for athletes. *Nutrition Reviews* 66(6):310–320.

Noakes, T. 2012. *Waterlogged: The serious problem of overhydration in endurance sports.* Champaign, IL: Human Kinetics.

Otis, C.L., and R. Goldingay. 2000. *The athletic woman's survival guide: How to win the battle against eating disorders, amenorrhea, and osteoporosis.* Champaign, IL: Human Kinetics.

Pfeiffer, B., T. Stellingwerff, A.B. Hodgson, R. Randell, K. Pottgen, and A.E. Jeukendrup. 2012. Nutritional intake and gastrointestinal problems during competitive endurance events. *Medicine and Science in Sports and Exercise* 44(2):344–351.

Putukian, M., and C. Potera. 1997. Don't miss gastrointestinal disorders in athletes. *The Physician and Sportsmedicine* 25:80–94.

Probiotics: Are enough in your diet? 2005. *Consumer Reports,* July, 34–35.

Raban, A., B. Keins, E.A. Richter, L.B. Rasmussen, B. Svenstrup, S. Micic, and P. Bennett. 1992. Serum sex hormones and endurance performance after a lacto-ovo vegetarian and a mixed diet. *Medicine in Science in Sports and Exercise* 24:1290–1297.

Ramano-Ely, B.C., M. Kent Todd, M.J. Saunders, and T. St. Laurent. 2006. Effect of an isocaloric carbohydrate-protein antioxidant drink on cycling performance. *Medicine and Science in Sports and Exercise* 38(1):608–616.

Rawson, E.S., and P. Clarkson. 2003. Scientifically debatable: Is creatine worth its weight? *Sports Science Exchange* 16(4):1–4.

Rehrer, N.J. 2001. Fluid and electrolyte balance in ultra-endurance sport. *Sports Medicine* 31(10):701–15.

Reid, S. et al. 2005. Consensus statement of the first international exercise-associated hyponatremia consensus development conference, Cape Town, South Africa. *Clinical Journal of Sports Medicine* 15:208–213.

Rock, C.L et al. 2012. Nutrition and physical activity guidelines for cancer survivors. *CA: A Cancer Journal for Clinicians* 62(4):242–274.

Rollo, I., C. Williams, and M. Nevill. 2011. Influence of ingesting versus mouth-rinsing a carbohydrate solution during a one hour run. *Medicine and Science in Sports and Exercise* 43:468–475.

Saunders, M.J., M. Kane, and M.K. Todd. 2004. Effects of a carbohydrate-protein beverage on cycling endurance and muscle damage. *Medicine and Science in Sports and Exercise* 36:1233–1238.

SCAN. 2010. *Sports nutrition: A practice manual for professionals,* eds. C. Rosenbloom and E. Coleman. Chicago: American Dietetics Association.

Sedlock, D.A. 2008. The latest on carbohydrate loading: A practical approach. *Current Sports Medicine Reports* 7(4):209–213.

Seyler, J., and D.K. Layman. 2012. The role of protein in overall health: Quality, quantity and timing considerations. *SCAN's Pulse* 31(3):4–6.

Shephard, R.J. 1993. Metabolic adaptations to exercise in the cold. *Sports Medicine* 16(4): 266–289.

Sims, S., N.J. Rehrer, M.L. Bell, and J.D. Cotter. 2007. Preexercise sodium loading aids fluid balance and endurance for women exercising in the heat. *Journal of Applied Physiology* 103(2):534–541.

Slater, G.J. et al. 2005. Body-mass management of Australian lightweight rowers prior to and during competition. *Medicine and Science in Sports and Exercise* 37(5):860–866.

Soles, C. 2002. *Climbing: Training for peak performance.* Seattle: The Mountaineers.

Sports Nutrition: The role of carbohydrates in endurance sports. *Peak Performance.* www.ppon-line.co.uk/encyc/sports-nutrition-the-role-of-carbohydrates-in-endurance-sports-42171.

Swanson, A., and L. Makowski. 2012. Physiologic and metabolic responses during vigorous exercise: Why recovery nutrition is indispensible. *SCAN's Pulse* 31(2):1–5.

Sykora, C., C.M. Grilo, D.E. Wilfley, and K.D. Brownell. 1993. Eating, weight, and dieting disturbances in male and female lightweight and heavyweight rowers. *International Journal of Eating Disorders* 14:203–211.

Tarnopolsky, M. 2004. Protein requirements for endurance athletes. *Nutrition* 20:662–668.

———. 2008. Nutritional consideration in the aging athlete. *Clinical Journal of Sport Medicine* 18(6):531–538.

Tarnopolsky, M., C. Zawada, L.B. Richmond, S. Carter, J. Shearer, T. Graham, and S. M. Phillips. 2001. Gender differences in carbohydrate loading are related to energy intake. *Journal of Applied Physiology* 91(1):225–230.

Tone, C. Nutrition guidance for winter athletes. *Today's Dietitian Health and Nutrition Center.* www.todaysdietitian.com/news/exclusive0211.shtml.

Tribole, E., and E. Resch. 2003. *Intuitive eating: A revolutionary program that works.* New York: St. Martin's Griffen.

Tussing-Humphreys, L., C. Pustacioglu, E. Nemeth, and C. Braunschweig. 2012. Rethinking iron regulation and assessment in iron deficiency, anemia of chronic disease, and obesity: Introducing hepcidin. *Journal of the Academy of Nutrition and Dietetics* 112:391–400.

U.S. Preventive Services Task Force draft recommendations. Vitamin D and calcium supplementation to prevent cancer and osteoporotic fractures. Comment period from June 12 to July 10, 2012. www.uspreventiveservicestaskforce.org

Van Essen, M., and M.J. Gibala. 2006. Failure of protein to improve time trial performance when added to a sports drink. *Medicine and Science in Sports and Exercise* 38(1):476–483.

von Dullivard, S.P. et al. 2004. Fluids and hydration in prolonged endurance performance. *Nutrition* 20:651–656.

Wismann, J., and D. Willoughby. 2006. Gender differences in carbohydrate metabolism and carbohydrate loading. *Journal of the International Society of Sports Nutrition* 3(1):28–34.

Yeo, S.E. et al. 2005. Caffeine increases exogenous carbohydrate oxidation during exercise. *Journal of Applied Physiology* 99(3):844–850.

INDEX

Note: The italicized *f* and *t* following page numbers refer to figures and tables, respectively.

ABOUT THE AUTHOR

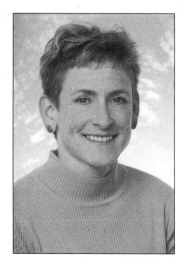

Suzanne Girard Eberle, MS, RDN, CSSD, is a board-certified sports dietitian and Intuitive Eating coach who counsels active people of all shapes, sizes, and athletic abilities on mastering high-performance eating habits. She's a lifelong carrot cake connoisseur, too. Girard Eberle's first career was as an elite professional runner. She's a USA Track and Field 5,000-meter track champion with a mile PR of 4:28, and she represented the United States on three national teams. Today, she includes competitive road cycling and hiking among her favorite sports. Girard Eberle has reached the summits of Mount Blanc, the highest mountain in the Alps, and Mount Kilimanjaro, the highest mountain in Africa. In her next life, she plans to be a sport psychologist and further her passion of assisting disordered eaters and compulsive exercisers in reestablishing a positive relationship with food and their bodies.

Girard Eberle is currently serving as the first-ever nutrition columnist for *Coach and Athletic Director* magazine. She also has been a contributing editor for *Running Times,* and her articles and nutrition advice have appeared in *USA Today, Newsweek, Runner's World, Environmental Nutrition, Men's Fitness, Self, Shape, Women's Running,* and *Marathon & Beyond.* As an adjunct professor at Portland State University, she taught sports nutrition through the School of Chemistry. Her client list includes Columbia Sportswear, Intel, Multnomah Athletic Club, Nike, Portland Timbers Soccer Academy, and the Oregon Beef Council.

Girard Eberle is the founder of Eat, Drink, Win! She holds a master's degree with distinction in nutrition from Boston University. She is a longtime member of the Academy of Nutrition and Dietetics, Academy for Eating Disorders, and SCAN (Sports, Cardiovascular, and Wellness Nutrition). Girard Eberle is an invited member of the United States Olympic Committee Sport Dietitian Network as well as a former SCAN representative to the Female Athlete Triad Coalition.

Girard Eberle lives and plays in Portland, Oregon, with her husband, John, and her whippet, Asa Babu. Find her at www.eatdrinkwin.com.

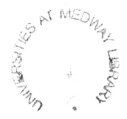